Controversial issues in cardiac pathophysiology

Supplement to
Basic Research in Cardiology, Vol. 81 Suppl. 1 (1986)
Editors:
R. Jacob (Tübingen) Th. Kenner (Graz) and W. Schaper
(Bad Nauheim)

R. Jacob (ed.)

Controversial issues in cardiac pathophysiology

Erwin Riesch Symposium, July 12/13, 1985

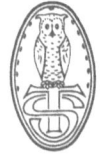

Springer-Verlag Berlin Heidelberg GmbH

CIP-Kurztitelaufnahme der Deutschen Bibliothek

Controversial issues in cardiac pathophysiology /
Erwin Riesch Symposium, July 12/13, 1985. R. Jacob
(ed.).
  (Supplement to "Basic research in cardiology" ;
  Vol 81,1)
  ISBN 978-3-662-11376-9   ISBN 978-3-662-11374-5 (eBook)
  DOI 10.1007/978-3-662-11374-5

NE: Jacob, Ruthard [Hrsg.]; Erwin-Riesch-Symposium
< 1985, Starzach > ; Basic research in cardiology /
Supplement

Indexed in Current Contents Basic Res. Cardiol.

Foreword

The past years have witnessed considerable progress in the field of fundamental research in cardiology. Nevertheless, numerous problems and controversial concepts remain. Some of these controversies concern relatively simple issues, e. g. the question of the extent to which a common length-tension or pressure-volume relationship exists independent of type of contraction and preload. The present volume is a compendium of an Erwin Riesch symposium held July 12–13, 1985, with the aim of critically analysing generally accepted concepts and theories as well as current trends in cardiology. In common with previous Erwin Riesch symposia, priority was given to issues concerning chronic reactions of the heart, although basic principles of normal myocardial contraction and ventricular dynamics as well as clinical aspects were also discussed.

We are greatly indebted to the Erwin Riesch-Stiftung for the invaluable generosity which enabled us to hold the symposium.

R. Jacob

Contents

IV. Chronic reactions of the myocardium – Determinants of hypertrophy development and regression

V. Morphology and pathophysiology of the failing heart

I. Contractile elementary processes: Cross-bridge theory and excitation-contraction coupling

The cross-bridge cycle in muscle.
Mechanical, biochemical, and structural studies on single skinned rabbit psoas fibers to characterize cross-bridge kinetics in muscle for correlation with the actomyosin-ATPase in solution*

B. Brenner

Institute of Physiology II, University of Tübingen (F.R.G.) and Laboratory of Physical Biology, National Institute of Arthritis, Diabetes, and Digestive and Kidney Diseases, NIH, Bethesda, Maryland (U.S.A.)

Summary

A characteristic and important feature of myocardium is the modulation of tension when stimulated or possibly even when unstimulated. In addition, resistance to stretch and its variation in unstimulated heart muscle is an important factor in myocardial function. These features may occur in some new light when viewed from some recent advances in understanding of cross-bridge action and regulation of muscle. For this reason we give a short review of such advances. Firstly, we summarize some of our earlier results obtained in experiments designed to see whether and to what extent actomyosin ATPase data obtained in solution might apply in muscle. Secondly, we present a recently developed experimental approach to estimate the rate constants that determine the cycling of cross-bridges between weak-binding, 'non-force-generating' states and strong-binding, 'force-generating' states. The estimated rate constants confirm the prediction of cross-bridge models derived from in vitro studies that the step which is rate-limiting in solution also determines the rate of force-generation in the cross-bridge cycle in muscle. Experiments at various Ca^{++} concentrations imply that a major mechanism of regulation is the control of the transition from the weak-binding, 'non-force-generating' states to the strong-binding, 'force-generating' states while the number of activated interaction sites appears unchanged and always at its maximum. This implies that changes in the force-pCa relation cannot be interpreted without detailed analysis of cross-bridge kinetics, and that factors other than Ca^{++} may have the potential to modulate muscle activity, both in stimulated and unstimulated muscle, by affecting cross-bridge kinetics.

Key words: cross-bridge cycle, actomyosin ATPase, skinned rabbit psoas fibers, fiber stiffness, force redevelopment

Introduction

Contraction of striated muscle occurs when actin and myosin filaments slide past each other (20, 23) and it is generally accepted that this process is driven by cross-bridges which extend from the myosin filaments and cyclically interact with the actin filaments while splitting ATP (21, 25). The cyclic interaction between the two sets of filaments results in maximum isometric force when the filaments are held at a fixed position (isometric

---

* Supported by the Deutsche Forschungsgemeinschaft; Br 849/1-1

contraction) or in muscle shortening when the filaments are allowed to slide past each other (isotonic contraction). In studying the detailed mechanism of this cyclic interaction, several approaches are used. In biochemistry, actin and soluble fragments of myosin, e. g., myosin subfragment one (S-1) or heavy meromyosin (HMM), are used to define the various states and the kinetics of the cyclic interaction of these proteins in solution. In physiology, by measuring force, speed of shortening, fiber stiffness, or fiber ATPase, an attempt is made to define the states and kinetics of the actin-myosin interactions while the proteins are assembled in the three-dimensional contractile system. Finally, using X-ray diffraction, for example, it is attempted to define the structure of the various cross-bridge states. The final goal, however, is the reconstruction of the detailed mechanism of the cross-bridge cycle by correlating the biochemical, physiological, and structural studies.

A key difference between the biochemical studies done in solution and physiological or structural studies both done with the assembled contractile system are the constraints the filament lattice imposes on cross-bridge actions such as changes in configuration. Such changes in cross-bridge configuration can occur unimpaired in solution but in muscle, where cross-bridges are fixed to both actin and myosin filaments, the changes in configuration might be restrained and directed by the filament lattice; a factor which eventually leads to generation of isometric force or directed shortening. Deformation of the cross-bridges and resulting strain will have effects on the kinetics of the cross-bridge cycle. These effects, however, are not observable with the proteins in solution. For this reason, experiments were performed to see whether and to what extent the characteristics of the in vitro actomyosin ATPase also apply for the cross-bridge cycle in muscle, and what differences, if any, may exist.

Kinetic schemes of the actomyosin ATPase cycle in solution

The various states and kinetics of the actomyosin ATPase, observed in solution, are summarized in the kinetic schemes of the actomyosin ATPase cycle. One possible scheme that accounts for the steady state and presteady state data is shown in Fig. 1 (34, 35). In this

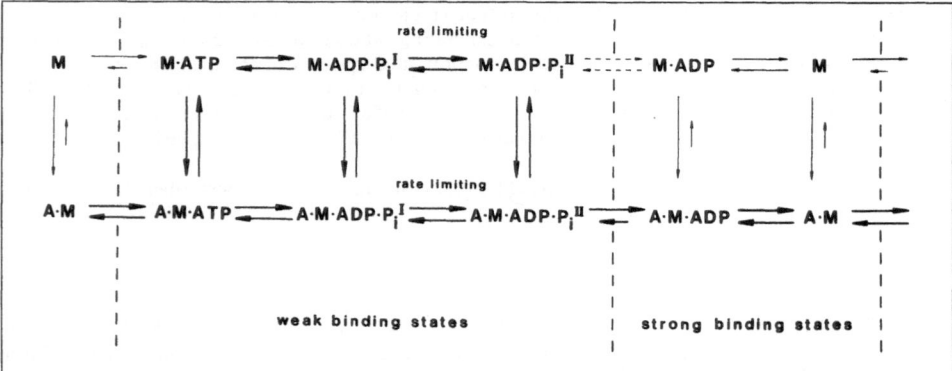

Fig. 1. A kinetic scheme of the in vitro actomyosin ATPase (34, 35). This '6-state model' includes six states with ATP or the hydrolysis products (ADP + P_i) bound to the myosin heads. The heavy solid arrows indicate the predominant pathway for the cycling system in the presence of actin. The dashed arrows represent the rate-limiting step in the absence of actin. The relative length of the forward and reverse arrows qualitatively indicate the change in free energy across the corresponding step. A = actin, M = myosin subfragment-1.

6-state model, six states have ATP or the hydrolysis products $(ADP + P_i)$ bound to the myosin heads. Other schemes such as 4-state models have been discussed where only 4 states have ATP or the hydrolysis products bound to the myosin heads (33, 35, 39). Besides the ongoing discussion concerning the minimum number of states with ATP or $ADP + P_i$ bound to the myosin heads required to account for all the experimental data, all the proposed kinetic schemes for the actomyosin ATPase cycle in solution have some common features: firstly, two groups of states are found; one group with low affinity to actin, called the 'weak-binding states', and another group with high affinity to actin, called the 'strong-binding states'. During each cycle, while splitting ATP, S-1 or HMM is believed to cycle between the weak-binding states and the strong-binding states. Secondly, all the biochemical schemes have a rate-limiting step, located either within the weak-binding states (33, 35), or possibly representing the transition from the weak-binding states to the strong-binding states (39). However, independent of the exact location, this rate-limiting step determines the transition from the weak-binding states to the strong-binding states when the system is cycling. Thirdly, a major mechanism of regulation appears to be the control of the transition from the weak-binding states to the strong-binding states since, in the presence of MgATP but without Ca^{++}, S-1 or HMM still bind to actin but do not show significant ATPase activity (10, 11, 37, 38).

Weak-binding states in muscle and some of their characteristics determined by mechanical and X-ray diffraction experiments

The work of Marston (28, 29) showed that in relaxed muscle fibers either ATP or the hydrolysis products $(MgADP + P_i)$ are bound to the cross-bridges. This finding suggests that cross-bridges in relaxed fibers might represent a pure population of cross-bridge states that are the equivalent of the weak-binding states of the in vitro system. In the case of an analogy between muscle fiber and solution where binding of the myosin fragments to regulated actin was found even in the absence of Ca^{++}, one should expect cross-bridge attachment to actin in relaxed fibers, unless actin affinity is too weak for significant cross-bridge attachment to occur. To optimize conditions for possible cross-bridge attachment in relaxed fibers, experiments were performed at an ionic strength of 0.02 M since in vitro actin affinity increases when ionic strength is lowered. To probe for possible cross-bridge attachment in relaxed fibers we used two parameters, previously shown to give information about cross-bridge attachment; apparent fiber stiffness (14, 22) and equatorial X-ray diffraction patterns (7, 18, 24, 41).

As shown in Fig. 2, apparent stiffness of relaxed fibers at low ionic strength is a significant fraction ($1/2$ to $2/3$) of the stiffness observed in fully Ca^{++}-activated fibers. Furthermore, it was found that apparent fiber stiffness of relaxed fibers at low ionic strength (0.02 M) is very closely proportional to filament overlap (2). This supports the interpretation that the observed stiffness is the result of cross-bridge attachment. Therefore, these data suggest that, at least at ionic strength of 0.02 M, a significant number of cross-bridges is attached in relaxed fibers without producing net axial force.

This, in turn, predicts that under the same conditions, the mass associated with the actin filaments should be significantly greater than the mass of the actin filaments alone. This prediction was tested by recording equatorial X-ray diffraction patterns from the same single skinned rabbit psoas fibers. The reconstructed 2-D electron density maps did show much more mass associated with the actin filaments than could be accounted for by the actin filaments alone. The observed mass associated with the thin filaments in relaxed fibers at low

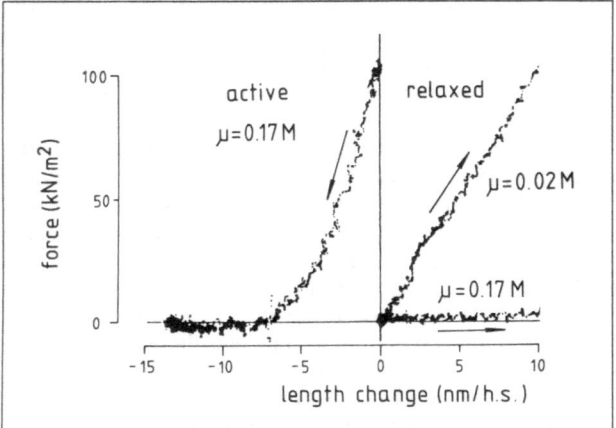

Fig. 2. Apparent fiber stiffness of relaxed and activated skinned rabbit psoas fibers. Force and changes in sarcomere length were recorded during length changes applied to one end of the fibers. Apparent fiber stiffness is defined as the resulting slope when force is plotted vs. change in sarcomere length. Stiffness in relaxing medium is measured while applying a stretch, in Ca^{++}-activating solution during a release (see arrows).

Coordinates: Abscissa, length change in nm/half-sarcomere; ordinate, force in kN/m^2. Temperature 5° C, ionic strength (μ) as indicated for each plot. Speed of applied length change 2.5–5 × 10^4 (nm/half-sarcomere) s^{-1}. Note the effect of ionic strength on apparent fiber stiffness in relaxed fibers and the substantial magnitude of apparent fiber stiffness at low ionic strength ($1/3$–$1/2$ of the active stiffness at $\mu = 0.17$ M). From (2).

ionic strength is approximately as large as in fully Ca^{++}-activated fibers (5). Therefore, both stiffness and equatorial X-ray diffraction data are consistent with the idea of significant cross-bridge attachment in relaxed fibers at low ionic strength, analogous to the binding of S-1 or HMM to regulated actin under the same conditions in solution.

Another typical feature of the weak-binding states as described for the in vitro system is the rapid equilibrium between association and dissociation of the soluble myosin fragments to and from actin (34, 40). We therefore tested whether cross-bridges, attached to actin in relaxed fibers at low ionic strength, also show evidence of a rapid equilibrium between attachment and detachment. Rapid detachment and reattachment would be expected to occur also during the changes in length which were applied to measure apparent fiber stiffness, resulting in a 'loss' of force observed during the changes in length. Consequently, apparent fiber stiffness, that is the slope when force is plotted vs. the change in sarcomere length during the applied stretches, is expected to decrease when the speed of stretch is reduced. This effect might be enhanced by a possible increase in the detachment rate when cross-bridges are strained during the length changes. Figure 3 shows measurements of apparent fiber stiffness at various speeds of stretch. In rigor fibers (Fig. 3, filled circles) where the probability of cross-bridge detachment is small, apparent fiber stiffness changes only by about 1–15% when the speed of stretch is varied over almost 6 orders of magnitude, up to about 10^4 (nm/half-sarcomere) s^{-1}. In contrast, relaxed fibers at low ionic strength show a very significant effect of speed of stretch on apparent fiber stiffness for speeds up to about 10^5 (nm/half-sarcomere) s^{-1} (Fig. 3, open circles). An estimate of the underlying rate constants for detachment and reattachment can be obtained in the following way; firstly, since a significant fraction, but most likely not all of the cross-bridges, is attached at low ionic

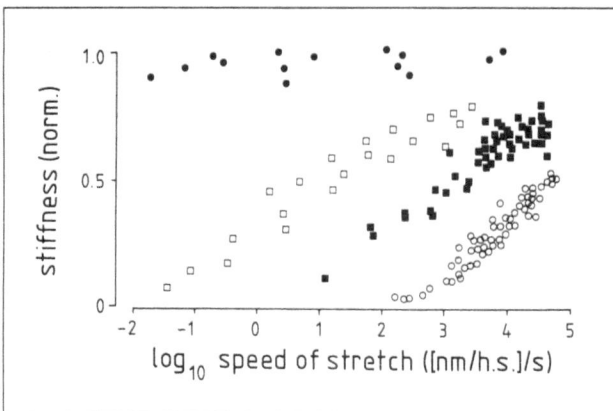

Fig. 3. Effect of speed of stretch on apparent fiber stiffness under various conditions. For all conditions, stiffness is normalized to the apparent fiber stiffness measured in rigor during stretches with a speed of about 10^4 (nm/half-sarcomere) s^{-1}.

(●)   fiber in rigor, ionic strength 0.12 M.

(○)   fiber relaxed at ionic strength 0.02 M.

(□)   stiffness in the presence of 4 mM MgPP$_i$ at ionic strength 0.12 M. At this ionic strength apparent in vitro binding constant for S-1 · PP$_i$ to regulated actin is similar to the binding constant of S-1 · ATP to regulated actin at ionic strength of 0.02 M.

(■)   apparent fiber stiffness of Ca^{++}-activated fibers at an ionic strength of 0.17 M.

Note that in rigor, apparent fiber stiffness is almost unaffected by the speed of stretch in the range of examined speeds. Under all the other conditions apparent fiber stiffness does depend on speed of stretch, implying that cross-bridges detach and possibly reattach during the stiffness measurements until a range of speeds is reached where apparent fiber stiffness is no longer affected by the speed of stretch. In the presence of MgPP$_i$, such a range appears to be approached around 10^3 (nm/half-sarcomere) s^{-1}. In Ca^{++}-activated fibers such a range may just be approached around 10^4 (nm/half-sarcomere) s^{-1}. In contrast, for relaxed fibers at low ionic strength no such range has been reached even with the fastest stretches we could apply. No conclusion could be drawn for relaxed fibers at ionic strength of 0.17 M. The low apparent stiffness at 0.17 M (Fig. 2) could either indicate that only few cross-bridges are attached or simply mean that the fastest speeds of stetch, attained in this study, were too slow to pick up any apparent fiber stiffness due to too fast rates for detachment and reattachment. The different position of the speed profiles in the presence of MgPP$_i$, during Ca^{++}-activation, and when relaxed at low ionic strength could be taken as evidence that detachment and/or reattachment rate constants are different for the three conditions.

strength under relaxing conditions, the apparent binding constant has to be around unity; i. e., the rate constants for attachment and detachment have to be of the same order of magnitude. Secondly, the time period for detachment and reattachment to occur is the time required to move the filaments by a distance approximately equal to the range of action of the cross-bridges, which is approximately 10 nm. For the fastest stretches the filaments slide relative to each other by 10 nm in about 10^{-4} s. Since cross-bridges apparently still detach and reattach during the fastest stretches we were able to apply (stiffness still increases with speed of stretch), attachment and detachment have to occur with rate constants up to at least 10^4s^{-1}. This suggests that in muscle, the same as in solution, the weak-binding states are characterized by a rapid equilibrium between attachment and detachment.

A third characteristic feature of the weak-binding states observed in vitro is the decrease in actin affinity with increasing ionic strength (17). To see whether a similar decrease in actin affinity occurs in muscle, we recorded apparent fiber stiffness and equatorial X-ray diffraction patterns of relaxed fibers at different ionic strengths. Since apparent fiber stiffness was found to be sensitive to the speed of stretch up to the fastest stretches we could apply, the observed decrease in apparent fiber stiffness with increasing ionic strength (Fig. 2, μ = 0.02 M and 0.17 M) could, at least partly, be due to increased rate constants for detachment and reattachment rather than to only less cross-bridge attachment. However, equatorial X-ray diffraction experiments, unaffected by rapid detachment and reattachment of cross-bridges during the measurements, showed some decrease in mass associated with the actin filaments when ionic strength is increased (5). This is consistent with less cross-bridge attachment at higher ionic strengths.

Thus, stiffness and equatorial X-ray diffraction experiments suggest that cross-bridges can attach in relaxed fibers and that these cross-bridge states have similar qualities as descibed for the weak-binding states of the in vitro actomyosin ATPase.

Strong-binding states in muscle and some of their characteristics determined from mechanical and X-ray diffraction experiments

The strong-binding states of the in vitro actomyosin ATPase, assumed to be the equivalent of the main force-generating states in muscle (35), are characterized by a much higher actin affinity at the same ionic strength and a slower equilibrium between association and dissociation to and from actin when compared with the weak-binding states (27, 30). Further characteristic features of the strong-binding states are the effect of Ca^{++} on the binding of S-1 to actin and the cooperativity of binding, especially prominent in the absence of Ca^{++} (16).

To see whether states with properties characteristic for these strong-binding states can also be found in muscle fibers, we first studied apparent fiber stiffness and equatorial X-ray diffraction patterns in the presence of $MgPP_i$ since this condition is believed to represent an analogue of the strong-binding states. Here, we are dealing with a pure population of strong-binding states, whereas in active muscle, with cycling cross-bridges, both weak- and strong-binding states are expected to coexist. Both approaches, stiffness and equatorial X-ray diffraction, showed that with $MgPP_i$, cross-bridge attachment is stronger than in relaxed fibers since ionic strength has to be increased much more so as to observe comparable cross-bridge attachment as observed in relaxed fibers at low ionic strength (μ = 0.02 M). In fact, less than 100% attachment can only be achieved by both raising ionic strength and lowering temperature to at least 5° C (3). Concerning the possible equilibrium between attachment and detachment in the presence of $MgPP_i$, speed of stretch has quite a different effect on apparent fiber stiffness than observed in the relaxed system. The profile of apparent fiber stiffness vs. speed of stretch is shifted by approximately 3 orders of magnitude toward slower speeds (Fig. 3, open squares). This implies that the rate constants required for detachment and reattachment to occur during the length changes are about 3 orders of magnitude smaller than required for the relaxed system at low ionic strength.

To see whether cross-bridge states of similar properties can be found in active muscle, apparent fiber stiffness was again measured at various speeds of stretch. The ionic strength in these experiments (0.17 M) was chosen such that possible cross-bridge attachment in states equivalent to the weak-binding states would not be detected with the stiffness measurements. As shown in Fig. 2, at an ionic strength of 0.17 M no significant fiber stiffness was found to originate from cross-bridges in the weak-binding states. Apparent fiber stiffness of fully Ca^{++}-activated fibers, measured at various speeds of stretch, are shown in Fig. 3 (filled squares). Comparison with the data of relaxed fibers at low ionic strength (open circles) implies that the necessary rate constants for detachment and reattachment are again slower by more than one order of magnitude.

These results imply that in the assembled contractile system we not only can find cross-bridge states equivalent to the weak-binding states of the in vitro actomyosin ATPase but also states with similar qualities as described for the strong-binding states. In fact, besides the similarities reported above, cross-bridges in the presence of MgPP$_i$ show very similar effects of ionic strength on attachment in the presence and absence of Ca^{++}, including similar cooperativity, as found in vitro (3).

Kinetics of the cross-bridge cycle derived from measurements of force, force redevelopment, and isometric ATPase

I Relation between cross-bridge kinetics and experimental parameters

The first quantitative model that allowed to relate experimental parameters to kinetics of the proposed cross-bridge cycle was put forward by A. F. Huxley in 1957 (21). In this model two states, one attached, force-generating state and one detached, non-force-generating state were included (Scheme I). Two rate constants were incorporated to define the kinetics of the cycling cross-bridges; the rate constant that determines cross-bridge attachment, called 'f', and the rate constant 'g' that determines cross-bridge detachment. Since only two cross-bridge states were incorporated, attachment and detachment are equivalent to the transition from the non-force-generating state to the force-generating state and back to the non-force-generating state. By proposing 'f' to be moderate and 'g' to be smaller than 'f' when filament sliding is prevented (isometric contraction) but larger (g$_2$) when the end of the working distance is reached when filament sliding can occur (isotonic contraction), it was possible to account for the observed force-velocity relation and the flattening off of the increase in the rate of energy liberation with speed of shortening (19). The relations between these two rate constants and isometric force, rate constant of force redevelopment, and isometric fiber ATPase are summarized in Scheme I.

Scheme I

$$
g \left(\begin{array}{c} M \\ \\ AM \end{array} \right) f \quad
\begin{array}{ll}
\text{isometric force} & \propto f/(f + g) \\
k_{redevelopment} & = f + g \\
\text{isometric ATPase} & \propto fg/(f + g)
\end{array}
$$

In this scheme M represents the detached, non-force-generating state and AM represents the attached, force-generating state. 'f' is the forward rate constant for the transition from the detached, non-force-generating state to the attached, force-generating state ('attachment rate constant'). 'g' is the forward rate-constant for the transition from the attached, force-generating state to the detached, non-force-generating state ('detachment rate constant').

Following the proposal of this model, experimental results have indicated that more than just two states exist in a cross-bridge cycle and that the non-force generating states can also attach to actin. Thus, attachment and detachment are no longer equivalent with the transitions from the non-force-generating states to the force-generating states or from the force-generating states back to the non-force-generating states. However, for these more complex cross-bridge models, including several weak-binding, non-force-generating states and several

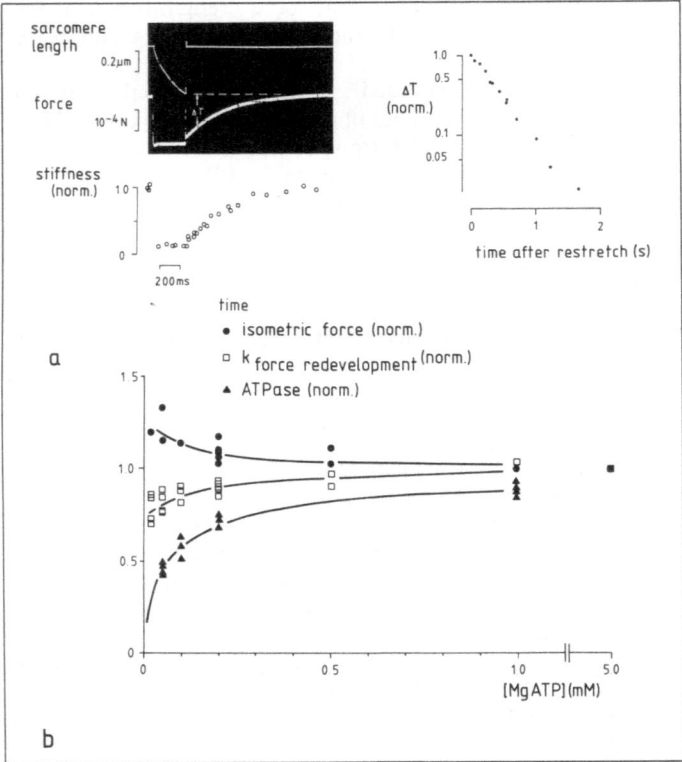

Fig. 4. (a) Experimental protocol to measure rate of force redevelopment. Following a period of 330 ms of isotonic shortening at near-zero load fibers are restretched to their original sarcomere length and subsequent redevelopment of force is recorded. Measurements of apparent fiber stiffness under conditions where only stiffness from cross-bridges in the strong-binding states is detected show that during the period of isotonic shortening at near-zero load the number of cross-bridges in the strong-binding states decreases to less than $1/5$ compared to the isometric steady state. The reincrease in force following the restretch is paralleled by a reincrease in apparent fiber stiffness. This suggests that the reincrease in force reflects the reincrease in the number of cross-bridges in the strong-binding, force generating states. Plotting ΔT, the difference between instanteneous and steady state tension, vs. time after restretch yields a rather straight relation when ΔT is plotted on a logarithmic scale. This means that force redevelopment is well described by a single exponential function. The rate constant of force redevelopment (k) was determined from the slope of the linearized relation. From (6).

(b) Effect of MgATP on force redevelopment, isometric force, and fiber ATPase. Since force redevelopment had to be measured in sarcomere-length-controlled feedback (4, 6, 9) which could not be done in the small chamber used for ATPase measurements (120 µl), the data were collected in parallel measurements. Data of 5 fibers (ATPase) and 8 fibers (isometric force and force redevelopment) are summarized. All three parameters were normalized to the values observed in the presence of 5 mM MgATP. Lines are drawn by eye.

Isometric ATPase was measured using a coupled enzyme system; pyruvate kinase converts ADP + phosphoenole pyruvate to ATP and pyruvate, and the second system converts pyruvate + NADH to lactate + NAD by lactate dehydrogenase. Thus, following NAD production at 340 nm allows monitoring of fiber ATPase (26).

strong-binding, force-generating states, apparent rate constants can be defined for the transition from the weak-binding, non-force-generating states to the strong-binding, force-generating states and for the transition back to the former states via release of hydrolysis products ($MgADP + P_i$) and rebinding of MgATP. Assuming that the forward rate constants for these two transitions are on average significantly greater than the corresponding reverse rate constants, an assumption which is consistent with the expected large decrease in free energy across these two steps during isometric contraction, then the two apparent forward rate constants are related to the experimental parameters (isometric force, isometric fiber ATPase, and rate constant of force redevelopment) in the same way as shown in Scheme I for the 2-state model of (21). For this reason, the two apparent rate constants are designated '$f_{app.}$' and '$g_{app.}$'. They describe the transition from the weak-binding, non-force-generating states to the strong-binding, force-generating states ('$f_{app.}$') as well as the transition from the stong-binding, force-generating states back to the weak-binding, non-force-generating states via product release and rebinding of MgATP ('$g_{app.}$'). Since it was demonstrated that at least under certain conditions weak-binding, non-force-generating states can also bind to actin (2), the two rate constants no longer describe attachment and detachment, respectively.

The relations between the three experimental parameters and the two apparent rate constants ($f_{app.}$ and $g_{app.}$), analogous to the relations given for 'f' and 'g' in Scheme I, allow to experimentally determine the two apparent rate constants for various conditions. Figure 4a summarizes an experimental approach for simultaneous measurements of isometric force and rate constant of force redevelopment following free or lightly loaded isotonic shortening (4, 6, 9). For some details in the ATPase measurements see Fig. 4b.

II Effect of MgATP on isometric force, force redevelopment and isometric ATPase

Figure 4b shows the effect of MgATP concentration on the three experimental parameters isometric force, rate constant of force redevelopment, and isometric fiber ATPase. The product of the rate constant of force redevelopment times the corresponding isometric tension is proportional to '$f_{app.}$'. This product was derived from the data shown in Fig. 4b and found to be independent of the MgATP concentration within the accuracy of the experiments. This implies that MgATP mainly affects the transition from the force-generating states back to the non-force-generating states ('$g_{app.}$'). Using the values for the rate constants of force redevelopment and the corresponding normalized rate constants of the isometric ATPase shown in Fig. 4b, '$f_{app.}$' and '$g_{app.}$' can be calculated. At 5 mM MgATP '$f_{app.}$' is found approximately 3 × greater than '$g_{app.}$'. However, it should be pointed out that the ATP regenerating system used in the ATPase measurements might cause some ATP depletion at low MgATP concentrations, leading to a more pronounced decrease in observed isometric ATPase with decrease in MgATP concentration. This, however, leads to a larger value for the apparent K_m of the ATPase (15), which is 50–60 µM in Fig. 4b. Using the procedure suggested by Glyn and Sleep (15) to estimate the true K_m of the ATPase, we found a value for K_m of about 30 µM. Using this K_m value or the 20 mM reported by Glyn and Sleep (15), '$f_{app.}$' is found to be 2–3 times greater than '$g_{app.}$' in the presence of 5 mM MgATP. At 5° C and with 5 mM MgATP, the rate of force redevelopment is found to be 4.5 ± 1.9 s^{-1} (mean $\pm$ S. D., n = 13), yielding '$f_{app.}$' of 3–3.5 s^{-1} and '$g_{app.}$' of 1–1.5 s^{-1}.

From these values for the two apparent rate constants it follows that under the experimental conditions 2/3 to 3/4 of the cycling cross-bridges are in the force-generating states at any given time. Under the same conditions, we found stiffness of fully Ca^{++} activated skinned rabbit psoas fibers to be 0.71 ± 0.12 (mean $\pm$ S. D., n = 7) of the rigor stiffness, both stiffnesses measured at 5° C and at an ionic strength of 0.17 M. Since active stiffness was again measured under conditions where cross-bridge attachment in states equivalent to the weak-binding states of relaxed fibers does not contribute, the measured apparent fiber stiffness should only orginate from cross-bridges in strong-binding states. Since presumably all cross-bridges are attached in rigor (12) and assuming that stiffness per cross-bridge in rigor is the same as in active fibers, these data imply that all cross-bridges have to be recruited in active muscle with 2/3 to 3/4 attached in strong-binding, force-generating states to account for a stiffness of about 70% of the rigor stiffness.

At higher temperatures, we observed an increased isometric force; at 15° C isometric tension is 1.83 ± 0.06 (mean ± S. D., n = 6) times greater than that observed at 5° C. At 20° C isometric tension is found to be 2.31 ± 0.31 (mean ± S. D., n = 4) times the isometric tension at 5° C. Obviously, the increase in isometric force with temperature cannot be accounted for by only an increased number of cross-bridges in the force-generating states. The actual increase in number of cross-bridges in the force-generating states at 15° C can be estimated from our preliminary parallel measurements of both force redevelopment and fiber ATPase at 15° C. For 'f_{app}.' and 'g_{app}.' we found values in the range of $12 \, s^{-1}$ and $2 \, s^{-1}$ respectively, indicating that about 85% of the cycling cross-bridges are in the force-generating states. Thus, only a small part of the increase in force with temperature can be accounted for by the increased fraction of cross-bridges in the force-generating states. An additional increase in average force per cross-bridge has therefore to be postulated. However, there is need of further experiments to decide whether force produced in a force-generating state is affected by temperature or whether the required increase in average force per cross-bridge might reflect temperature dependence of an equilibrium between at least two force-generating states producing low and high force respectively.

The rate constant of force redevelopment and the in vitro actomyosin ATPase (9) show almost parallel behaviour when temperature is increased. The agreement is even closer when 'f_{app}.' is compared with the in vitro actomyosin ATPase instead of k_{redev}.(Table 1). This close

Table 1. Comparison of the rate constant for force redevelopment, f_{app}., g_{app}., and the cross-linked acto-S-1 ATPase activity

Temperature	k_{redev}. (s^{-1})	'f_{app}.'(s^{-1})	'g_{app}.' (s^{-1})	ATPase (s^{-1})#
5° C	4.5 ± 1.9*	3–3.5	1–1.5	1.92
15° C	14.5 ± 2.4	~ 12	~ 2	11.41

Maximum actin activated acto-S-1 ATPase measured under the same conditions as the mechanical parameters ($\mu = 0.17$ M) by using S-1 cross-linked to actin (31, 36). From (9).
* mean ± SD

agreement between actomyosin ATPase in solution and 'f_{app}.' (or the rate of force redevelopment since this rate is dominated by 'f_{app}.', especially at high temperature) suggests that both 'f_{app}.' and in vitro actomyosin ATPase are determined by the same parameters. This implies that the same mechanism which is rate-limiting in vitro also determines the rate of force generation in the cross-bridge cycle, i. e., governs the transition from the weak-binding, non-force-generating states to the strong-binding, force-generating states.

III Effect of sarcoplasmic Ca++ concentration on cross-bridge kinetics

Isometric force, force redevelopment and isometric ATPase were measured at various sarcoplasmic Ca++ concentrations. In Fig. 5 a the observed rate constant of force redevelopment is plotted vs. isometric force. We found that firstly, the rate constant of force redevelopment is affected by the sarcoplasmic Ca++ concentration, indicating that Ca++

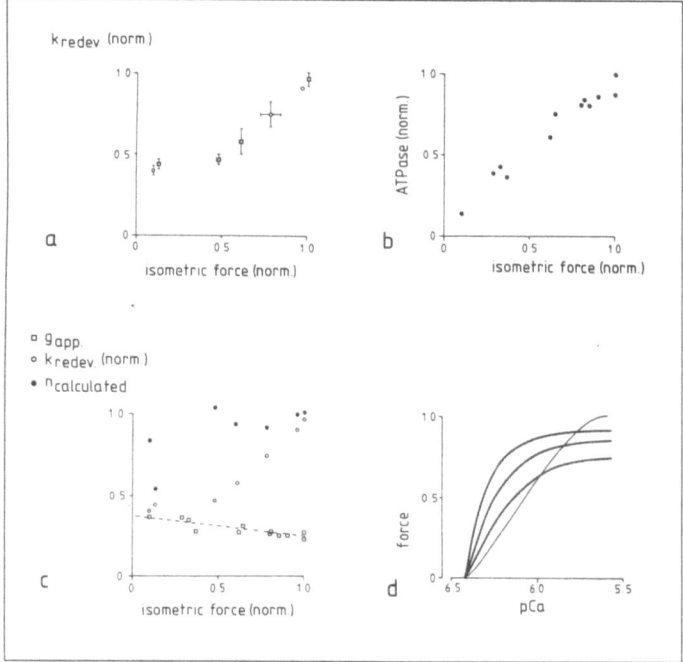

Fig. 5. Effect of sarcoplasmic Ca^{++} concentration on isometric force, force redevelopment, and isometric fiber ATPase.

(a) Rate constant of force redevelopment vs. isometric force
   Abscissa, isometric force (normalized); ordinate rate constant of force redevelopment (normalized). Symbols represent means $\pm$ SEM.

(b) isometric fiber ATPase vs. isometric force
   Abscissa, isometric force (normalized); ordinate isometric ATPase (normalized).

(c) $k_{redevelopment}$ (open circles). The symbols are the means shown in (a)
   '$g_{app.}$' (open squares) is given as fraction of $k_{redev.}$ at full Ca^{++} activation. This fraction is calculated from ATPase/force which is proportional to '$g_{app.}$' and the finding that at 5 mM MgATP '$g_{app.}$' is between $1/4$ to $1/3$ of $k_{redev.}$ (see experiments at various MgATP concentrations). Dashed line represents the linear least squares fit to the data.
   n (fraction of activated interaction sites, filled circles). n at the various Ca^{++} concentrations is proportional to force/('$f_{app.}$'/('$f_{app.}$' + '$g_{app.}$')) since force is proportional to n('$f_{app.}$'/('$f_{app.}$' + '$g_{app.}$')), see Scheme 1, with '$f_{app.}$' = $k_{redev.}$ − '$g_{app.}$'.

(d) '$f_{app.}$' and isometric force ($\propto$ '$f_{app.}$'/('$f_{app.}$' + '$g_{app.}$')) vs. pCa (schematic).
   The thin solid line represents the effect of pCa on '$f_{app.}$'. The heavy solid lines represent the effect on isometric force when the absolute magnitude of $f_{app.}$ was varied ($4.5\ s^{-1}$, $2 \times 4.5s^{-1}$, $4 \times 4.5s^{-1}$) while '$g_{app.}$' ($1.5s^{-1}$) and the effect on Ca^{++} on '$f_{app.}$' were left unchanged.

does affect kinetics of the cross-bridge cycle. Secondly, with force approaching zero the rate constant of force redevelopment approaches a value that is 25–30% the value of the rate constant measured at full Ca^{++} activation. Thirdly, compared with the relative increase in isometric force, the rate constant of force redevelopment has a steeper increase at the higher degrees of activation than at low levels of activation. In Fig. 5b isometric ATPase is plotted vs. isometric force. At low levels of activation the relative increase in fiber ATPase is somewhat larger than the relative increase in tension while at the higher levels of activation the situation is reversed. It is, however, not clear whether this behaviour might at least partly be caused by some deterioration of the fibers at the high degrees of activation. In fibers with pronounced disorder on the sarcomere level at high degrees of activation, we found ATPase to be more suppressed than isometric force. On the other hand, the slight non-linearity might indicate a slight effect of Ca^{++} on '$g_{app.}$' which is proportional to the ratio of isometric ATPase/isometric force.

From the experiments with MgATP we derived that at full Ca^{++} activation '$g_{app.}$' is about $^1/_3-^1/_2$ of '$f_{app.}$'. From Fig. 6 b we can derive the maximum effect of Ca^{++} on '$g_{app.}$'. By combining the two results, we can obtain an estimate for '$f_{app.}$' ($k_{redev.}-$'$g_{app.}$'). It is found that at low Ca^{++} concentrations '$f_{app.}$' approaches zero, indicating that the effect of Ca^{++} on this rate constant can play an important role in regulation of muscle contraction. From the calculated values for '$f_{app.}$' and '$g_{app.}$' at different Ca^{++} concentrations we then can determine the fraction of time during which cycling cross-bridges remain in the force-generating states ('$f_{app.}$'/['$f_{app.}$' + '$g_{app.}$']). Since isometric force is proportional to the product of the number of cycling cross-bridges, times the fraction of time during which the cycling cross-bridges remain in the force-generating states, the comparison of isometric force with the calculated fraction of time makes it possible to estimate the proportion of cycling cross-bridges. As demonstrated in Fig. 5 c the number of cycling cross-bridges increases very rapidly at low Ca^{++} concentrations. In fact, it cannot be ruled out that the number of cycling cross-bridges is always maximal, implying that not the number of cycling cross-bridges is regulated but rather the kinetics of the cycling cross-bridges.

The Ca^{++} effects on $f_{app.}$ could be caused by effects of Ca^{++} on either an unfavourable equilibrium prior to the transition from the weak-binding states to the strong-binding states or on the rate constant for this transition directly. For example, Wagner (38) found an approximately 5-fold increase in binding of HMM in the weak-binding states when Ca^{++} was present. In addition, in vitro (Fig. 1) the transition to the strong-binding states is very much faster when S-1 or HMM are bound to actin. Assuming analogy between muscle and solution, one could postulate that an increase in cross-bridge attachment in the weak-binding states when Ca^{++} is present might be the cause for the increase in the observed rate constant for the transition from the weak-binding states to the strong-binding states. However, when we lowered the ionic strength in relaxed fibers which was shown to increase cross-bridge attachment in the weak-binding states (2, 5), we did not observe any cross-bridge cycling, e. g., force generation, unless again Ca^{++} had been added (2). This suggests that very likely it is not simply an increase in cross-bridge attachment in the weak-binding states which increases the apparent rate constant for the subsequent transition to the strong-binding states, but probably the rate constant for this transition itself is affected.

The observed effect of Ca^{++} on cross-bridge kinetics has important implications for the interpretation of observed force-pCa relations (Fig. 5 d). The light solid line represents the pCa effect on '$f_{app.}$'. The heavy solid lines represent effects of pCa on observed isometric force when '$g_{app.}$' and the effect of pCa on '$f_{app.}$' are kept constant and only the absolute magnitude of '$f_{app.}$' is changed. This demonstrates that without analysis of cross-bridge kinetics, neither slope nor midpoint of the force-pCa relation, in themselves, allow any conclusions to be made about cooperativity in muscle regulation or Ca^{++} binding to TnC or about alterations in these parameters when the force-pCa relation has changed. This further demonstrates that changes in cross-bridge kinetics may play an important role in modulation of muscle activity which is an important feature of myocardium. In studying and interpreting modulation of activity of myocardium, analysis of cross-bridge kinetics ought to be included.

Conclusion and implications

From the present results the following features have to be incorporated in kinetic schemes of the cross-bridge cycle in muscle, and should be considered in interpreting regulation and modulation of muscle activity.

(1) A group of cross-bridge states which is characterized by (a) low affinity to actin, (b) binding to actin even in the absence of Ca^{++}, and (c) a rapid equilibrium between attachment and detachment. These states very likely represent the equivalent of the weak-binding states described in the kinetic schemes of the in vitro actomyosin ATPase. Because of the rapid equilibrium between attachment and detachment, cross-bridges attached to actin in the weak-binding states will not present significant resistance to stretch of relaxed muscle on a slow or moderate time scale.

(2) A group of cross-bridge states with (a) higher affinity to actin, (b) a slower equilibrium between attachment and detachment, and (c) cooperative binding to actin. These states very likely represent the equivalent of the strong-binding states of the kinetic schemes of the in vitro actomyosin ATPase. The slower equilibrium between attachment and detachment can result in an increased resistance to stretch when cross-bridges attached in these states are present in muscle.

(3) Kinetics of the cycling cross-bridges ('f_{app}.' and 'g_{app}.') are affected by MgATP almost exclusively via 'g_{app}.', the apparent rate constant for the transition from the strong-binding, force-generating states back to the weak-binding, non-force-generating states after product release and subsequent rebinding of MgATP.

(4) The relative magnitude of 'f_{app}.' and 'g_{app}.' is such that in fully Ca^{++} activated fibers at $5°$ C, $2/3$ to $3/4$ of the cross-bridges are in the strong-binding states. At higher temperatures, this fraction increases slightly whereas force can increase several fold. This implies that a mechanism has to be engaged that allows the average force per cross-bridge to change with temperature.

(5) The experiments at various Ca^{++} concentrations indicate that Ca^{++} affects the apparent rate constant for the transition from the weak-binding, non-force-generating states to the strong-binding, force-generating states. The number of activated interaction sites derived at various Ca^{++} concentrations implies that possibly all interaction sites are available at all Ca^{++} concentrations and that regulation of muscle activity occurs via regulation of cross-bridge kinetics ('f_{app}.'). The observed effect of Ca^{++} on 'f_{app}.' is not inconsistent with the observation that Ca^{++} has only a small if any effect on the maximum speed of shortening (1, 8, 13, 32) since this parameter is mainly determined by 'g_{app}.' which is only slightly affected by Ca^{++} or not at all.

(6) Factors which can affect cross-bridge kinetics via 'f_{app}.' or 'g_{app}.' can become important parameters for modulation of muscle activity. Such factors may affect the fraction of cross-bridges in the strong-binding, force-generating states not only when the muscle is stimulated but also in unstimulated muscle if 'f_{app}.' becomes significant. This is based on our observation that regulation of cross-bridge cycling may occur mainly via 'f_{app}.'. Such modulation of tension, in turn, requires detailed studying of cross-bridge kinetics if the effect of various parameters on muscle activity is analysed.

Acknowledgement

I would like to thank Drs. R. J. Podolsky, L. C. Yu, and M. Schoenberg for encouragement and support. I would especially like to thank Dr. E. Eisenberg for many suggestions and numerous stimulating discussions, and Dr. R. Jacob for his generous support, advice, and encouragement over many years.

14

References

1. Brenner B (1980) Effect of free sarcoplasmic Ca^{2+} concentration on maximum unloaded shortening velocity: measurements on single glycerinated rabbit psoas fibres. J Muscle Res Cell Mot 1: 409–428
2. Brenner B, Schoenberg M, Chalovich JM, Greene LE, Eisenberg E (1982) Evidence for cross-bridge attachment in relaxed fibers at low ionic strength. Proc Natl Acad Sci USA 79: 7288–7291
3. Brenner B, Yu LC, Green LE, Eisenberg E, Schoenberg M, Podolsky RJ (1983) Cooperative crossbridge formation in skinned rabbit psoas fibers in the presence of $MgPP_i$. Biophys J 41: 33 a
4. Brenner B (1984) The rate of force redevelopment in single skinned rabbit psoas fibers in the presence of $MgPP_i$. Biophys J 45: 155 a
5. Brenner B, Yu LC, Podolsky RJ (1984) X-ray diffraction evidence for cross-bridge formation in relaxed muscle fibers at various ionic strengths. Biophys J 46: 299–306
6. Brenner B (1985) Correlation between the cross-bridge cycle in muscle and the actomyosion ATPase cycle in solution. J Muscle Res Cell Mot 6: 659–664
7. Brenner B, Yu LC (1985) Equatorial X-ray diffraction from single skinned rabbit psoas fibers at various degrees of activation. Changes in intensities and lattice spacing. Biophys J 48: 829–834
8. Brenner B (1986) The necessity of using two parameters to describe isotonic shortening velocity of muscle tissues: the effect of various interventions upon initial shortening velocity (v_i) and curvature (b). Basic Res Cardiol 81: 54–69
9. Brenner B, Eisenberg E (1986) Rate of force generation in muscle: Correlation with actomyosin ATPase activity in solution. Proc Natl Acad Sci USA 83: 3542–3546
10. Chalovich JM, Chock PB, Eisenberg E (1981) Mechanism of action of troponin-tropomyosin J Biol Chem 256: 575–578
11. Chalovich JM, Eisenberg E (1982) Inhibition of actomyosin ATPase activity by troponin-tropomyosin without blocking the binding of myosin to actin. J Biol Chem 257: 2431–2437
12. Cooke R, Franks K (1980) All myosin heads form bonds with actin in rabbit rigor skeletal muscle. Biochemistry 19: 2265–2269
13. Ferenczi MA, Goldman YE, Simmons RM (1984) The dependence of force and shortening velocity on substrate concentration in skinned muscle fibres from Rana Temporaria. J Physiol Lond 350: 519–543
14. Ford LE, Huxley AF, Simmons RM (1981) The relation between stiffness and filament overlap in stimulated frog muscle fibres. J Physiol Lond 311: 219–249
15. Glyn H, Sleep J (1985) Dependence of adenosine triphosphatase activity of rabbit psoas muscle fibres and myofibrils on substrate concentration. J Physiol Lond 365: 259–276
16. Greene LE, Eisenberg E (1980) Cooperative binding of myosin subfragment-1 to the actin-troponin-tropomyosin complex. Proc Natl Acad Sci USA 77: 2616–2620
17. Greene LE, Sellers JR, Eisenberg E, Adelstein RS (1983) Binding of gizzard smooth muscle myosin subfragment-one to actin in the presence and absence of ATP. Biochemistry 22: 530–535
18. Haselgrove JC, Huxley HE (1973) X-ray evidence for radial cross-bridge movement and for the sliding filament model in actively contracting skeletal muscle. J Mol Miol 77: 549–568
19. Hill AV (1938) The heat of shortening and the dynamic constants of muscle. Proc R Soc B 126: 136–195
20. Huxley AF, Niedergerke R (1954) Interference microscopy of living muscle fibres. Nature Lond 173: 971–973
21. Huxley AF (1957) Muscle structure and theories of contraction. Prog Biophys Biophys Chem 7: 255–318
22. Huxley AF, Simmons RM (1971) Proposed mechanism of force generation in striated muscle. Nature 233: 533–538
23. Huxley HE, Hanson J (1954) Changes in the cross-striations of muscle during contraction and stretch and their interpretation. Nature Lond 173: 973–976
24. Huxley HE (1968) Structural differences between resting and rigor muscle. Evidence from intensity changes in the low-angle equatorial X-ray diagram. J Mol Biol 37: 507–520
25. Huxley HE (1969) The mechanism of muscular contraction. Science NY 164: 1356–1366
26. Loxdale HD (1976) A method for continuous assay of picomole quantities of ADP released from glycerol-extracted skeletal muscle fibers on MgATP activation. J Physiol Lond 260: 4 P

27 Lymn RW, Taylor EW (1971) Mechanism of adenosine triphosphate hydrolysis by actomyosin. Biochemistry 10: 4617–4624

28. Marston SB, Tregear RT (1972) Evidence for a complex between myosin and ADP in relaxed muscle fibers. Nature New Biol 235: 23–24

29. Marston SB (1973) The nucleotide complexes of myosin in glycerol-extracted muscle fibers. Biochim Biophys Acta 305: 397–412

30. Marston SB (1982) The rates of formation and dissociation of actin-myosin complexes. Biochem J 230: 453–460

31. Mornet D, Bertrand R, Pantel P, Audemard E, Kassab R (1981) Structure of the actin-myosin interface. Nature, Lond 292: 301–306

32. Podolsky RJ, Teichholz LE (1970) The relation between calcium and contraction kinetics in skinned muscle fibres. J Physiol Lond 211: 19–35

33. Rosenfeld SS, Taylor EW (1984) The ATPase mechanism of skeletal and smooth muscle acto-sub-fragment 1. J Biol Chem 259: 11 908–11 919

34. Stein LA, Schwarz RP, Chock PB, Eisenberg E (1979) Mechanism of actomyosin adenosine triphosphatase. Evidence that adenosine 5'-triphosphate hydrolysis can occur without dissociation of the actomyosin complex. Biochemistry 18: 3895–3909

35. Stein LA, Chock PB, Eisenberg E (1984) The rate-limiting step in the actomyosin adenosinetriphosphatase cycle. Biochemistry 23: 1555–1563

36. Stein LA, Greene LE, Chock PB, Eisenberg E (1985) Biochemistry 24: 1357–1363

37. Wagner PD, Giniger E (1981) Calcium-sensitive binding of heavy meromyosin to regulated actin in the presence of ATP. J Biol Chem 256: 12647–12650

38. Wagner PD (1984) Effect of skeletal muscle myosin light chain 2 on the Ca^{2+}-sensitive interaction of myosin and heavy meromyosin with regulated actin. Biochemistry 23: 5950–5956

39. Webb MR, Trentham DR (1981) The mechanism of ATP hydrolysis catalyzed by myosin and actomyosin using rapid reaction techniques to study oxygen exchange J Biol Chem 256: 10910–10916

40. White HD, Taylor EW (1976) Energetics and mechanism of actomyosin adenosine triphosphatase. Biochemistry 15: 5818–5826

41. Yu LC, Hartt JE, Podolsky RJ (1979) Equatorial X-ray intensities and isometric force levels in frog sartorius muscle. J Mol Biol 132: 53–67

Author's address:

Dr. B. Brenner, Physiologisches Institut II, Gmelinstr. 5, D-7400 Tübingen (F.R.G.)

Calcium sensitivity of myofilaments in cardiac muscle – effect of myosin phosphorylation

I. Morano and J. C. Rüegg

II. Physiologisches Institut, Universität Heidelberg, Heidelberg (F. R. G.)

Summary

We investigated the influence of the extent of phosphorylation of the myosin P-light-chain on the calcium sensitivity of skinned heart fibres. Treatment of skinned heart fibres with PCM-phosphatase decreased the phosphorylation level of P-light-chain from 0.3 mol P/mol LC-2 and 0.2 mol P/mol LC-2* to 0.16 mol P/mol LC-2 and 0.14 mol P/mol LC-2*. Isometric tension development decreased by 34 % at submaximal Ca^{2+}-concentration (pCa 5.5) after incubation with PCM-phosphatase while tension achieved at maximum Ca^{2+}-concentration (pCa 4.3) was not affected. The effect of desensitization on skinned fibres could be reversed by washing out the phosphatase or by addition of myosin light chain kinase.

Key words: cardiac skinned fibres, P-light-chain phosphorylation, Ca^{2+} effects, myosin phosphatase, Ca^{2+}-sensitivity

Introduction

In cardiac muscle the free calcium concentration attained during systole is about 1 μM (1). This is sufficient to induce about halfmaximal activation (12). The heart, therefore, has a large contractile reserve which can be mobilized under conditions which further raise the intracellular calcium ion concentration, such as application of catecholamines. The decisive parameter of force development is, however, not the calcium concentration per se but the calcium occupancy of troponin. Hence force may be altered even at constant calcium occupancy of troponin by altering the calcium affinity. Such changes may lead to a shift in the relationship of force and calcium concentration in living muscle (1) and in skinned or demembranated muscle fibres (for review see [20]). In skinned fibres the calcium ion concentrations surrounding the myofilaments may be altered at will and clamped at the desired levels by means of CaEGTA-buffers.

In view of the fact that the calcium sensitivity may be altered after pharmacological interventions (10) and under pathological conditions, e. g. hypoxia (2) and atrial hypertrophy (3), it is important to learn more about the biochemical mechanisms which are capable of influencing calcium sensitivity.

One such mechanism is phosphorylation of the regulatory light chain (designated as LC-2 or P-light-chain) by myosin light chain kinase (MLCK) and calmodulin (18), which has been also shown to increase Ca^{2+}-sensitivity of skeletal muscle (19). In skeletal muscle a correlation between myosin P-light-chain phosphorylation and potentiation of the isometric twitch tension has been observed (15, 16).

Here we show that the sensitization of skinned cardiac fibres for calcium ions by

MLCK-induced phosphorylation of the myosin P-light-chain (LC-2) could be reversed by dephosphorylation of the light-chain. The phosphatase used here has already been reported to accept myocardial P-light-chains as a substrate for the dephosphorylation reaction (5). As the activity of this enzyme may be modulated by polycationic effectors (e. g. polylysine) the enzyme is called "polycationic modulable phosphatase", abbreviated PCM-phosphatase (4, 10). Dephosphorylation of the myosin P-light-chain with PCM-phosphatase also decreased the calcium sensitivity in and accelerated relaxation of chemically skinned chicken gizzard (4). These results are in accordance with the concept that P-light-chain phosphorylation is involved in the activation of smooth muscle contraction (14) but its significance in the regulation of cardiac and skeletal muscle (19) is still controversial.

Materials and methods

Trabecula fibre bundles of the right ventricle of pigs were chemically skinned in a solution containing 50% glycerol, 20 mM imidazole, 10 mM NaN_3, 5 mM ATP, 5 mM $MgCl_2$, 4 mM EGTA, 2 mM DTE, pH 7.0 at $+4°$ C for 1 hour and then in the same solution including 1% Triton X-100 at $+4°$ C for 12 hours. The fibres were washed and stored at $-20°$ C in the first solution without detergent for three days before starting the experiments.

The chemically skinned ventricular fibres were mounted isometrically and attached to a force transducer (AME 801, Aksjeselskapet, Horten, Norway). The relaxation and contraction solutions both contained an ATP-regeneration system. The relaxation solution contained 10 mM ATP, 12.5 mM $MgCl_2$, 5 mM EGTA, 20 mM imidazole, 5 mM NaN_3, 10 mM phosphocreatine, and 380 U/ml CPK (Boehringer, Mannheim, F. R. G.), pH 6.7. The contraction solution had the same composition as the relaxation solution except that EGTA was substituted by 5 mM CaEGTA. The free Ca^{2+}-concentration was adjusted by mixing the relaxation and contraction solution as described in (18) using an apparent stability constant for CaEGTA of $10^6 M^{-1}$. To 1 ml solution either 80 μl/ml PCM-phosphatase (160 U/ml dissolved in a "phosphatase-buffer" containing 50% glycerol, 20 mM TRIS/HCl, 0.5 mM DTT, pH 7.4) or 80 μl "phosphatase-buffer" were added. One phosphatase unit (U) is the amount of enzyme releasing 1 nmol ^{32}P per minute of phosphorylated myocardial light chains at 30° C. PCM-phosphatase, extracted and purified from bovine aorta (10), was obtained from J. Di Salvo (Cincinnati, USA) and C. Bialojan (Heidelberg, F. R. G.). Contraction and relaxation were induced by raising and lowering the calcium ion concentration. After a contraction cycle at a suboptimal pCa the fibres were then incubated for 30 min in relaxation solution containing 160 U/ml PCM-phosphatase. In control experiments the PCM-phosphatase was inactivated by thawing and freezing, a procedure which is known to destroy PCM-phosphatase activity (Bialojan, personal communication). After a contraction-relaxation cycle and subsequent incubation (30 min) of the fibres with phosphatase (160 U/ml relaxation solution) a second contraction was elicited. The inhibition could be reversed in two different ways. Firstly, the phosphatase was washed out for 90 min by changing the relaxation solution serveral times. In a second approach fibres were first treated with PCM-phosphatase as described and then activated with Ca^{2+} (pCa 5.5) in the presence of cardiac myosin light chain kinase (12.4 μg/ml bathing solution, cf. 18) and calmodulin (4.2 μM).

Myosin light chain phosphorylation of skinned fibres was determined by two-dimensional gel electrophoresis (9). Fibres were treated exactly as in the mechanical experiments: They were either incubated for 30 min in relaxation solution containing 160 U/ml of PCM-phosphatase, or "phosphatase-buffer" in the control experiments. The fibres were then denatured with icecold trichloroacetic acid (15%) containing 2% pyrophosphate, washed with 20 mM imidazole-buffer (pH 6.7) and stored for no longer than 7 days at $-20°$ C. The fibres were then homogenized in 44 mM NaH_2PO_4, 6 mM KH_2PO_4, 10 mM DTE, 1% SDS, pH 7.5 and mixed with glycerol and ampholine. Isolelectric focussing was performed over night in gels composed of 6.8% acrylamide, 1.7% Triton X-100, 9 M urea, 20% ampholine at 400 V. Ampholines were in the pH-range 4–6 (LKB, S) or 4.5–5.4 (Pharmacia, S). The second dimension was run as described (17).

The spots representing the P-light-chain were evaluated densitometrically with a "model 1650 scanning densitometer" (Bio-Rad, F. R. G.). The degree of P-light-chain phosphorylation was expressed in % of the total amount of P-light-chain areas. Values are expressed as means ± SE and a Student's t-test was used for the significance analysis.

Results

Mechanical experiments. Incubation with PCM-phosphatase decreased the isometric force at submaximal Ca^{2+}-concentration (pCa 5.5) (Fig. 1) and led to a shift of the calcium-tension curve to higher calcium-concentrations (Fig. 2). Isometric force at maximum calcium concentration (pCa 4.3) was not affected (Fig. 1). To exclude unspecific effects the same

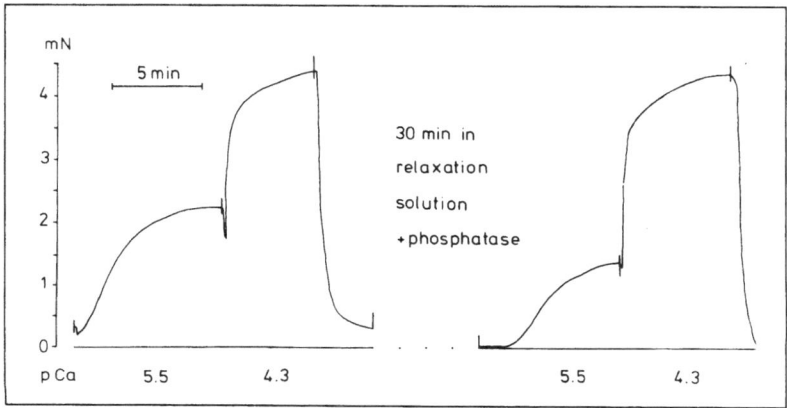

Fig. 1. Isometric force of chemically skinned right trabecula fibres of pigs at submaximal (pCa 5.5) and maximal Ca^{2+} (pCa 4.3) respectively. The fibres were incubated in relaxation solution for 30 min in the presence of 160 U/ml PCM-phosphatase and then a second contraction was elicited at pCa 5.5 and 4.3.

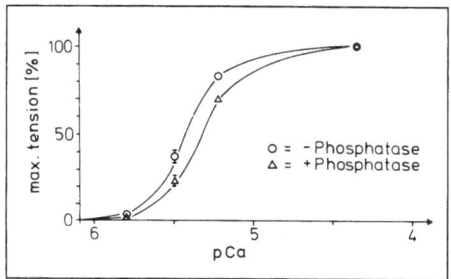

Fig. 2. Tension development of chemically skinned cardiac fibres (in % of maximum tension) plotted versus pCa before (0) and after (Δ) incubation with 160 U/ml PCM-phosphatase for 30 min in relaxation solution. 7 fibres were investigated at pCa 5.5 (mean values ± SE).

experiments were performed with inactivated PCM-phosphatase. No change of the isometric tension at submaximal or maximal Ca^{2+}-concentrations could be detected after 30 min of incubation with inactivated PCM-phosphatase (Fig. 3). As shown in Table 1, isometric force achieved at pCa 5.5 induced 42.7 ± 5.1% of the isometric tension achieved at maximum activation. After 30 min of incubation with phosphatase in relaxation solution the mean isometric tension decreased to 28.9 ± 5.3% of the tension achieved at pCa 4.3. This decrease is statistically significant at p < 0.001-level. Comparing directly the force generation

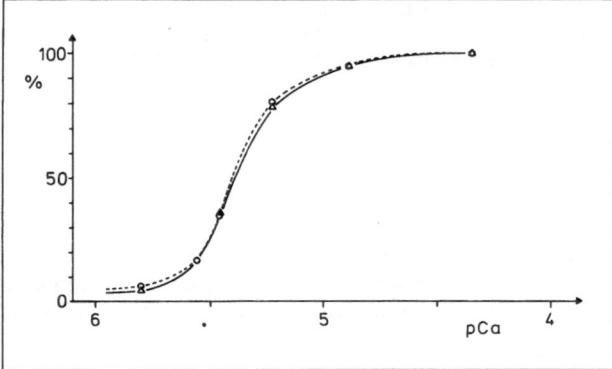

Fig. 3. Tension development of 3 chemically skinned cardiac muscle fibres expressed as % of maximum tension plotted versus pCa before (0) and after (Δ) incubation with 160 U/ml inactivated PCM-phosphatase for 30 min in relaxation solution.

Table 1. Isometric force achieved at submaximal Ca²⁺-concentration (pCa 5.5) and P-light-chain phosphorylation before (A) and after phosphatase incubation (B) of chemically skinned right trabecula fibres of pigs for 30 min in relaxation solution with 160 U/ml PCM-phosphatase.
Isometric force at pCa 5.5 is expressed in % of isometric tension achieved at maximum Ca²⁺-concentration (pCa 4.3). The areas of the different components of LC-2 were expressed as per cent of the total regulatory light chain (LC-2).
Values are mean ± SE with the number of fibres in parentheses.

Conditions pCa phosphatase	Isometric tension (%)	Myosin light chain phosphorylation		
		LC-2	"P-LC-2"	LC-2*-P
A 5.5 0	42.7 ± 5.1 (7)	50.4 ± 2.2 (6)	44.6 ± 2.2 (6)	5.0 ± 1.9 (6)
B 5.5 160 U/ml	28.9 ± 5.3 (7)	60.8 ± 2.8 (6)	35.6 ± 2.9 (6)	3.7 ± 0.7 (6)

Table 2. Reversibility of phosphatase effects

Cycle	Conditions	Force (%)	
		(A)	(B)
1	Before phosphatase	35	35
2	With phosphatase	28	27
3	+ MLCK	34	26*
4	Wash out of phosphatase	–	34

Force development of skinned trabecula fibres at pCa 5.5 in % of maximal tension (at pCa 5). Sequence of 4 contraction cycles elicited by increasing and lowering free calcium ion concentration:
cycle 1 before addition of phosphatase;
cycle 2 after incubation (30 min) with myosin phosphatase, 160 U/ml);
cycle 3 incubation with myosin light chain kinase (12.4 μg/ml) in imidazole buffer restores calcium responsiveness (3A);
    * in the contrary, the addition of a control buffer has no effect (3B);
cycle 4 after washing out the phosphatase with relaxing solution for 90 min: restoration of calcium responsiveness in fibre A.

of the fibres at pCa 5.5 before and after incubation with PCM-phosphatase, the phosphatase-induced decrease of the isometric tension at pCa 5.5 was 34.3 ± 4.6% (mean ± SE of 7 fibres).

This inhibitory effect produced by the dephosphorylation of the myosin P-light-chain could be reversed by two different methods: Firstly, by washing out the phosphatase and secondly by phosphorylation of the myosin P-light-chain with Ca^{2+}/calmodulin activated myosin light chain kinase (MLCK) (Table 2). In the first case a prolonged washing out period of 90 min was necessary to reverse the desensitization caused by PCM-phosphatase action. The second case MLCK-treatment of the desensitized fibres led within minutes to a resensitization of the fibres for Ca^{2+}.

Phosphorylation of the myosin P-light-chain. Three spots representing the P-light-chain of chemically skinned right trabecula fibres of pigs were visible after two-dimensional electrophoresis using the pH-range 4–6 in the first dimension (Fig. 4). These spots have been

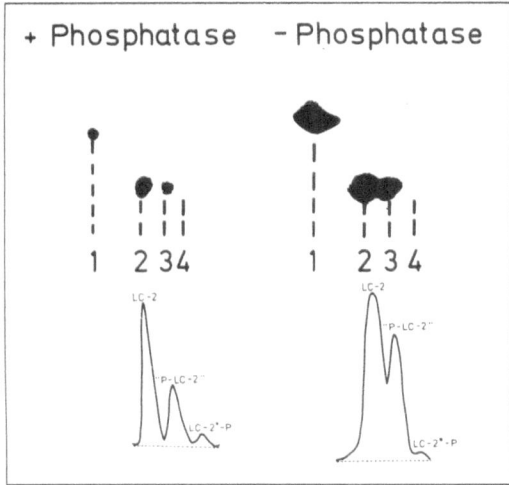

Fig. 4. Two-dimensional gel electrophoresis of chemically skinned right trabecula fibres incubated for 30 min with 160 U/ml PCM-phosphatase or the appropriate volume of phosphatase-buffer in relaxation solution with ($+$) phosphatase or without ($-$) phosphatase respectively. A pH-range of 4–6 was used in the first dimension (isoelectric focussing).

top: light chains after coommassie-staining;

bottom: densitometrical scans of the P-light-chain spots;

$1 = $ LC-1; $2 = $ LC-2; $3 = $ "P-LC-2"; $4 = $ LC-2*-P;

"P-LC-2" consists of 2 components (cf. Fig. 5).

designated in this article as LC-2, "P-LC-2" and LC-2*-P. Incubation of chemically skinned heart fibres with PCM-phosphatase decreased the phosphorylation level of the P-light-chain: Whereas in the untreated fibres "P-LC-2" amounted to $44.6 \pm 2.2\%$ of total LC-2, it decreased to $35.6 \pm 2.9\%$ in the PCM-phosphatase treated fibres. This decrease was statistically significant at the $p < 0.005$ level. However, by using a narrow pH-range in the first

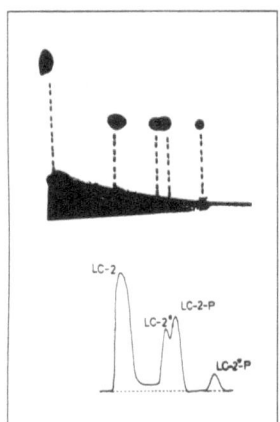

Fig. 5. Two-dimensional gel electrophoresis of chemically skinned right trabecula fibres of pigs. First dimension (isoelectric focussing) was carried out with the pH-range 4.5–5.4.

top: coommassie-stained spots;

bottom: densitometrical scan of the P-light-chain spots;

$1 = $ LC-1; $2 = $ LC-2; $3 = $ LC-2*; $4 = $ LC-2-P; $5 = $ LC-2*-P;

LC-2* and LC-2-P correspond to "P-LC-2" in Fig. 4

(* designates light chain isoform);

LC-2-P and LC-2*-P are the phosphorylated forms of LC-2.

dimension (pH 4.5–5.4) the "P-LC-2-spot" could be resolved into two components, LC-2* and LC-2-P, the latter only being phosphorylated (7, 12). The densitometrical evaluation of the different forms of the P-light-chain areas lead to the following results: LC-2: 50.4 ± 0.9%, LC-2*: 22.4 ± 1.9%, LC-2-P: 22.2 ± 2%, LC-2*-P: 5.1 ± 0.9%. Values are means ± SE of 4 different fibre bundles and are expressed as % of total P-light-chain areas (Fig. 5).

Discussion

The results presented in this article demonstrate that PCM-phosphatase from bovine aorta not only dephosphorylates purified cardiac light chains but also accept the myosin P-light-chain of chemically skinned heart fibres as substrate.

The assessment of the phosphorylation level of myosin P-light-chain by determination of the amount of the P-LC-2-spot has already been discussed (18). Here it could be shown that the spot designated in this article as "P-LC-2" indeed consists of two components: LC-2* (the extra phosphorylatable P-light-chain) and LC-2-P (the phosphorylated form of LC-2). Taking into account that on the average 22.4% of the whole P-light-chain areas represent the extra phosphorylatable P-light-chain (LC-2*) (see results), the relative amount of the phosphorylated form of LC-2 (called LC-2-P) is approximately 22% of the whole P-light-chain. This means that the phosphorylation level of light chains is about 0.3 mol P/mol LC-2 and 0.2 mol P/mol LC-2*. Treatment with PCM-phosphatase decreased these values to 0.16 mol P/mol LC-2 and 0.14 mol P/mol LC-2*. The finding of a second type of a phosphorylatable myosin P-light-chain in the pig ventricle supports the observation that the ventricular myosin P-light-chain of several species exists in two forms (21, 22). In accordance with this notice we found that an incorporation of ^{32}P after MLCK-treatment of skinned pig ventricular fibres appeared only in the LC-2-P and LC-2*-P spot.

Incubation with PCM-phosphatase desensitized the chemically skinned cardiac fibres for calcium. This is in accordance with our previous findings that MLCK-treatment sensitized skinned fibres of cardiac (18) and skeletal muscle (19) to Ca^{2+}-ions. It has been suggested that the phosphate content of the myosin-P-light-chain of fast skeletal muscle is implicated in the phenomenon of "isometric twitch potentiation" (16).

In conclusion then, our results show that contraction of cardiac muscle may be varied over a wide range by phosphorylation and dephosphorylation of the myosin P-light-chain. Thus, addition of MLCK increases force by 146.5 ± 10% and of phosphatase decreased force of skinned fibres to 65.7 ± 4.6% of control contractions elicited by pCa 5. Our studies suggest that phosphorylation/dephosphorylation of the myosin P-light-chain is involved in the modulation of cardiac contractility and calcium sensitivity. It is interesting to note that alpha$_1$-adrenoceptor stimulation increased calcium sensitivity of cardiac myofibrils (11) and that ischemia enhanced myocardial alpha$_1$-adrenoceptor density (8) and myosin P-light-chain phosphorylation (21, 6). The question arises then whether P-light-chain phosphorylation is involved in modulating the calcium sensitivity of myofilaments in vivo in particular during α-adrenergic stimulation and/or ischemia.

Acknowledgements

We are grateful to Isolde Berger for editing and typing the manuscript, and to Drs. J. Di Salvo and C. Bialojan for the gift of myosin phosphatase and F. Hofmann for myosin light chain kinase. This work was supported by Deutsche Forschungsgemeinschaft and Fonds der Chemischen Industrie.

References

1. Allen DG, Kurihara S (1980) Calcium transients in mammalian ventricular muscle. Eur Heart J 1: 5–15
2. Allen DG, Orchard CH (1983) Intracellular calcium concentration during hypoxia and metabolic inhibition in mammalian ventricular muscle. J Physiol (London) 339: 107–122
3. Arndt H, Katus HA, Mall G, Rüegg JC (in press) Calcium sensitivity of human left atrial muscle. Pflügers Arch
4. Bialojan C, Merkel L, Rüegg JC, Gifford D, Di Salvo J (1985) Prolonged relaxation of detergent-skinned smooth muscle involves decreased endogenous phosphatase activity. Proc Soc Exp Biol Med 178: 648–652
5. Bialojan C, Rüegg JC, Di Salvo J (1985) Phosphatase-mediated modulation of actin-myosin interaction in bovine aortic actomyosin and skinned porcine carotid artery. Proc Soc Exp Biol Med 178: 36–45
6. Cummins P, Crome R, Yellon DM, Hearse DJ (1981) Changes in myosin light chain phosphorylations during regional myocardial ischemia. J Mol Cell Cardiol 13: 18
7. Cummins P, Price KM, Littler WA (1980) Foetal myosin light chain in human ventricle. J Muscle Res Cell Mot 1: 357–366
8. Corr PB, Shayman JA, Kramer JB, Kipnis RJ (1981) Increased α-adrenergic receptor in ischemic Ca-myocardium. J Clin Invest 67: 1232–1236
9. Di Salvo J, Gruenstein E, Silver PJ (1979) Ca^{2+} dependent phosphorylation of Ca^{2+} sensitive aortic actomyosin. Proc Soc Exp Biol Med 162: 337–341
10. Di Salvo J, Gifford D, Kokkinakis A (1984) Modulation of aortic protein phosphatase activity by polylysine. Proc Soc Exp Med 177: 24–32
11. Endoh M, Blinks JR (1984) Regulation of the intracellular Ca^{2+} transient and Ca^{2+}-sensitivity of myofibrils via α and β-adrenoceptors in the rabbit papillary muscle. Cell Calcium 5: 301
12. Fabiato A (1983) Calcium-induced calcium release from the sarcoplasmic reticulum. Eur J Physiol 245: C1–C14
13. Frearson N, Perry VS (1975) Phosphorylation of the light-chain components of myosin from cardiac and red skeletal muscles. Biochem J 151: 99–107
14. Gagelmann M, Mrwa U, Bostrom S, Rüegg JC, Hartshorne D (1984) Effect of Ca^{2+}-independent myosin light chain kinase in different skinned smooth muscle fibres. Pflügers Arch 401: 107–109
15. Houston ME, Green HJ, Stull JT (1985) Myosin light chain phosphorylat-on and isometric twitch potentiation in intact human muscle. Pflügers Arch 403: 348–352
16. Klug G, Boltermann B, Stull JT (1982) The effect of low frequency stimulation on myosin light chain phosphorylation in skeletal muscle. J Biol Chem 257: 4688–4690
17. Laemmli UK, Favre M (1973) Maturation of the head of bacteriophage T4. I. DNA packaging events. J Mol Biol 80: 575–611
18. Morano I, Hofmann F, Zimmer M, Rüegg JC (in press) The influence of P-light-chain phosphorylation by myosin light chain kinase on the calcium sensitivity of chemically skinned heart fibres. FEBS Lett.
19. Persechini A, Stull JT, Cooke R (1985) The effect of myosin phosphorylation on the contractile properties of skinned skeletal muscle fibres. Biophys J 47: 63 a
20. Rüegg JC (1985) Modulation of calcium sensitivity in cardiac muscle cells. Basic Res Cardiol 80, Suppl. 2: 79–82
21. Westwood SA, Perry SV (1981) The effect of adrenaline on the phosphorylation of the P-light-chain of myosin and troponin. Biochem J 197: 185–193
22. Westwood SA, Perry SV (1982) Two forms of the P-light chain of myosin in rabbit and bovine heart. FEBS Lett 142: 31–34

Authors' address:

Dr. I. Morano, II. Physiologisches Institut, Universität Heidelberg, Im Neuenheimer Feld 326, D-6900 Heidelberg (F. R. G.)

Ca-pools involved in the regulation of cardiac contraction under positive inotropy. X-ray microanalysis on rapidly-frozen ventricular muscles of guinea-pig

Maria F. Wendt-Gallitelli

Physiologisches Institut II Universität Tübingen, Tübingen (F. R. G.)

Summary

Electron probe microanalysis of rapidly-frozen small ventricular trabeculae of guinea-pig demonstrates that 1. the distribution of total intracellular calcium varies under positive inotropy depending on the type of inotropic intervention. 2. The sarcoplasmic reticulum (SR) (or part of it) localized at the level of the z-lines reveals high calcium accumulation at the end of diastole whenever a stimulus is followed by a contraction with a short time to peak of force. After paired pulse stimulation, *only* this cell compartment accumulates calcium at the end of diastole. Since this cell compartment is "Ca-empty" in muscles frozen during contraction, SR is considered to be the source of activator Ca. 3. In several cases of inotropy (after application of ARL, caffeine or after lowering the extracellular Na^+ concentration), calcium is also detectable on the mitochondria, suggesting that these organelles participate in slow regulation of cytosolic calcium. 4. In some cases, total calcium located on the sarcomeres is increased. The interpretation of this finding is intriguing and requires the assumption of supplementary cytosolic Ca-sinks as yet unknown.

Key words: calcium pools, positive inotropy, electron probe X-ray microanalysis, excitation-contraction coupling

Introduction

The experiments described in this paper are part of a study undertaken to identify the calcium pools involved in the various mechanisms of inotropy in heart muscle. Some of the data have been published already (8–12).

In planning the experiments it was first assumed that under normal conditions most of the calcium responsible for full activation in the mammalian heart is released at the beginning of the action potential essentially from intracellular stores and is not of direct extracellular origin (merely entering to the cell through the cell membrane via the inward calcium current). This assumption is supported by a large body of experimental evidence (1–4, 6, 7, 13). Given that these stores exist, they must be filled with calcium – at least in the cases of maximal force development – at a time when an electrical stimulus would depolarize the cell membrane, that is at the end of diastole. Such conditions may exist following strongly positive inotropic interventions such as paired pulses stimulation, adminstration of caffeine, ouabain, ARL, or

Supported by the Deutsche Forschungsgemeinschaft grant We 879/3-1

when muscle contract at very low frequency in low-sodium or norepinephrine solution (rested state contractions).

Based on the established fact that in cardiac muscle the pattern of contraction (peak of force and time to peak) is variable, depending on the nature of the inotropic intervention, it was also assumed that, depending on the mechanisms leading to positive inotropy, various cell compartments could be involved in buffering and releasing activator calcium in a specific way. In other words, the calcium distribution in the cell should reveal the mode of action of inotropic agents. Moreover, changes in intracellular sodium concentration are also expected to occur in all the cases of intropy in which the Na^+/K^+ pump or/and the Na^+/Ca^{2+} exchange mechanism are involved. Based on this assumption, the aim of this study was to obtain direct evidence of the specific mode of action of cardiac active agents using energy dispersive electronprobe microanalysis and cryotechniques applied to working muscles. The effects of paired pulses stimulation, untoxic doses of ouabaine, low extracellular sodium on intracellular Ca-distribution in guinea-pig ventricular muscles were analysed.

Electron probe microanalysis permits the simultaneous localisation and quantification of most diffusible elements of biological interest even in small subcellular compartments, when observed in the electron microscope. The method, however, has limitations which should be stated in order to avoid misinterpretation or overinterpretation of the data: *firstly*, the minimal detectable concentrations of biologically interesting elements are in the range of about 1–2 mmol/kg dry weight (in other words corresponding to about 200–250 μmol/l, depending on the respective actual water content in the compartments). *Secondly*, only the total concentrations of elements can be determined, and it is not possible to distinguish free from bound elements. *Thirdly*, when analyzing a small structure even with an adequately focused electron beam, one can hardly avoid part of adjacent organelles being included in analysis; over- or underestimation of concentrations are thus possible when a given compartment has lower or higher concentration than the surroundings. This error is obviously unavoidable in all laboratories and we should bear in mind that electron probe data allow essentially *qualitative* statements.

Methods

Ventricular free-running trabeculae or small papillary muscles (diameter 100–300 μm) were rapidly frozen at exactly defined times of the contraction cycle after superfusion with a Tyrode solution of the following composition (in mmoles/l): NaCl 130; KCl 4.9; $MgCl_2$ 1.2; $CaCl_2$ 1.2; glucose 24; $NaHCO_3$ 20; NaH_2PO_4 0.85; pH 7.4. Low-sodium solution contained 15 mmol/l NaCl, 25 mmol/l $NaHCO_3$ and 200 mmol/l sucrose. The concentration of noradrenalin hydrochloride was 10^{-5} mol/l; ARL 115 300 μmol/l; caffeine 10 mmol/l.

The apparatus for triggered freezing and freeze-drying are described in detail in previous papers (9, 12). The freeze-dried cryosections were analyzed with a Siemens Elmiskop 102 electron microscope, equipped with a Kevex energy dispersive system (model 5100), and more recently with a full quantitative Link System (5), model 860–500. More details of calibration curves for quantitation of elements have been already published in previous papers (9, 12).

The preservation of the superficial cells in a small trabecula after freezing is illustrated in Fig. 1. For better visualization of morphology this muscle was freeze-substituted, after shock-freezing. No damage by ice crystals is detectable. All cellular organelles are indistinguishable from those of preparations conventionally fixed and embedded. The dense network of sarcoplasmic reticulum crossing the sarcomeres at the level of the Z-lines is characteristic for the muscles used. In such muscles t-tubuli are either rare or absent.

In Fig. 1 a scheme illustrates the dimensions of the beam respectively maximally focused as a circular spot, or astigmatically deformed to cover a surface of 7 nm width and one micron length.

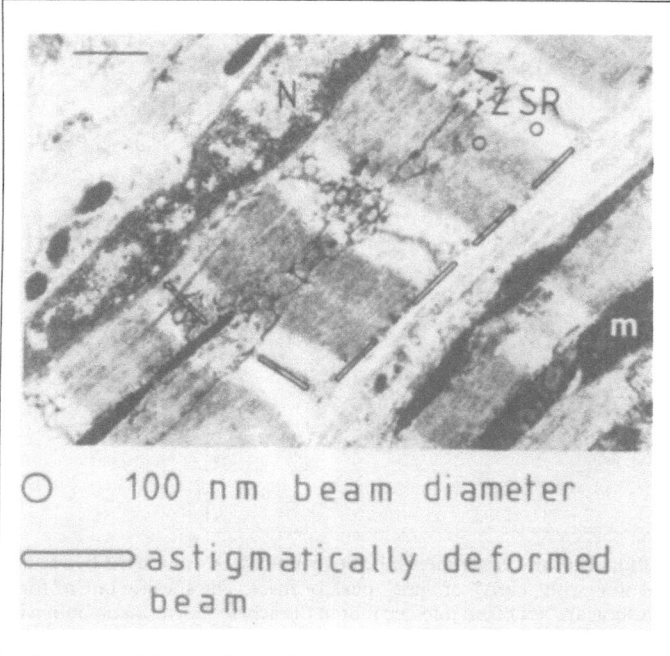

Fig. 1. Longitudinal section of a guinea-pig papillary muscle (200 μm diameter) rapdily frozen and freeze-substituted with acetone for 4 days at $-79°$ C, conventionally embedded and counterstained in order to better visualize the preservation of cellular structures. Note the well developed network of sarcoplasmic reticulum at the level of the Z-lines. o = diameter of the maximally focussed analyzing beam ⊂⊃ = astigmatically deformed beam, covering approximately the same area. Bar = 1μm.

In Fig. 2 the rationale of the experiments is illustrated. Positive inotropy in small guinea-pig trabeculae was induced (1) by varying the frequency and pattern of stimulation, applying paired pulse stimulation; or (2) by administering positive inotropic active drugs such as ARL 15, caffeine, ouabain, norepinephrine or changing the ionic composition of the extracellular medium; or (3) by simultaneously applying drugs and varying the frequency of stimulation, for instance by reducing the frequency of stimulation in the presence of norepinephrine or low sodium solution. In situations (1) and (2) the peak of contraction is reached within a short time as a consequence of positive inotropic interventions of various origins. In (3), maximal activation is markedly retarded. The freezing of the muscles at a moment at which a stimulus would induce a fast or slow contraction should reveal differences in the calcium distribution and one can for instance expect that calcium is released from internal stores located near the contractile machinery in the cases of fast developing contractions on the one hand and that activation is brought about by processes which involve diffusions-delay as Ca-current when contraction shows a retarded peak, on the other hand. In order to test whether a store assumed to be the source of activator calcium actually releases Ca during activation, muscles were also shock-frozen and analyzed at defined times after stimulation during contraction.

The elemental distribution, particularly that of calcium sodium and potassium on cytoplasm, Z-line (that is sarcoplasmic reticulum including free SR and elements or corbular SR), mitochondria and sites near the cell membrane (possibly incuding intracellular elements of peripheral SR as well as extracellular material), is compared using muscles frozen under different inotropic situations. Furthermore, it is compared with that found presystolically at the end of normal diastole and after negative inotropic interventions.

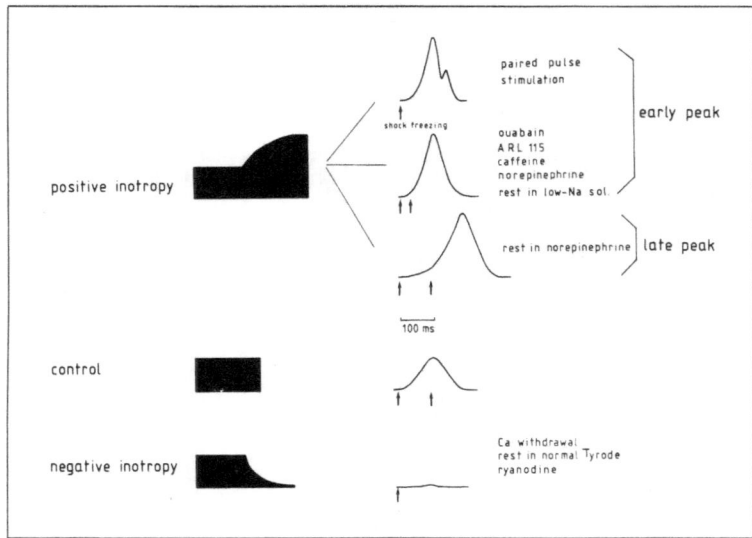

Fig. 2. Scheme illustrating the rationale of the experiments. Positive inotropy was induced by various interventions, resulting in contractions with "early" or "late" peak of force. The specific rate of force development and the rate of relaxation are not taken into account in the schematic mechanogram with "early" peak following application of non-toxic doses of ouabain, ARL 115, caffeine, norepinephrine, or rest in low-sodium solution. The arrows indicate the time at hwich muscles were frozen. Control msucles working in normal Tyrode solution and at 1 sec stimulation interval were frozen at the end of diastole and during contraction. For comparison muscles were also frozen after nearly complete force decline following negative inotropic interventions with various agents.

Results and discussion

In the case of positive inotropy induced by paired pulse stimulation Ca was clearly stored only in SR at the level of the Z-line (Fig. 3). Mitochondria and cytoplasm did not reveal any abnormal Ca accumulation, when compared with muscles frozen at the end of normal diastole. The calcium revealed at the "cell membrane" cannot be unequivocally attributed to sites located internally or externally (or both) to the plasmalemma, it corresponds also to the applied extracellular calcium concentration of 2 mmol/l. In the case of strong positive inotropy induced by paired pulse stimulation only the SR seems to be filled with calcium. All other cell compartments are "Ca-empty" like in control or under negative inotropy. Since these stores were found to be "Ca-empty" during contraction, it is legitimate to consider this SR component as the source of activator calcium. In the cases in which the peak of contraction is retarded, regardless whether contraction develops a low (normal Tyrode) or a high peak of force (norepinephrine) all cell compartments are "Ca-empty" (Fig. 3).

A different calcium distribution was found in muscles frozen after positive inotropic interventions with drugs applied in non-toxic doses (i. e. when diastolic tension was not increased). Under ouabain ($2 \cdot 10^{-7}$ molar) high Na concentrations were detected intracellularly on the cytoplasm but not in the mitochondria. Ca was increased not only on the Z-lines (SR) but also in cytoplasm and particularly on membrane-near sites (at the moment I am not

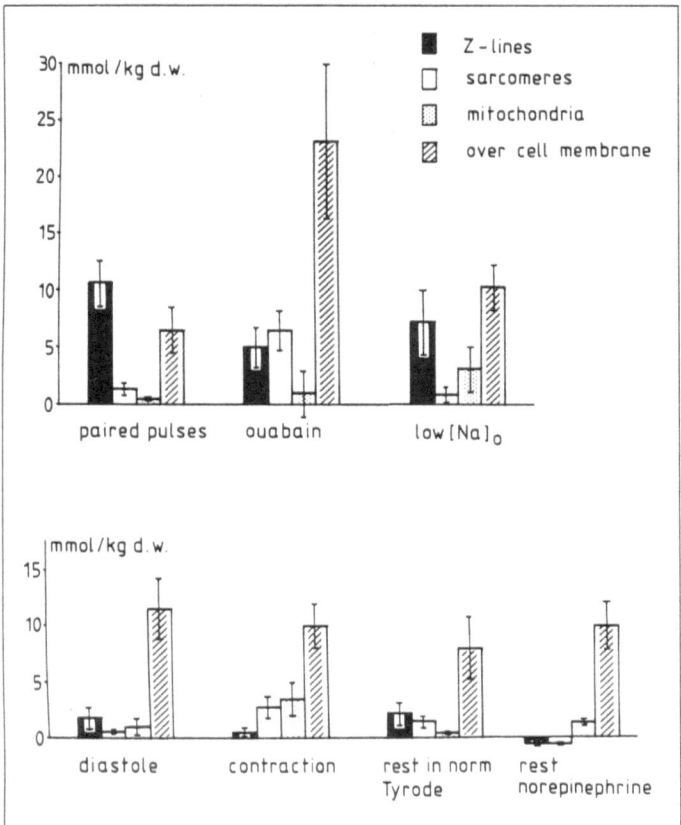

Fig. 3. Total calcium distribution in muscles frozen at the end of diastole after positive inotropic interventions leading to high contractions with "early" peak of force (upper group of experiments on muscles frozen after paired pulse stimulation, ouabain application or low extracellular sodium). For comparison, in the lower group, the calcium distribution is given in muscles frozen at the end of diastole or during contraction under normal conditions, as well as after prolonged rest in normal Tyrode solution (small "late" peak of force), and after prolonged rest in the presence of noradrenaline (high, "late" peak of force). Note that, regardless of whether contraction shows a high (rest in noradrenaline) or small peak (rest in normal Tyrode), in both cases of "late" contraction the SR-stores at the level of the Z-lines do not reveal any marked calcium accumulation. For statistical analysis see original studies (8–12).

able to differentiate whether this Ca is located on peripheral elements of SR or on extracellular membrane components). Ca concentration is not particularly high in the mitochondria. Taking into account the volume the cytoplasm occupies in the cell, this small increase indicates that a calcium overload occurs under non-toxic doses of ouabain, i. e. even when diastolic tension is normal. I cannot exclude that elements of longitudinal SR, filled with high Ca concentration and running parallel to the bundles of myofibrils, mask an existing lower Ca concentration over the contractile system. But, longitudinal SR is often easy to recognize in cryosection because it does not have a strongly parallel texture; furthermore, free SR is not abundant enough so as to mask *each* measurement. Moreover, the Ca concentration on the cytoplasm is as high as on the Z-lines. It is also possible that several cells in the multicellular preparations are already damaged, although the integrated diastolic tension does not reveal this fact (experiments are being planned with single cells to clarify this point). But it is just as possible that the total cytoplasmic calcium is increased under ouabain but not the free calcium, which would otherwise lead to enhanced diastolic tension: this would imply the presence of buffer systems in cytoplasm which respond to drugs in a specific manner. The increase in sarcoplasmic calcium as well as sodium can be regarded as a consequence of inhibition of the Na^+/K^+ pump.

The intracellular Ca distribution in resting muscles superfused with low-sodium solution is different from that found after application of digitalis. At low extracellular sodium the intracellular total calcium concentration increases even in the absence of the Ca inward current (since the muscles were not stimulated for the time of superfusion with the low sodium solution before freezing: i. e. 10 minutes). Mitochondria accumulate Ca, the cell membrane and the cytoplasm to much lesser degrees than under ouabain. The reduced gradient of sodium between extra- and intracellular compartments is probably responsible for the calcium shift via sodium/calcium exchange. Electron probe data show that inhibition of the Na^+/K^+ pump or the Na^+/Ca^+ exchange leads to specific intracellular calcium distribution and that under non-toxic doses of ouabain the elevated intracellular total calcium concentration is primarily a consequence of inhibition of the Na^+/K^+ pump, rather than of the Na^+/Ca^+ exchange.

The *sarcoplasmic reticulum* is found to be filled with calcium (Fig. 4) in all cases of potentiated contractions, regardless of the agent of inotropy, i. e. by using paired pulse stimulation as well as drugs, except when the full activation of contraction is substantially delayed (late peak). In this case another source of the activator calcium must exist, since the cell compartments, including SR, are presystolically Ca-empty. Since this compartment is also calcium-empty 80 ms seconds after stimulation, it is assumed that the activator calcium enters the cell membrane via the Ca inward current.

If we now compare the calcium distribution on the *mitochondria* in all experiments mentioned, we find that in all the positive inotropic situations induced by drugs, the mitochondria accumulate more calcium than under normal conditions or after paired pulse stimulation. Even when mitochondria are not involved in the beat to beat regulation of relaxation and contraction, it seems reasonable to speculate about their possible role in long-time regulation of cytoplasmic calcium, and not only in cases of toxicity. In contrast, with paired pulse stimulation, despite its strong positive inotropic effect, it was not possible to detect mitochondria that are loaded with calcium.

Total calcium is increased in the cytoplasm in muscles treated with non toxic doses of ouabain, ARL, and low-sodium in extracellular medium. The total concentrations detected are hardly reconciliable with normal diastolic tension. This finding suggests that in the cytoplasm soluble proteins or such that are an integral part of the contractile filaments may exist and thus act as calcium buffer under certain conditions, such as application of several drugs.

In conclusion, the results show that:

1. Under positive inotropy the distribution of total intracellular calcium varies depending on the type of inotropic agent.
2. The SR is filled with Ca wherever a stimulus is followed by a fast developing contraction, with a short time to peak of force. After paired pulse stimulation, *only* this cell compartment accumulates calcium.
3. Conversely, when a stimulus is followed by a slow developing contraction with retarded peak of force, SR and all other cellular stores are calcium-empty. Accordingly, I consider

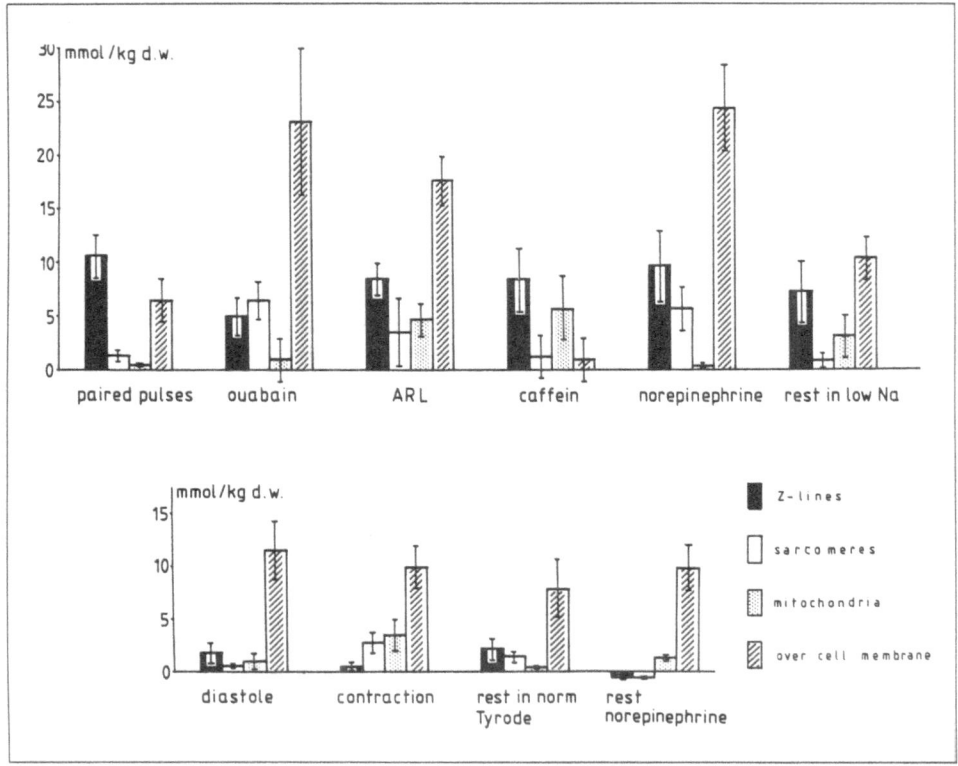

Fig. 4. Summary of experiments on calcium distribution on Z-lines, sarcomeres, mitochondria and membrane-near sites in muscles frozen after positive inotropic interventions leading to "early", high contractions (upper row). In the lower row the calcium distribution in control experiments as well as in experiments on muscles developing "late" contractions. For details see text.

SR to be the primary source of activator calcium in fast developing contractions whereas in slow developing contractions, the calcium that activates the contractile system is most probably of extracellular origin.

4. When positive inotropy is induced by application of drugs, or by changes in the composition of the extracellular medium, calcium is also detectable in several cases on the mitochondria. It is possible that the mitochondria participate to slow regulation of cytoplasmic calcium.

5. Total Ca is in some cases markedly increased in the cytoplasm. This finding is difficult to reconcile with complete relaxation of the muscle. Either a certain percent of the cells are possibly already damaged, with the whole multicellular preparation still showing normal diastolic tension, or proteins with calcium affinity which can be specifically influenced by drugs exist in the cytoplasm of heart muscle.

References

1. Antoni A, Jacob R, Kaufmann R (1969) Mechanische Reaktionen des Frosch- und Säugetiermyokards bei Veränderung der Aktionspotential-Dauer durch konstante Gleichstromimpulse. Pflügers Arch 306: 33–57
2. Chapman RA (1979) Excitation-contraction coupling in cardiac muscle. Prog Biophys Mol Biol 35: 1–52
3. Fabiato A and Fabiato F (1977) Calcium release from the sarcoplasmic reticulum. Circ Res 40: 119–129
4. Fabiato A (1983) Calcium-induced release of calcium from the cardiac sarcoplasmic reticulum. Am J Physiol 245 (Cell Physiol 14): C1–C4
5. Hall TA (1979) Biological X-ray microanalysis. J Microscopy 117: 145–163
6. Morad M, Goldman Y (1973) Excitation-contraction coupling in heart muscle: membrane control of development of tension. Prog Biophys Mol Biol 27: 257–313
7. Reuter H (1974) Exchange of calcium ions in the mammalian myocardium. Mechanisms and physiological significance. Circ Res 34: 599–605
8. Wendt-Gallitelli MF (1985) Presystolic calcium-loading of the sarcoplasmic reticulum influences time to peak force of contraction. X-ray microanalysis on rapidly frozen guinea-pig ventricular muscle preparations. Basic Res Cardiol 80: 617–625
9. Wendt-Gallitelli MF and Isenberg G (1985) Extra- and intracellular lanthanum: modified calcium distribution, inward currents and contractility in guinea pig ventricular preparations. Eur J Physiol 405: 310–322
10. Wendt-Gallitelli MF, Jacob R, Wolburg H (1982) Intracellular membranes as boundaries for ionic distribution. In situ elemental distribution in guinea pig heart muscle in different defined electromechanical coupling states. Z Naturforsch 37 c: 712–720
11. Wendt-Gallitelli MF, Jacob R (1984) Efects of non-toxic doses of ouabain on sodium, potassium, calcium distribution in guinea pig papillary muscle. Electronprobe microanalysis. In: Erdmann E (ed) Cardiac glycoside receptors and positive inotropy. Steinkopff Verlag, Darmstadt pp 79–86
12. Wendt-Gallitelli MF, Wolburg H (1984) Rapid freezing, cryosectioning, and X-ray microanalysis on cardiac muscle preparations in defined functional states. J Electron Microsc Technique 1: 151–174
13. Wood EH, Heppner RL, Weidman S (1969) Inotropic effects of electric currents. Circ Res 24: 409–445

Author's address:

Maria F. Wendt-Gallitelli, Physiologisches Institut II, Universität Tübingen, Gmelinstraße 5, D-7400 Tübingen (F. R. G.)

The contribution of Na channel block to the negative inotropic effect of antiarrhythmic drugs

P. Honerjäger

Institut für Pharmakologie und Toxikologie der Technischen Universität München, Munich (F. R. G.)

Summary

The specific Na channel blocker tetrodotoxin (TTX) produces a direct negative inotropic effect on the isolated guinea-pig papillary muscle stimulated at 1 Hz. The toxin is significantly more potent in reducing maximal upstroke velocity of the transmembrane action potential ($\dot{V}_{max}$, an index of the available Na conductance) than in reducing force of contraction (F_c), the IC50 for $\dot{V}_{max}$ divided by the IC50 for F_c being 0.23 (95% confidence interval, 0.16–0.43). This IC50 ratio defines the negative inotropic influence of Na channel blockade per se, because TTX has no known action other than blocking Na channels. $\dot{V}_{max}$-reducing to negative inotropic concentration ratios were also obtained for 5 widely used and 2 experimental antiarrhythmic agents belonging to the Na channel-blocking class (class 1). Five of these drugs (aprindine, CCI 22277, disopyramide, mexiletine, and quinidine) differed significantly from TTX in that the Na channel block was associated with a stronger negative inotropic effect. It is concluded that one or more mechanisms in addition to Na channel blockade are involved in the negative inotropic effect of these antiarrhythmic drugs. If the antiarrhythmic activity of class 1 agents depended solely on Na channel block, more selective agents with less negative inotropic action could conceivably be developed.

Key words: negative inotropic effect, myocardial sodium channels, tetrodotoxin, aprindine, disopyramide

Introduction

Szekeres and Papp, in a recent review on the discovery of antiarrhythmics (8), conclude: "As regards the future of antiarrhythmic drug therapy, more emphasis should be laid upon agents protecting against ventricular arrhythmias *without unduly depressing myocardial contractility*." This recommendation is based on the fact that life-threatening ventricular tachyarrhythmias occur often in association with myocardial failure (1) thus necessitating a prophylactic arrhythmia treatment that does not further depress cardiac function. It is of importance, therefore, to examine why most, though not all, antiarrhythmic drugs are negative inotropic agents.

According to their major cellular mechanism of action, antiarrhythmic drugs may be subdivided into Na channel blocking (class 1), β-adrenoceptor blocking (class 2), repolarization-prolonging (class 3), and Ca channel blocking (class 4) drugs (9). Negative inotropic effects are usually observed with class 1, 2 or 4, but not with class 3 agents. Class 2 drugs are cardiodepressant by antagonising the positive inotropic influence of sympathetic tone, class 4 drugs diminish the intracellular activator Ca by directly blocking the sarcolemmal Ca channels. The negative inotropic effect of class 1 drugs, on the other hand, is less well understood, although antiarrhythmics of this type are most often used clinically to combat ventricular arrhythmia.

In the study (5) which is briefly reviewed here, we have examined whether Na channel block, i. e., the mechanism by which class 1 drugs prolong the refractory period of the heart and, at least in part, exert their antiarrhythmic effect, can also account for the negative inotropic effect of class 1 agents. Block of Na channels decreases the amount of Na entering the cardiac cell. This action would be expected to shift the transmembrane distribution of Na und Ca ions maintained by the Na/Ca exchange (6) and thereby decrease the intracellular concentration of Ca, as shown schematically in Fig. 1. This possible mechanism of the

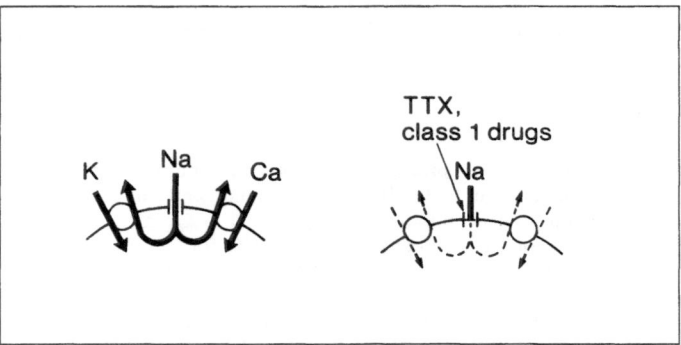

Fig. 1. Simplified scheme of sarcolemmal Na/K and Na/Ca exchange explaining a possible mechanism by which class 1 (Na channel blocking) antiarrhythmic drugs may decrease intracellular Ca and myocardial contractility.

negative inotropic effect of Na channel blocking antiarrhythmics has been repeatedly proposed (e. g., 2, 3, 10), but the quantitative relation between Na channel blocking and negative inotropic activities for individual drugs has not been previously presented in detail.

Methods

Right ventricular papillary muscles were excised from guinea-pig hearts and mounted in a two-chambered vessel with an internal circulation of 50 ml bath solution which contained (mmol/l): NaCl, 115; NaHCO$_3$, 25; KCl, 5.9; CaCl$_2$, 3.2; MgSO$_4$, 1.2; glucose, 10. Furthermore, 30 nmol/l TTX was added to the bath solution. This nerve-blocking concentration does not yet block guinea-pig myocardial Na channels. The precaution is necessary in order to avoid inotropic responses resulting from block of intracardiac adrenergic nerves rather than from block of myocardial Na channels. The solution was gassed and stirred continuously with 95 % O$_2$/5 % CO$_2$; temperature was maintained at 35° C; pH was 7.6. Stimulation frequency was 1 Hz, intensity twice threshold and pulse duration 2 or 5 ms. Isometric force was recorded by an inductive force transducer. Transmembrane electrical activity was recorded with conventional glass microelectrodes filled with 3 mol/l KCl and an electrometer amplifier providing capacity compensation. Maximal upstroke velocity of the action potential ($\dot{V}_{max}$) was measured by electronic differentiation. Drug concentrations reducing $\dot{V}_{max}$ or peak force of contraction (F$_c$) by 50 % (IC50) were evaluated from concentration-effect relationships obtained as follows. For effects on $\dot{V}_{max}$, a single drug concentration was applied to the preparation and allowed to act for 30 min during which time a steady-state effect was achieved. Only results from continuous microelectrode impalements were accepted. A given concentration was tested on 3 to 6 muscles, and 3 to 5 different concentrations of a given drug were examined. For effects on F$_c$, different preparations (n = 6 for each drug) were exposed to 4 cumulatively increasing drug concentrations allowing an equilibration time of 30 min for each concentration. Further methodological details are given in (5).

Results and discussion

The effects of TTX (10 μmol/l) on transmembrane action potential and $\dot{V}_{max}$ and the accompanying isometric contraction are illustrated in Fig. 2 A. TTX reduced $\dot{V}_{max}$ by 59%

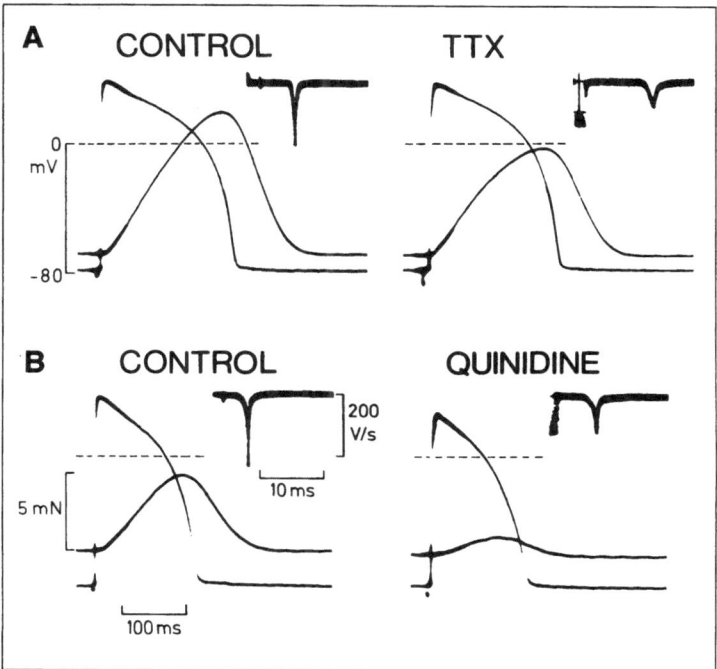

Fig. 2. Original records of transmembrane potential and isometric contraction of 2 guinea-pig papillary muscles. The tetrodotoxin (TTX) record (A) was taken 20 min after adding 10 μmol/l, the quinidine record (B) 30 min after adding 30 μmol/l. While being approximately equi-effective in reducing $\dot{V}_{max}$, quinidine produced a larger negative inotropic effect than TTX. 30 nmol/l TTX applied troughout these experiments. Stimulation frequency, 1 Hz. (P. Honerjäger and E. Loibl, unpublished).

and peak force of contraction, F_c, by 25%. For comparison, Fig. 2 B shows records from a different preparation where 30 μmol/l quindine affected $\dot{V}_{max}$ similarly. The antiarrhythmic drug reduced $\dot{V}_{max}$ by 50% and F_c by 77%. Thus, although quinidine induced slightly less Na channel block than TTX, its negative inotropic effect exceeded by far that of TTX.

Figure 3 shows the time course and reproducibility of these effects by comparing 4 experiments with TTX (A) to 4 experiments with quinidine (B). Evidently, TTX acted more rapidly on $\dot{V}_{max}$ and F_c than quinidine. TTX produced steady-state electromechanical effects within 7 min following bath application, the quinidine effect on $\dot{V}_{max}$ required about 30 min to reach a steady-state value. The negative inotropic quinidine effect was close (within 7%) to its steady-state value after 30 min equilibration. The relatively fast action of TTX conforms to its extracellular site of action and inability to penetrate through the plasmalemma (7), while the slowness of action of quinidine is compatible with the concept that local anaesthetic type Na channel blockers have to penetrate into and through the plasmalemma to reach their site of action (4).

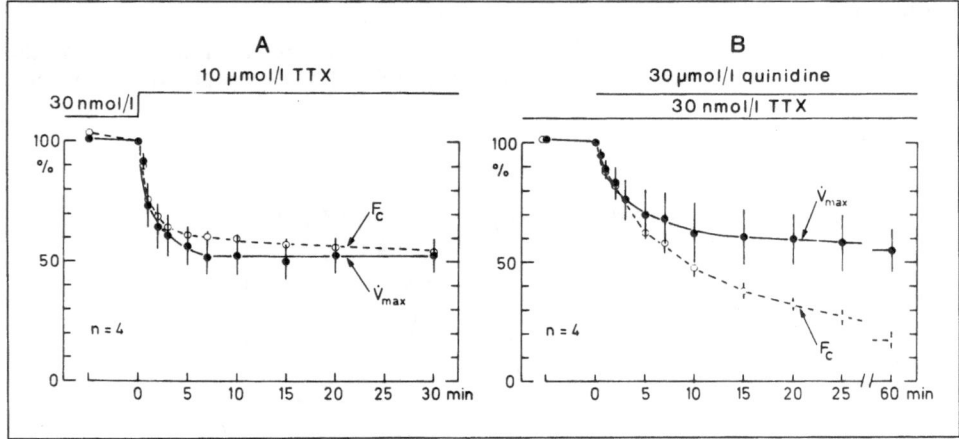

Fig. 3. Maximal upstroke velocity of action potential ($\dot{V}_{max}$) and peak force of contraction (F_c) as affected by time of incubation with tetrodotoxin (TTX, A) or quinidine (B). Mean values $\pm$ S. E. M. (as vertical bars) of 4 guinea-pig papillary muscles. Ordinate indicates % of pre-drug control value. Stimulation frequency, 1 Hz. (P. Honerjäger and E. Loibl, unpublished).

The results of Fig. 3 confirm the predominant negative inotropic action of quinidine as compared to its effect on $\dot{V}_{max}$ and the difference from TTX in this regard. TTX and quinidine were equieffective in reducing $\dot{V}_{max}$, but F_c was significantly smaller after a 25 min quinidine treatment ($27 \pm 3\%$ of control) than after a 30 min TTX treatment ($54 \pm 3\%$; $P < 0.001$).

Full concentration-effect relationships for $\dot{V}_{max}$ and F_c, respectively, were obtained as described in Methods. Table 1 lists the ratio IC50 ($\dot{V}_{max}$)/IC50 (F_c) for various drugs, where

Table 1. Relation between Na channel blocking and negative inotropic potency for tetrodotoxin (TTX) and various antiarrhythmic drugs as defined by the ratio IC50 ($\dot{V}_{max}$)/IC50 (F_c)

Drug	IC50($\dot{V}_{max}$)/IC50(F_c) (95% conf. interval)
TTX	0.27 (0.16–0.43)
Sparteine	0.23 (0.12–0.39)
AR-LH 31	0.31 (0.20–0.46)
Aprindine	0.87 (0.60–1.28)
Mexiletine	1.24 (0.91–1.66)
CCI 22277	1.48 (0.94–2.30)
Quinidine	1.86 (0.97–3.65)
Disopyramide	2.21 (1.66–3.05)

Data taken from (5).
AR-LH 31 is 8-(3-diethylaminopropyl)-6,6-dimethyl-2-phenyl-1H-imidazo-(4,5-h)isoquinoline-7,9-(6H,8H)dione dihydrochloride.
CCI 22277 is methyl 2β-ethoxy-3α-hydroxy-11α-(3-methyl-butyl-amino)-5α-androstane-17β-carboxylate hydrochloride.

values smaller than 1 indicate predominant Na channel blocking activity and values larger than 1 indicate predominant negative inotropic activity.

All the antiarrhythmic drugs listed in Table 1 possess negative inotropic activity in guinea-pig myocardium. Two subgroups can be distinguished, however, with regard to their simultaneous effect on maximal upstroke velocity of the action potential. Sparteine and AR-LH 31 are more potent in reducing $\dot{V}_{max}$ (over F_c) and do not differ significantly from TTX in this regard. The 5 remaining antiarrhythmic agents differ significantly from TTX in being either similarly or more potent in reducing F_c (over $\dot{V}_{max}$).

In conclusion, the experiments with TTX show that Na channel block per se exerts a negative inotropic influence on guinea-pig ventricular myocardium. It is therefore predictable that class 1 antiarrhythmic agents in general, if they depress $\dot{V}_{max}$ (or widen the QRS complex in the electrocardiogram) at the examined heart rate, produce a cardiodepressive influence that is caused by and therefore inseparable from their Na channel blocking effect. The negative inotropic effect of some antiarrhythmic drugs, including aprindine, mexiletine, quinidine and disopyramide, even exceeds the extent expected from the reduction of $\dot{V}_{max}$ (or Na channel block) alone. A negative inotropic mechanism separate from and in addition to Na channel block has to be postulated to explain these findings. If class 1 antiarrhythmic drugs owe their antiarrhythmic effectiveness exclusively or mainly to the Na channel blocking action (and not to additional cardiodepressive actions), more selective antiarrhythmic agents could conceivably be developed in which the ratio of Na channel blocking to cardiodepressant activity is improved beyond that of aprindine, mexiletine, quinidine or disopyramide.

Acknowledgement

This work was supported by the Deutsche Forschungsgemeinschaft (Ho 705/6).

References

1. Bigger JT (1984) Identification of patients at high risk for sudden cardiac death. Am J Cardiol 54: 3D–8D
2. Eisner DA, Lederer WJ, Sheu S-S (1983) The role of intracellular sodium activity in the anti-arrhythmic action of local anaesthetics in sheep Purkinje fibres. J Physiol (Lond) 340: 239–257
3. Fozzard HA, Wasserstrom JA (1985) Voltage dependence of intracellular sodium and control of contraction. In: Zipes DP, Jalife E (eds) Cardiac electrophysiology and arrhythmias. Grune & Stratton, Orlando, pp 51–57
4. Hille B (1977) Local anesthetics: Hydrophilic and hydrophobic pathways for the drug-receptor reaction. J Gen Physiol 69: 497–515
5. Honerjäger P, Loibl E, Steidl I, Schönsteiner G, Ulm K (1986) Negative inotropic effects of tetrodotoxin and 7 class 1 antiarrhythmic drugs in relation to sodium channel blockade. Naunyn-Schmideberg's Arch Pharmacol 332: 184–195
6. Mullins LJ (1981) Ion transport in heart. Raven Press, New York
7. Narahashi T, Anderson NC, Moore JW (1966) Tetrodotoxin does not block excitation from inside the nerve membrane. Science 153: 765–767
8. Szekeres L, Papp JG (1984) The discovery of antiarrhythmics. In: Parnham MJ, Bruinvels J (eds) Discoveries in pharmacology, vol 2: Haemodynamics, hormones & inflammation. Elsevier Science Publishers BV, pp 185–215
9. Vaughan Williams EM (1984) A classification of antiarrhythmic actions reassessed after a decade of new drugs. J Clin Pharmacol 24: 129–147
10. Wasserstrom JA, Ferrier GR (1982) Effects of phenytoin and quinidine on digitalis-induced oscillatory afterpotentials, aftercontractions, and inotropy in canine ventricular tissues. J Mol Cell Cardiol 14: 725–736

Author's address:

Prof. Dr. P. Honerjäger, Institut für Pharmakologie und Toxikologie der Technischen Universität München, Biedersteiner Straße 29, D-8000 München 40 (F. R. G.)

II. Myocardial mechanics and ventricular dynamics

Cardiac oxygen consumption and systolic pressure volume area

H. Suga, Y. Igarashi, O. Yamada, and Y. Goto

Department of Cardiovascular Dynamics, National Cardiovascular Center (NCVC), Osaka (Japan)

Summary

Since we found that the total mechanical energy generated by ventricular contraction could be represented by a specific area (PVA) in the pressure-volume diagram, we have been studying the correlation between myocardial oxygen consumption (Vo_2) per beat and PVA in dog left ventricles. Vo_2 was found to be closely and linearly correlated with PVA under a variety of loading, heart rate, and contractile conditions. The regression of Vo_2 on PVA was given by $Vo_2 = A \times PVA + B$. A was 1.8×10^{-5} ml O_2/(mm Hg ml) on the average and was relatively constant despite the changes in loading, heart rate, and contractile conditions. B was 0.02 ml O_2/beat/100 g on the average in control contractile state and was relatively constant despite the changes in loading and heart rate conditions. However, B increased by 50–80% with 70–80% increases in Emax by epinephrine or calcium infused into the coronary circulation. After both Vo_2 and PVA were expressed in J/beat/100 g, the inverse of the slope coefficient A indicated that the energy conversion efficiency of PVA from the excess Vo_2 above the Vo_2 of the mechanically unloaded contraction was relatively constant at 40%, independent of the loading, heart rate, and contractile conditions.

Key words: dog heart, left ventricle, pressure-volume relation, myocardial energetics

Introduction

Although many cardiodynamic variables and indices have been proposed as the major determinants of myocardial oxygen consumption, there has been no agreement as to which is the best (3, 5, 6). Among them, peak ventricular pressure, pressure time integral, peak ventricular wall force, and force time integral have been considered to be best correlated with myocardial oxygen consumption or energy utilization, and the contribution of stroke work to oxygen consumption has been controversial (3, 5, 6). However, most of the pressure or tension based determinants of oxygen consumption do not have dimensions of energy and their coefficients cannot directly indicate the mechanical efficiency (3, 5, 6).

Partly supported by Research Grants (53C-2 and 56C-5) for Cardiovascular Diseases from the Ministry of Health and Welfare of Japan, and Grants in Aid (422031, 557026, 57123109, 59570047) for Scientific Research from the Ministry of Education, Science and Culture of Japan

While we were investigating the ventricular mechanics in terms of the ventricular systolic pressure-volume relationship (13), we found a method to assess the total mechanical energy generated by ventricular contraction (10). The method is based on energetics of the time-varying elastance model which can simulate the ventricular pressure-volume relationship. Since then, we have carried out a series of experiments on dog left ventricles to examine how such a total mechanical energy is correlated with myocardial oxygen consumption. This paper summarizes our major new findings that have been already published in detail in a series of original papers (8, 14–21, 23, 24).

Methods

Since the details of our experimental methods have been described in our previous papers (8, 14–21, 23, 24), we will describe them briefly in this paper. We used the excised cross-circulated heart preparation of the adult dog. Under anesthesia with pentobarbital sodium (30 mg/kg i. v.) or a mixture of alpha-chloralose (50 mg/kg i. v.) and urethane (500 mg/kg i. v.), a heart lung section was isolated from the systemic circulation in one dog and its left subclavian artery and right ventricle via the right atrium were connected to the common carotid artery and the external jugular veins, respectively, of the other dog. After the pulmonary hili were ligated, the cross-circulated heart was excised from the chest. There was no stoppage of coronary flow during the preparation.

The left atrium was opened and all the chordae tendineae were cut. A thin balloon tied on a connector (11 mm ID) was placed within the left ventricle and the cable of a Konigsberg P-7 miniature pressure gauge placed inside the apical end of the balloon was pulled out of the ventricle through a stab incision at the apex. The balloon was connected to our custom-made volume servo pump (8, 14–21, 23, 24) and the balloon and the pump were primed with water. The servo pump enabled us to precisely control and accurately measure left ventricular volume.

From ventricular pressure and volume signals, we on-line computed a specific area in the pressure-volume diagram that we considered to represent the total mechanical energy generated by ventricular contraction (18–21, 23, 24). This specific area is the area circumscribed by the end-systolic pressure-volume line, end-distaolic pressure-volume curve, and the systolic segment of the pressure-volume trajectory. Figure 1 schematically illustrates this area. This area is called the "systolic pressure-volume area" and is abbreviated to PVA (10). The physical meaning of PVA was first given in the time-varying elastance model of the ventricle (10). The area under the systolic segment of the pressure-volume trajectory is the external mechanical work, or stroke work, and the area of PVA on the origin side of the external work is considered to represent elastic potential energy generated during systole and stored at end-systole (10). PVA and its two parts were determined on-line with a digital computer (NEC San-ei,

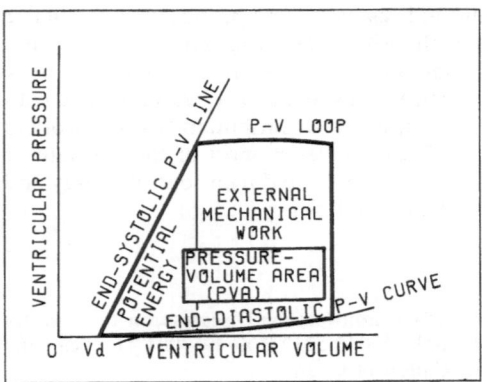

Fig. 1. Schematic illustration of ventricular pressure-volume diagram and systolic pressure-volume area (PVA).

7T17). PVA was determined in terms of mm Hg ml/beat, and normalized for 100 g left ventricle. PVA in mm Hg ml was converted to PVA in J as needed with a physical conversion of 1 mm Hg ml = 0.000133 J.

Myocardial oxygen consumption (Vo_2) was determined as the product of coronary flow and coronary arteriovenous oxygen content difference. Coronary flow was measured with an electromagnetic flowmeter in the middle of the tubing draining hydrostatically the right ventricle which was receiving all the coronary venous return. Coronary arteriovenous oxygen content difference was continuously measured with an AVOX oximeter (9), which was calibrated against a Lex 02 Con oxygen content analyzer in each experiment. Both coronary flow and oxygen content difference signals were processed with the digital computer to obtain Vo_2 in ml O_2/beat after being divided by heart rate. Vo_2 was normalized for 100 g myocardium. Vo_2 in ml O_2 was converted as needed to Vo_2 in J with a biological conversion of 1 ml O_2 = 20 J (3, 5, 6). The measured Vo_2 contained oxygen consumption of the right ventricle which was kept mechanically unloaded. The unloaded right ventricular oxygen consumption was estimated by proportioning Vo_2 that was obtained when both ventricles were mechanically unloaded to the weight ratio of the left ventricle (including the septum) and the right ventricular free wall. This ratio was 1 to 0.37 ± 0.04 (SD). The left ventricular unload Vo_2 was therefore 27% less than the total unload Vo_2 that was documented in our previous papers (8, 14–21, 23, 24).

The details of experimental protocols were described in our individual papers (8, 14–21, 23, 24). Briefly, in control contractile state, namely, without any inotropic interventions to the preparation, we changed the mode of contraction between isovolumic and ejecting, and widely varied end-diastolic volume, afterload pressure, and stroke volume. Under each of various loading conditions, we waited for a steady state, which was usually reached 2–3 min after each change of loading conditions. Both PVA and Vo_2 were determined only in steady-state contractions.

Heart rate was widely varied by electric pacing of the atrium in a stable contractile state and both PVA and Vo_2 were determined in steady-state contractions.

Ventricular contractile state was enhanced with either epinephrine or calcium, and depressed with propranolol or verapamil while heart rate was kept constant by electric pacing.

Results

Figure 2A shows a correlogram between Vo_2 on the ordinate and PVA on the abscissa of isovolumic contractions (o) and ejecting contractions (•) in one dog left ventricle. The correlation was very good and linear, as shown by the high correlation coefficient and the regression line. The regression of Vo_2 on PVA was formulated by

$$Vo_2 = A \times PVA + B \qquad (1)$$

where A is the regression coefficient, or slope of the regression line and B is the regression constant, or Vo_2 axis intercept of the regression line. In the case shown in Fig. 2A,

A = 0.000017 (ml O_2/[mm Hg ml])

and

B = 0.016 (ml O_2/beat/100 g)

On the average of 10 dog left ventricles (4),

A = 0.000016 ± 0.000004 (SD) (ml O_2/[mm Hg ml])

and

B = 0.017 ± 0.002 (ml O_2/beat/100 g)

B was not statistically different from the directly measured Vo_2 of the mechanically unloaded contraction with zero PVA.

Correlation coefficient between Vo_2 and PVA was

R = 0.923 ± 0.023

These results indicate that in a given stable contractile state Vo_2 was closely and linearly correlated with PVA in each dog left ventricle regardless of the mode of contraction whether

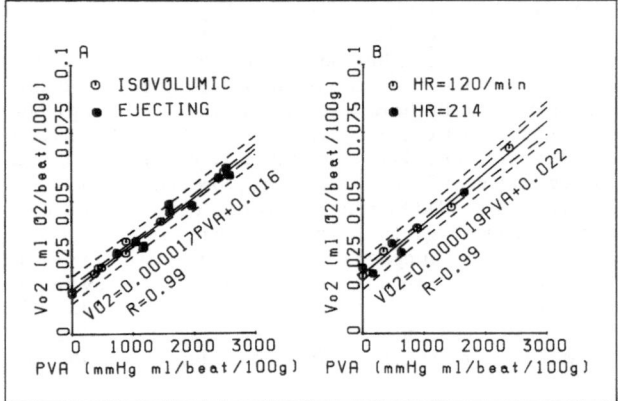

Fig. 2. Correlation and regression between left ventricular oxygen consumption (Vo₂) and systolic pressure-volume area (PVA). Panel A shows data of isovolumic contractions and ejecting contractions in a stable contractile state in one dog left ventricle. Panel B shows data of contractions at control and a higher heart rate in one dog left ventricle. The solid diagonal line represents the linear regression line. The inner pair of dashed curves are the 95% confidence limits of the regression line. The outer pair of dashed curves are the 95% confidence limits of the sampled data points. The equation indicates the linear regression line. R value indicates correlation coefficient.

it was isovolumic or ejecting. In other words, Vo₂ was uniquely correlated with the size or magnitude of PVA independent of the shape of PVA.

To confirm the above contention, we compared the oxygen cost of external mechanical work (EW) and that of potential energy (PE), of which PVA consists (namely, PVA = EW + PE). We applied multiple regression analysis to a set of Vo₂, EW and PE of isovolumic and ejecting contractions in a stable contractile state, and determined A_1, A_2, and C of

$$Vo_2 = A_1 \times EW + A_2 \times PE + C$$

in each dog left ventricle. On the average of seven dog left ventricles (15),

$$A_1 = 0.000017 \pm 0.000004 \, (ml \, O_2/[mm \, Hg \, ml])$$

$$A_2 = 0.000017 \pm 0.000005 \, (ml \, O_2/[mm \, Hg \, ml])$$

and

$$C = 0.018 \pm 0.005 \, (ml \, O_2/beat/100 \, g)$$

A_1 and A_2 were not different from each other. This result indicates that the oxygen cost of external mechanical work was identical with the oxygen cost of potential energy. Because PVA = EW + PE, the result implies that Vo₂ is correlated with PVA as a whole, independent of the relative magnitudes of EW and PE.

We also corroborated the above contention in a different experiment (21). We measured Vo₂ and PVA of ejecting contractions where the systolic segment of the pressure-volume trajectory and hence the shape and size of PVA were kept unchanged whereas the relaxation and diastolic segment of the pressure-volume trajectory was markedly shifted. In other words, the relative magnitudes of EW and PE were changed within the PVA. As the result, Vo₂ remained unchanged despite the marked change in EW/PE ratio. This result corroborates our contention that Vo₂ is uniquely correlated with PVA, which is determined by the end of systole and is independent of how PVA is re-divided into EW and PE during the following ventricular relaxation.

We then studied the effect of heart rate on the Vo_2-PVA relationship. Although Vo_2 per min for a given PVA increased significantly with increases in heart rate by pacing, Vo_2 per beat for a given PVA remained unchanged over a wide range of heart rate. Figure 2 B shows a representative correlogram of Vo_2-PVA data at control heart rate and a higher paced heart rate pooled together. The correlation was good and linear as shown by the high correlation coefficient and the linear regression line. The regression of Vo_2 on PVA was also expressed by Eq. (1), and on the average of 15 dog left ventricles (19)

$A = 0.000017 \pm 0.000004$ (ml O_2/[mm Hg ml])

and

$B = 0.022 \pm 0.008$ (ml O_2/beat/100 g)

at control heart rate of 124 ± 17 beats/min,

and

$A = 0.000018 \pm 0.000007$ (ml O_2/[mm Hg ml])

and

$B = 0.023 \pm 0.008$ (ml O_2/beat/100 g)

at a higher paced heart rate of 193 ± 23 beats/min. A and B values between the lower and higher heart rates in individual dog left ventricles were not different from each other. Thus, changes in heart rate by electric pacing did not affect the Vo_2-PVA relationship on a per beat basis. Emax, the slope of the end-systolic pressure-volume relation line, increased only by 10% from 6.4 ± 1.9 mm Hg/(ml/100 g) to 7.0 ± 1.7 mm Hg/(ml/100 g), indicating that ventricular contractile state was little increased by the pacing.

We studied the effect of changes in ventricular contractile state on the Vo_2-PVA relationship period Figure 3 A shows the effect of epinephrine (EPI). The solid circles are control

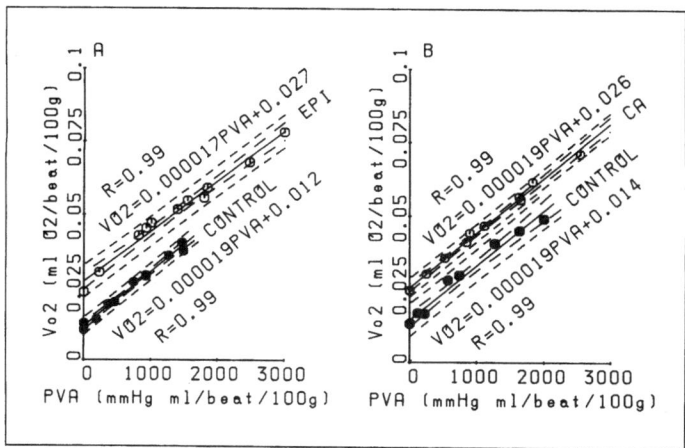

Fig. 3. Correlation and regression between left ventricular oxygen consumption (Vo_2) and systolic pressure-volume area (PVA). Panel A shows data of contractions in control and an epinephrine (EPI)-enhanced contractile state in one dog left ventricle. Panel B shows data of contractions in control and a calcium (CA)-enhanced contractile state in one dog left ventricle. The solid diagonal line represents the linear regression line. The inner pair of dashed curves are the 95% confidence limits of the regression line. The outer pair of dashed curves are the 95% confidence limits of the sampled data points. The equation indicates the linear regression line. R value indicates correlation coefficient.

data points, and the open circles are data points obtained in an enhanced contractile state with epinephrine (1 ug/min/kg, i. v.). Heart rate was fixed by electric pacing at 170 ± 17 beats/min. The Vo_2-PVA regression line parallel shifted upward with epinephrine. Both Vo_2-PVA regression lines were expressed by Eq. (1). On the average of nine dog left ventricles (18),

$A = 0.000018 \pm 0.000003$ (ml O_2/[mm Hg ml])

and

$B = 0.018 \pm 0.006$ (ml O_2/beat/100 g)

in control contractile states.

$A = 0.000020 \pm 0.000004$ (ml O_2/[mm Hg ml])

and

$B = 0.032 \pm 0.010$ (ml O_2/beat/100 g)

in enhanced contractile states with epinephrine. Thus, A remained unchanged, whereas B increased significantly. Emax increased by 80% from control value of 6.3 ± 1.4 mm Hg/(ml/100 g) to 11.3 ± 1.6 mm Hg/(ml/100 g) with epinephrine.

Similar results were obtained with calcium chloride (0.03 mEq/min/kg, i. v.), as shown in Fig. 3 B. On the average,

$A = 0.000019 \pm 0.000003$ (ml O_2/[mm Hg ml])

and

$B = 0.023 \pm 0.009$ (ml O_2/beat/100 g)

in control contractile states, and

$A = 0.000019 \pm 0.000005$ (ml O_2/[mm Hg ml])

and

$B = 0.036 \pm 0.009$ (ml O_2/best/100 g)

in enhanced contractile states with calcium. Heart rate was kept constant at 154 ± 18 beats/min. Emax increased by 70% from control values of 7.5 ± 2.1 mm Hg/(ml/100 g) to 12.9 ± 4.9 mm Hg/(ml/100 g). Thus, A remained unchanged whereas B increased significantly in individual dog left ventricles.

Although we have not made a systematic analzysis, the Vo_2-PVA relation tended towards a parallel downward shift with propranolol (1 mg/min into coronary artery) or verapamil (0.1 mg/min into coronary artery).

We analyzed the mechanism of the upward parallel shift of the Vo_2-PVA relation line as follows (18). Vo_2 of mechanically unloaded contraction with zero PVA was determined, which was called unload Vo_2. The leftmost column of Fig. 4 shows this value per min. Then, we continuously infused KCl solution (0.3 mEq/min) directly into coronary circulation of the unloaded heart and Vo_2 of the arrested heart was determined. This value is shown by the second column from the left in Fig. 4. There was a significant decrease in Vo_2 after arrest. This remaining Vo_2 under arrest represents basal metabolism of myocardium. The difference between the unload Vo_2 and the arrest Vo_2 was considered to be Vo_2 associated with myocardial activation, or excitation-contraction coupling. We then infused either epinephrine or calcium chloride directly into the coronary circulation at the same dose that was used in the beating left ventricles. However, neither epinephrine nor calcium increased Vo_2 under KCl arrest. From these results we speculated that the parallel upward shift of the Vo_2-PVA relation line was probably due to the increased Vo_2 component associated with the augmented activation, or excitation-contraction coupling in an enhanced contractile state.

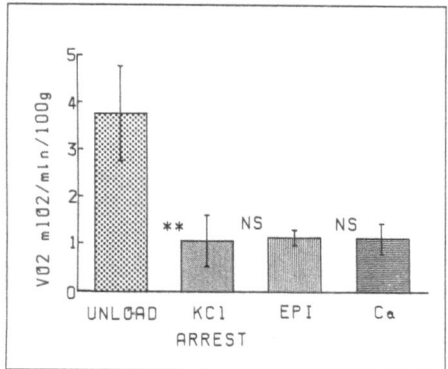

Fig. 4. Comparison among unload V_{O_2}, V_{O_2} under KCl arrest, arrest V_{O_2} with epinephrine (EPI), and arrest V_{O_2} with calcium cloride (Ca). ** indicates $P < 0.05$. NS indicates $P > 0.05$. SD is shown by the bar on each column.

We then analyzed the correlation between B values on the ordinate and Emax on the abscissa. As the result (24),

$$B = 0.0023 \times Emax + 0.004$$

with correlation coefficient of 0.65 ($P < 0.05$) under epinephrine, and

$$B = 0.0014 \times Emax + 0.015$$

with correlation coefficient of 0.57 ($P < 0.05$) under calcium. Because there was no statistically significant difference between these two regression lines by the analysis of covariance, we pooled both epinephrine and calcium data and obtained a single regression line:

$$B = 0.0018 \times Emax + 0.010 \tag{2}$$

with correlation coefficient of 0.61 ($P < 0.05$).

Combining Eqs. (1) and (2) with a control A value, we obtain

$$V_{O_2} = 0.000017 \times PVA + 0.0018 \times Emax + 0.010 \tag{3}$$

This equation will be used to predict V_{O_2} from PVA and Emax.

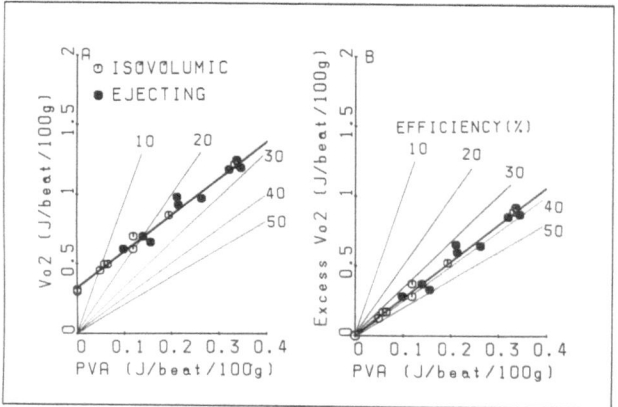

Fig. 5. Iso-efficiency lines and V_{O_2}-PVA data in isovolumic and ejecting contractions in one dog left ventricle in a stable contractile state. Panel A shows PVA/V_{O_2} efficiency, whereas Panel B PVA/(excess V_{O_2}) efficiency.

Next, we treated Vo₂-PVA data after the dimensions of them were converted to J/beat/100 g (14, 18, 19, 23). Figure 5 A shows the same Vo_2-PVA data points as in Fig. 2 A. The ordinate shows Vo_2 in J/beat/100 g, and the abscissa shows PVA in J/beat/100 g. The family of diagonal lines diverging from the origin are the iso-efficiency lines, indicating the energy conversion efficiency from Vo_2 to PVA. Vo_2 is the total energy (or enthalpy) input to myocardium, and PVA is the total mechanical energy output of the myocardium. Figure 5 A indicates that the PVA/Vo_2 efficiency increases as PVA increases regardless of the mode of contraction. Figure 5 B shows the same data points after unload Vo_2 was subtracted from all Vo_2 data. Thus, the ordinate shows the excess Vo_2 above unload Vo_2. The excess Vo_2 was considered to be the Vo_2 component that was primarily used for mechanical contraction because the unload Vo_2 was considered to represent the Vo_2 component associated with such non-mechanical activities of myocardium as the basal metabolism and the activation. In Figure 5 B, the iso-efficiency lines indicate the efficiency of energy conversion from the excess Vo_2 to PVA, which we considered primarily reflecting the energy conversion efficiency of the contractile machinery. All data points gathered along an iso-efficiency line of about 40%. This indicates that the PVA/(excess Vo_2) efficiency was independent of the mode of contraction and the loading conditions. The PVA/(excess Vo_2) efficiency was about 40% on the average in 10 dog left ventricles (14, 23).

We obtained the PVA/Vo_2 and PVA/(excess Vo_2) efficiencies of contractions at control and higher heart rates in the same way as above. Although PVA/Vo_2 efficiency increased with increases in PVA, PVA/(excess Vo_2) efficiency was relatively constant at 40% despite changes in PVA and heart rate (9, 23).

Figure 6 A plots Vo_2-PVA data in control, epinephrine-enhanced, and calcium-enhanced contractile states. In either control or enhanced contractile state, the PVA/Vo_2 efficiency increased with increases in PVA. For a given PVA, however, Vo_2 was greater and the PVA/Vo_2 efficiency was lower in the enhanced contractile state. Figure 6 B plots excess Vo_2-PVA data in these respective contractile states. They were gathered along an iso-efficiency line of about 40%. On the average, the PVA/(excess Vo_2) efficiency was about 35%, independent of contractile states and inotropic agents (18, 23). All these efficiency data

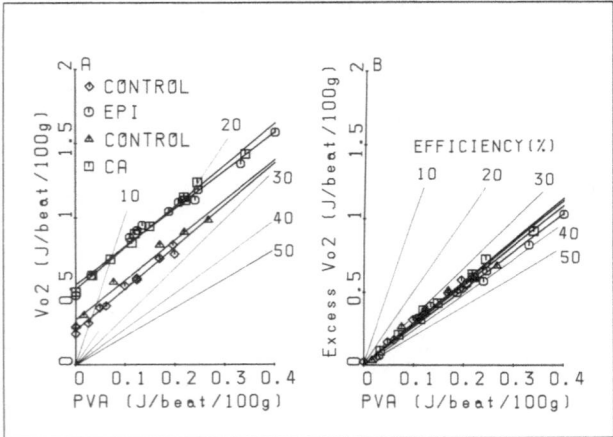

Fig. 6. Iso-efficiency lines and VO₂-PVA data in control and enhanced contractile states in one dog left ventricle. Panel A shows PVA/Vo₂ efficiency, whereas Panel B PVA/(excess Vo₂) efficiency.

together indicate that the PVA/(excess V_{O_2}) efficiency remained relatively constant at 35–40% regardless of marked changes in loading, heart rate, and contractile conditions.

Discussion

The unique feature of our study resides in the analysis of the relationship between cardiac mechanics and energetics by using PVA which represents the total mechanical energy generated by contraction. Because PVA has dimensions of energy, we were able to analyze the V_{O_2}-PVA relation in an energetically meaningful way, i. e., in terms of energy conversion efficiency. The relation between V_{O_2} and a mechanical variable or index cannot simply be analyzed in terms of efficiency unless this mechanical variable or index has dimensions of energy. Although the relatively linear relation between V_{O_2} and ventricular wall force, or between V_{O_2} and myocardial tension, and its parallel upward shift with various positive inotropoc agents have been reported (3, 5, 6), one cannot discuss the mechanical efficiency from these relations under the respective conditions. Instead, the shift of the V_{O_2}-force relation has been associated with economy of force generation. However, the economy of force generation is a vague and qualitative term, and can serve only as an indirect index of mechanical efficiency of myocardium.

Despite the relatively clear-cut conclusions mentioned above, we have depended on some basic assumptions. First, we assumed that PVA of the real ventricle represented the total mechanical energy generated by ventricular contraction as in the time-varying elastance model. The physical and physiological meaning of PVA was derived from the time-varying elastance model of the ventricle, but this does not guarantee that the PVA of the real ventricle has the same meaning as in the model. External mechanical work is real in both the ventricle and the model. However, potential energy part of PVA in the real ventricle may not be mechanical potential energy. Therefore, in a separate study (11, 12), we attempted to extract as much external work as possible from the potential energy part of PVA in the real ventricle. As the result, we were able to extract as much as 70% of the potential energy part in the form of actual external work. This result made the possibility more likely that the potential energy part of PVA was actually potential energy if it was not used as work.

A second assumption in the discussion of the PVA/(excess V_{O_2}) efficiency is that the same amount of V_{O_2} as unload V_{O_2} was needed for non-mechanical activities of myocardium in loaded contractions regardless of the mode of contraction and the magnitude of PVA in a given stable contractile state. We verified this assumption as follows. We compared V_{O_2} of a contraction starting from a high end-diastolic volume but ejecting against a near zero pressure load with V_{O_2} of the unloaded contraction. Although the former contraction was highly loaded at the onset of systole, it was nearly unloaded during systole and hence PVA was close to zero. We found that V_{O_2}s of both contractions were comparable (22). This result implied that V_{O_2} for the non-mechanical activities was not significantly affected by the preload per se. We also compared V_{O_2}s of the isovolumic and the ejecting contractions that had the same PVA (16). Although the preloaded end-diastolic volumes and the afterloaded ventricular pressures were different between the two contractions, V_{O_2}s of these contractions were the same. This implied that V_{O_2} for the non-mechanical activities was independent of the preload and afterload.

The assumption of the constancy of V_{O_2} for the non-mechanical activities in a given contractile state may appear to be contradictory to the recent concept of the length-dependent activation of myocardium (1, 7). Namely, myocardial activation is augmented at longer muscle lengths. Then, we would expect a greater V_{O_2} for the non-mechanical activities in contractions with near zero PVA starting from a greater end-diastolic volume. However, our results did not match this expectation (22), implying that Vo_2 for activation was virtually independent of preload.

If Vo_2 for the non-mechanical activities changed with PVA rather than preload or afterload, then our method is not able to detect it because Vo_2 for a finite PVA cannot be divided into Vo_2 for the non-mechanical activities and the excess Vo_2 exclusively for PVA. At present, we cannot either affirm this possibility or deny it.

Our results have shown a sensitive dependence of the unload Vo_2 on contractile state measured in Emax. This dependence has been shown to result from the dependence of Vo_2 associated with activation or excitation-contraction coupling on ventricular contractile state (18, 24). Therefore, if contractile state changed as a function of PVA even under a stable inotropic background, the Vo_2-PVA regression line obtained under a stable inotropic background would become a composite Vo_2-PVA relation and the excess Vo_2 for mechanical contraction cannot be equal to total Vo_2 minus unload Vo_2. If Vo_2 for the non-mechanical activities had increased with PVA, the excess Vo_2 would have been overestimated and the PVA/(excess Vo_2) efficiency underestimated. At present we do not know whether this situation existed or not in our experiments.

A third assumption is that the unloaded contraction with zero PVA is truly unloaded mechanically. The unloaded ventricle has zero external mechanical work and zero PVA. Although the unloaded ventricle contracting isovolumically at Vd is not generating any positive pressure, it is still changing ventricular shape with contraction. We assumed that ventricular wall force was zero or slightly negative and therefore regional myocardial mechanical work was also zero or nearly zero despite the shortening. This assumption seems common when ventricular pressure and wall force are related theoretically (2).

We consider that the PVA/(excess Vo_2) efficiency would reflect the efficiency of the contractile machinery. PVA/(excess Vo_2) efficiency is the product of Vo_2-to-ATP efficiency and ATP-to-PVA efficiency. Although Vo_2 has an enthalpy of 20 J/ml O_2, all Vo_2 is not converted to ATP. The ATP/Vo_2 efficiency may be about 70% because 6 mols of ATP are produced from 1 mol of O_2 in oxidative phosphorylation and the free energy of ATP is assumed to be -57 KJ (4). If this metabolic efficiency is constant despite changes in loading, heart rate, and contractile conditions, the constant PVA/(excess Vo_2) efficiency would imply that the mechanical efficiency of the contractile machinery converting the free energy in ATP to total mechanical energy, i. e., PVA, would also be constant at about 57% ($= 40/70$). However, this efficiency is not the thermodynamic efficiency of the contractile machinery because in the latter its numerator must be external work. Since external work is a variable fraction of PVA depending on loading, heart rate, and contractile conditions, we would consider that PVA/(excess Vo_2) reflects the maximal limit of the thermodynamic efficiency of the contractile machinery (4).

The mechanical efficiency of the heart is given by the ratio of external work to total Vo_2 or Vo_2 minus basal metabolism (3–6). This efficiency will be variably smaller than the PVA/(excess Vo_2) of about 40% because external work is a variable fraction of PVA and Vo_2 for activation is a sizable amount as compared to the excess Vo_2. The PVA/(excess Vo_2) efficiency can be considered to indicate the maximal limit that the mechanical efficiency of the heart cannot exceed.

To summarize, we have shown major experimental findings on the relationship between left ventricular oxygen consumption and systolic pressure-volume area, which we consider represents the total mechanical energy generated by ventricular contraction. Taking the advantage of the pressure-volume area, we analyzed the oxygen consumption vs. pressure-volume area relation in terms of energy conversion efficiency.

Acknowledgment

We thank Eisai Co., Ltd., for providing us with 40 ampoules of verapamil solution (5 mg/2 ml) free of charge.

References

1. Allen DG, Kurihara S (1982) The effects of muscle length on intracellular calcium transients in mammalian cardiac muscle. J Physiol 327: 79–94
2. Beyar R, Sideman S (1984) A computer study of the left ventricular performance based on fiber structure, sarcomere dynamics and transmural electrical propagation velocity. Circ Res 55: 358–375
3. Braunwald E, Ross J, Sonnenblick EH (1976) Mechanisms of Contraction of the Normal and Failing Heart, 2nd ed. Little, Brown and Co, Boston, pp 169–199
4. Chapman JB (1983) Heat production. In: Cardiac Metabolism, edited by AJ Drake-Holland, MIM Noble. John Wiley and Sons, Chichester, pp 239–256
5. Elzinga G (1983) Cardiac oxygen consumption and the production of heat and work. In: Drake-Holland AJ Noble MIM (eds) Cardiac Metabolism. John Wiley and Sons, Chichester, pp 173–194
6. Gibbs CL (1979) Cardiac energetics. In: Handbook of Physiology. The Cardiovascular System. The Heart. American Physiological Society, Washington, DC, pp 775–804
7. Jewell BR (1977) A re-examination of the influence of muscle lengzj on myocardial performance. Circ Res 40: 221–230
8. Khalafbeigui F, Suga H, Sagawa K (1979) Left ventricular systolic pressure-volume area correlates with oxygen consumption. Am J Physiol 237: H 566–H 569
9. Shepherd AP, Burger CG (1977) A solid-state arteriovenous oxygen difference analyzer for flowing whole blood. Am J Physiol 232: H437–H440
10. Suga H (1979) Total mechanical energy of a ventricle model and cardiac oxygen consumption. Am J Physiol 236: H498–H505
11. Suga H (1979) External mechanical work from relaxing ventricle. Am J Physiol 236: H494–H497
12. Suga H (1980) Relaxing ventricle performs external mechanical work greater than quickly released elastic energy. Eur Heart J 1 (Suppl A): 131–137
13. Suga H, Sagawa K (1974) Instantaneous pressure-volume relationships and their ratio in the excised supported canine left ventricle. Circ Res 35: 117–126
14. Suga H, Hayashi T, Shirahata M (1981) Ventricular syslic to pressure-volume area as predictor of cardiac oxygen consumption. Am J Physiol 240: H39–H44
15. Suga H, Hayashi T, Shirahata M, Hisano R (1981) Regression of cardiac oxygen consumption on ventricular pressure volume area in dog. Am J Physiol 240: H320–H325
16. Suga H, Hayashi T, Suehiro S, Hisano R, Shirahata M, Ninomiya I (1981) Equal oxygen consumption rates of isovolumic and ejecting contractions with equal systolic pressure volume area in canine left ventricle. Circ Res 49: 1082–191
17. Suga H, Hisano R, Hirata S, Hayashi T, Ninomiya I (1982) Mechanism of higher oxygen consumption rate: pressure-loaded vs. volume-loaded heart. Am J Physiol 242: H942–H948
18. Suga H, Hisano R, Goto Y, Yamada O, Igarashi Y (1983) Effect of positive inotropic agents on the relation between oxygen consumption and systolic pressure volume area in canine left ventricle. Circ Res 53: 306–318
19. Suga H, Hisano R, Hirata S, Hayashi T, Yamada O, Ninomiya I (1983) Heart rate independent energetics and systolic pressure-volume area in dog heart. Am J Physiol 244: H206–H214
20. Suga H, Yamada O, Goto Y (1984) Energetics of ventricular contraction as traced in the pressure-volume diagram. Fed Proc 43: 2411–2413
21. Suga H, Goto Y, Yamada O, Igarashi Y (1984) Independence of myocardial oxygen consumption from pressure-volume trajectory during diastole in canine left ventricle. Circ Res 55: 734–739
22. Suga H, Yamada O, Goto Y, Igarashi Y (1984) Oxygen consumption and pressure-volume area of abnormal contractions in canine heart. Am J Physiol 246: H154–H160
23. Suga H, Yamada O, Goto Y, Igarashi Y, Ishiguri H (1984) Constant mechanical efficiency of contractile machinery of canine left ventricle under different loading and inotropic conditions. Jpn J Physiol 34: 679–698

24. Suga H, Igarashi Y, Yamada O, Goto Y (1985) Mechanical efficiency of the left ventricle as a function of preload, afterload, and contractility. Heart an Vessels, 1:3–8

Authors' address:

Dr. Hiroyuki Suga, National Cardiovascular Center, Fujishirodai, Suita, Osaka, 565 (Japan)

The concept of "end-systolic" pressure-volume and length-tension relations of the heart from a muscle physiologist's point of view

R. W. Gülch

Institute of Physiology II, University of Tübingen (F. R. G.)

Summary

End-systolic length-tension relationships were measured on ultrathin isolated heart preparations of rat (mean diameter ± S. D. = 96 μm ± 45 μm). Independent of contractile state being changed by variation in extracellular Ca^{++}-concentration no unique end-systolic length-tension relation was found when varying pre- and afterload over a wide range. It is more likely that rectilinear end-systolic curves can be obtained under a low contractile state than under a high one. Thus, the muscle physiological basis is withdrawn from the E_{max}-concept for which a single end-systolic pressure-volume relation is typical.

Key words: end-systolic pressure-volume relation, length-tension diagram, end-systolic length-tension curve, rat myocardium, force-frequency relation

Introduction

Progress in method over the past decades has made available to today's cardiologist in situ data which facilitate a quantitative description of heart mechanics. Thus, the pump function of the heart can, in principle, be expressed at any moment of pressure and volume changes in terms of the so-called working diagram. Nevertheless, complete pressure-volume diagrams, as synopsis of the most important mechanical parameters of ventricular contractions, are only obtainable when preload and afterload are varied over a wide range. This is often not realizable or justifiable in patients. Thus, there is a great need in the clinics for alternative parameters that are independent of pre- and afterload, but are suitable for characterizing the contractile activity of the heart.

Sagawa (17, 18) and Suga (20, 21) presented a concept that came very close to meeting these requirements. This is illustrated schematically in Fig. 1. For a given contractile state, all end-systolic pressure-volume data of ejecting ventricles obey one single rectilinear end-systolic pressure-volume relationship, which can be described by equation (1):

$$P_{ES} = E_{max}(V_{ES} - V_d)$$ (1)

Irrespective of whether preload A or afterload B is changed, the left upper corner C of the three pressure-volume loops lies very close to the end-systolic line. According to the authors' opinion, the slope of the straight line is a direct measure of the contractile state of the heart or myocardium.

Changes in ventricular contractility will only affect the slope E_{max} without changing V_d, the volume intercept, which is called "dead volume". V_d should be clearly distinguished from the unstressed ventricular volume V_o which is obtained as the volume intercept of the resting

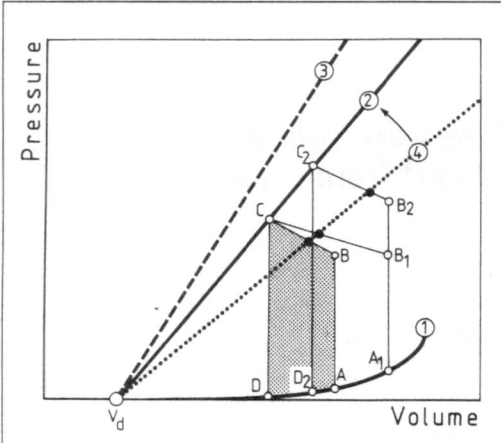

Fig. 1. Schematic pressure-volume diagram. 1 = diastolic pressure-volume curve, 2 = end-systolic pressure-volume relation, 3 = end-systolic pressure-volume relation under elevated contractile state, 4 = instantaneous pressure-volume relation. The arrow indicates that the instantaneous relations move anti-clockwise towards the end-systolic curve as a function of the time of estimation after the onset of contraction. The trajectory ABCD expresses a complete pressure-volume loop of the ejecting ventricle. Three different loops are selected: ABCD = control loop, A_1B_1CD = pressure-volume loop under higher preload A_1 but unchanged afterload B_1, $A_1 B_2 C_2 D_2$ = pressure-volume loop under higher preload and afterload B_2.

pressure-volume curve. Extension of equation (1) to an entire systole of a cardiac cycle leads to instantaneous pressure-volume relations (2):

$$P(t) = E(t)[V(t) - V_d(t)] \qquad (2)$$

These straight lines represent the pressure-volume data specified at a particular time t after the onset of contraction. The slope $E(t)$ increases with time, reaching the maximum E_{max} at end-systole. $V_d(t)$ proves to be virtually time-invariant (24).

$E(t)$ has the dimension of volume elastance. Thus it can be interpreted as a time-varying volume elastance which "waxes" with time during systole and "wanes" during diastole (22).

This so-called E_{max}-concept was rapidly adopted by cardiologists. In fact, on patients, end-systolic pressure-volume relations can only be obtained based on very few pressure-volume points, e. g. on two points in the study of Grossman et al. (7). Thus, the numerous clinical studies (for references see [18]) cannot be considered to verify the E_{max}-concept. On the other hand, there are studies on laboratory animals clearly contradicting it (6, 11, 12, 16).

Irrespective of the pros and cons in the clinical use of the E_{max}-concept, the latter must be equally applicable to linear heart muscle strips, since E_{max}, as an index of contractility, is supposed to render information about the state of cardiac contractility, based on data from the whole heart. Furthermore, the area below the linear end-systolic pressure-volume relationship has meanwhile (22, 23) been analyzed as a predictor of oxygen consumption of the ejecting heart, thus, also in this respect, the E_{max}-concept must be founded on the elementary mechanisms of myocardium. Previous studies on isolated heart muscle are partly contradictory. The group of Sonnenblick (3) and that of Paulus et al. (15) found an uniform rectilinear end-systolic length-tension relationship. Other groups (2, 8–10) described totally separate isotonic and isometric maxima curves. The present experiments on the rat, which has become the preferred laboratory animal with respect to topics in chronic alterations in the heart, were designed mainly to complement previous studies and results on the cat (8–10). Furthermore, the E_{max}-concept will be examined under altered contractility since our previous studies have indicated that rectilinear, maximum curves in length-tension diagram are more likely found under reduced contractility.

Methods and material

The experiments were performed on isolated right ventricular trabeculae and papillary muscles of rat heart. The Wistar rats were sacrificed at the age of 15–17 weeks weighing 330 ± 29 g (mean ± S. D.; n = 8). The hearts were rapidly excised under ether anesthesia and prepared in a temperature-controlled bath superfused with carbogen-equilibrated Tyrode bathing solution. The Tyrode bathing solution had the following composition in mmol/l: NaCl 130, NaHCO$_3$ 20, NaH$_2$PO$_4$1.2, KCl 4.1, MgCl$_2$ 1.2, CaCl$_2$ 1.1 (when not otherwise stated), glucose 23. In a temperature-controlled muscle bath (temperature 27° C) which was superfused with carbogen-equilibrated Tyrode solution at a sufficiently rapid rate, one end of the isolated heart preparations was attached to a piezoresistive force transducer (AE 801 ame, resonance frequency 3 kHz) the other to an isotonic electrically controlled lever system consisting of a rebuilt dc microservomotor (M 915L, Portescap). The non-ferrous rotor coil of the motor to which a small balsa wood lever was attached was pivoted in jewel bearings so that friction could be neglected. The effective mass of the moving part of the lever system was < 10 mg. The attachment of the preparations to the set-up was achieved with 2 mm long tips of glass micropipettes pulled out from glass capillary tubes. Via the electric field of a pair of platinum electrodes, the heart muscles were stimulated with 1 ms squarewave pulses at a frequency of 0.25 Hz and an amplitude 10% above threshold.

The vital statistics of the heart muscles are:
mean optimum length = 2.5 ± 0.7 mm, mean cross-sectional area = 0.0081 ± 0.0065 mm^2 ($\bar{x}$ ± S. D.; n = 8).

All measurements, following variations in extension of the preparations, were made under strictly stationary conditions of the isometrically beating heart muscles (9).

Results and discussion

The almost inertia-free and frictionless isotonic lever system made it possible to perform measurements of lenght-tension diagrams on ultrathin heart muscles. In this series of study, the thinnest preparation had a diameter of 50 μm, the thickest that of 170 μm, the mean diameter was 96 μm ± 45 μm ($\bar{x}$ ± S. D.). To demonstrate the optimum diffusion conditions existing in such thin preparations, their frequency-tension behaviour is briefly shown. Fig. 2 demonstrates a typical steady state frequency-tension curve, measured at 37° C and 1.1 mmol/l Ca^{++}. In contrast to the current opinions (4, 5), in support of a negative staircase

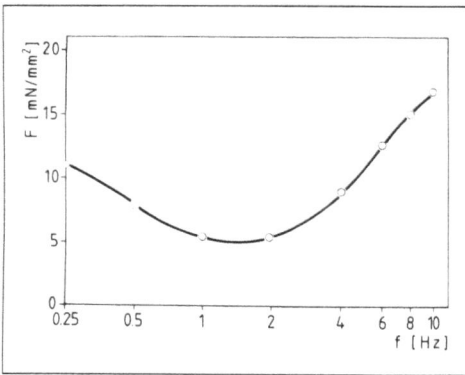

Fig. 2. Representative steady-state tension-frequency curve. The stimulation frequency was increased from 0.25 Hz to 10 Hz in steps according to the abscissa of the data points. The muscle bath temperature was 37° C.

phenomenon for the rat model, these thin heart muscle preparations show, similarly to the myocardium of other warm-blooded animals, a positive staircase, i. e. within the range of physiological frequency > 2 Hz, the force increases with increasing frequency. These findings correspond well to those of Meijler (14) who also described the positive staircase phenomenon in perfused isolated rat heart.

Complete length-tension diagrams were constructed from isometric and afterloaded isotonic contractions at 27° C and 0.25 Hz. Typical oscilloscope recordings of these contractions are documented in Fig. 3. All measurements are related to the isometrically beating

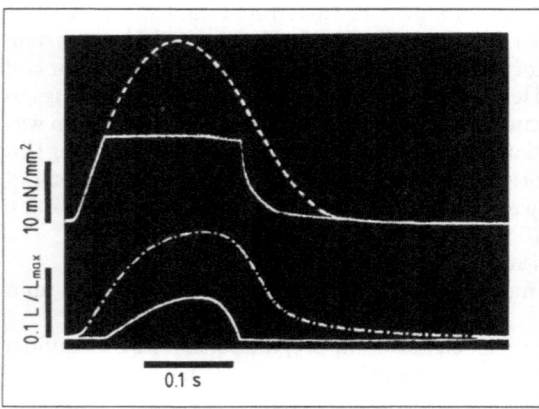

Fig. 3. Oscilloscope recordings of an isometric (-----), isotonic (-.-.-) and an afterloaded isotonic contraction (_____). The upper trace shows the time course of force, the lower trace of shortening. (Temperature 27° C, stimulation frequency 0.25 Hz).

heart muscle under steady state conditions, i. e. after a train of stable isometric contractions, only the first nonisometric contraction was considered for further analysis when changing loading conditions. This procedure guaranteed absolutely reproducible results, although qualitatively similar diagrams result if all measurements were related to steady state of the isotonically beating heart muscle.

Qualitatively, two different types of length-tension diagrams were obtained as can be seen from Fig. 4. Although in the region of higher extension, both diagrams show distinctly separate isometric maxima curve and afterloaded isotonic maxima curves, in diagram 4b – in contrast to 4a – a separate course of the curve is no longer guaranteed under low preload. As a rule, even under external isometric conditions, no single sarcomere contracts in a purely isometric manner due to unavoidable intrinsic extensibility, mainly caused by damaged regions in the vicinity of the suspensions. Probably, the more marked relative decrease in developed isometric tension as compared to isotonic shortening with decreasing preload is due to this fact, since under less extension this extensibility, which solely falsifies the isometric contraction, becomes more serious. The preparation shown in diagram 4b revealed, under microscopic control, a more marked extensibility, giving rise to the more accentuated decrease in active tension under decreasing preload. When the isometric maxima curve is corrected by taking the same preload-dependency as for isotonic shortening (Fig. 4d), then an isometric maxima curve results (diagram 4b), which, also in the region of low preloads, is clearly separate from the afterloaded isotonic maxima curves. The auxotonic shortening of certain cardiac areas at the cost of others even during isolvolumic contraction of the heart is most probably the decisive reason why in many studies on the whole heart, a single end-systolic pressure-volume relationship is described. Thus the isovolumic data are far from being representative of the isometric behaviour of the myocardium.

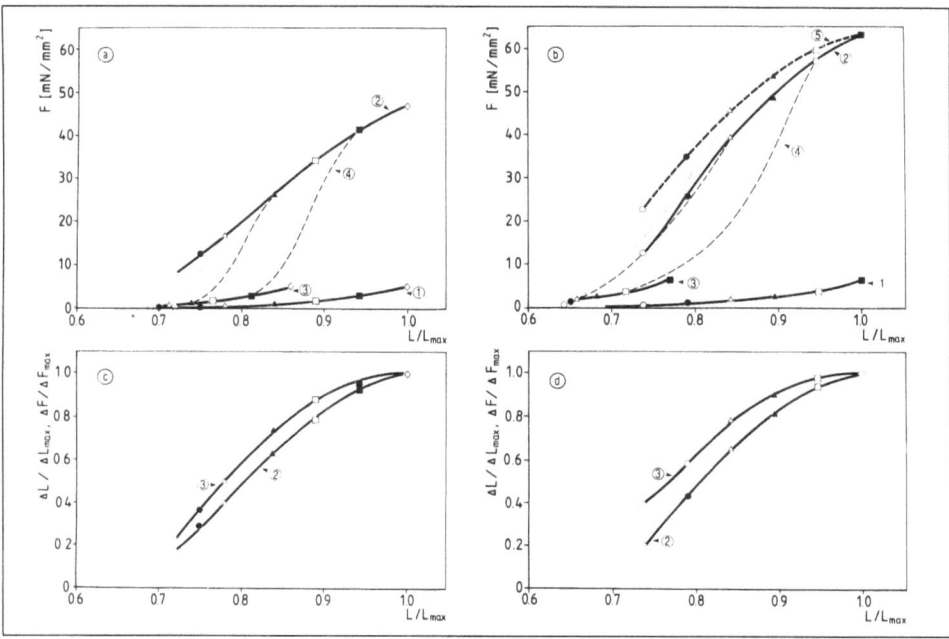

Fig. 4. Representative length-tension diagrams. In the upper part complete length-tension diagrams are shown. 1 = resting length-tension curve, 2 = isometric maxima curve, 3 = isotonic maxima curve, 4 = afterloaded isotonic maxima curve, 5 = corrected isometric maxima curve. In the lower part the respective active length-tension and length-shortening curves are demonstrated.
Diagram a is based on measurements on a heart preparation with low extensibility, diagram b refers to a heart muscle with higher extensibility. Assuming the same dependency on preload for the active isometric tension as for isotonic shortening by adapting curve 2 to 3 in Fig. 4d, then the corrected isometric maxima curve 5 results in diagram 4b.

To test the sensitivity of end-systolic length-tension relations to variation in contractile state of the myocardium, length-tension diagrams were measured under a wide range of different extracellular Ca^{++}-concentrations. Figure 5a shows isometric maxima curves under four different Ca^{++}-concentrations. For the sake of clarity, the afterloaded and isotonic maxima curves have been omitted, which in each case followed distinctly separate courses as the respective isometric maxima curve. The linearity of end-systolic curves, which is absolutely necessary for the evaluation of contractility using E_{max}, is all the more difficult to attain the better the contractile state of the myocardium. The schematic presentation in Fig. 5b makes this phenomenon plausible. In this case, a strictly rectilinear isometric maxima curve is obtained by superimposing the active length-tension curve (broken line), under low contractile state, to the resting length-tension curve. Under high Ca^{++}-concentrations a mathematically similar but higher active length-tension can be assumed, as increasing the available activator Ca^{++}-ions will increase the number of activated actin-myosin cross-bridges in a proportional manner independent of instantaneous sarcomere length and thus of preload. If one superimposes this active length-tension to the same resting length-tension curve a clearly non-linear isometric maxima curve is obtained.
These present findings on rat myocardium as well as our previous studies on cat papillary

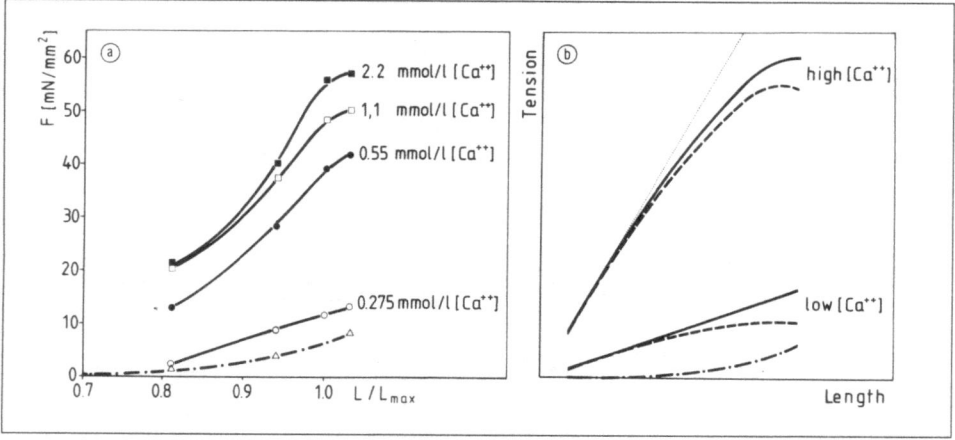

Fig. 5. Length-tension diagram under variations of the extracellular Ca^{++}-concentration. Only the resting length-tension and isometric maxima curves are demonstrated.

a) Representative diagram based on original data.

b) Schematic drawing illustrating that despite a rectilinear maxima curve under low Ca^{++}-concentration, a clearly nonlinear maxima relationship results under high Ca^{++}-concentration.

muscle (8–10) remove the muscle physiological basis that support the E_{max}-concept. Also in the range of minimal extension, the various end-systolic length-tension curves will most probably follow distinctly separate courses with better isometric conditions for each sarcomere. This statement also applies to the different contractile states.

There are two main reasons for the uniform linear end-systolic pressure-volume relation frequently described in whole hearts. Firstly, the heart musculature does not contract in an isometric manner, not even during the isovolumetric phase. Thus, there is the so-called transition phase during which the ventricle adopts more the form of a sphere at constant inner volume. Secondly, the range of preload alterations which is justifiable in patients is extremely narrow. Therefore, the range of end-systolic pressure-volume relations which can be obtained in clinics is rather limited with respect to both volume and pressure. Taking into account the great difficulties and considerable uncertainty in measurement involved in obtaining end-systolic pressure-volume data, it is not surprising that in clinical investigations, end-systolic data points are often approximated by a linear relationship. But it would be a mistake to overemphasize this relationship by taking the slope E_{max} as a measure of myocardial contractility. In my opinion, the E_{max}-value leads to an unnecessary reduction of data in that the more extensive information rendered by original pressure-volume data is lost. For example, in interindividual comparison of hearts of different sizes, the wall stress should definitely be included in the discussion, since the latter represents the real load that is imposed on heart muscle in ejecting hearts. This parameter is only obtainable from original pressure-volume data.

In conclusion, the high expectations clinicians placed in the E_{max}-concept as a measure of contractility cannot be met due to the aforementioned principal objections. Nevertheless, the discussion about this concept had a very positive effect. Cardiology has reverted to the analysis of pressure-volume diagrams of the heart, in issues pertaining to evaluation of contractility. This approach, which O. Frank recognized as early as 1898 (6), has been neglected for many years in favour of the maximum unloaded shortening velocity V_{max} as the unique index for evaluating myocardial contractility.

References

1. Alpert B, Benson L, Olley P (1980) E_{max} during exercise in children with left-sided cardiac disease. Amer J Cardiol 45: 467
2. Brady AJ (1967) Length-tension relations in cardiac muscle. Am Zool 7: 603–610
3. Downing SE, Sonnenblick, EH (1964) Cardiac muscle mechanics and ventricular performance: Force and time parameters. Am J Physiol 207: 705–715
4. Fabiato A (1981) Myoplasmic free calcium concentration reached during the twitch of an intact isolated cardiac cell and during calcium-induced release of calcium from the sarcoplasmic reticulum of a skinned cardiac cell from the adult rat or rabbit ventricle. J Gen Physiol 78: 457–497
5. Forester GV, Mainwood GW (1974) Interval dependent inotropic effects in the rat myocardium and the effect of calcium. Pflügers Arch 352: 189–196
6. Frank O (1898) Die Grundform des arteriellen Pulses. Z Biol 37: 483–526
7. Grossman W, Braunwald E, Mann T, McLaurin LP, Green LH (1977) Contractile state of left ventricle in man as evaluated from end-systolic pressure-volume relations. Circulation 56: 845–852
8. Gülch RW (1985) The "end-systolic" length-tension relation in mammalian myocardium. Basic Res Cardiol 80: 636–641
9. Gülch RW, Jacob R (1975) The effect of sudden stretches on the length-tension diagram and the force-velocity relations of mammalian cardiac muscle. Pflügers Arch 357: 335–347
10. Gülch RW, Jacob R (1975) Length-tension diagram and force-velocity relations of mammalian cardiac muscle under steady-state conditions. Pflügers Arch 355: 331–346
11. Jacob R, Weigand KH (1966) Die endsystolischen Druck-Volumenbeziehungen als Grundlage einer Beurteilung der Kontraktilität des linken Ventrikels in situ. Pflügers Arch 289: 37–49
12. Kissling G, Jacob R (1972) Begrenzende Faktoren für die Steigerungsfähigkeit des Schlagvolumens durch positive Inotropie. Pflügers Arch 335: 153–166
13. Marsh JD, Green LH, Wynne J, Cohn PF, Grossman W (1979) Left ventricular end-systolic pressure-dimension and stress length relation in normal human subjects. Amer J Cardiol 44: 1311–1317
14. Meijler FL (1962) Staircase, rest contractions, and potentiation in the isolated rat heart. Amer J Physiol 202: 636–640
15. Paulus WJ, Claes VA, Brutsaert DL (1980) End-systolic pressure-volume relation estimated from physiologically loaded cat papillary muscle contractions. Circulation Res 47: 20–26
16. Reichel H (1939) Die Beziehungen zwischen Länge und Spannung, Volumen und Druck des Herzmuskels. Z Biol 99: 63–79
17. Sagawa K (1978) The ventricular pressure-volume diagram revisited. Circulation Res 43: 677–687
18. Sagawa K (1981) The end-systolic pressure-volume relation of the ventricle: Definition, modifications and clinical use. Circulation 63: 1223–1227
19. Sagawa K, Suga H, Shoukas AA, Bakalar KM (1977) End-systolic pressure-volume ratio: a new index of contractility. Amer J Cardiol 40: 748–753
20. Suga H (1970) Time course of left ventricular pressure-volume relationship under various extents of aortic occlusion. Jpn Heart J 11: 373–378
21. Suga H (1971) Left ventricular pressure-volume ratio in systole as an index of inotropism. Jpn Heart J 12: 153–160
22. Suga H (1979) Total mechanical energy of a ventricle model and cardiac oxygen consumption. Amer J Physiol 5: H 498–H 505
23. Suga H (1986) Cardiac oxygen consumption and systolic pressure volume area. Basic Res Cardiology in press
24. Suga H, Sagawa K (1974) Instantaneous pressure-volume relationships and their ratio in the excised, supported canine left ventricle. Circulation Res 35: 117–126
25. Taylor RR (1970) Active length-tension relations compared in isometric, afterloaded and isotonic contractions of cat papillary muscle. Circulation Res 26: 279–288

Author's address:

Prof. Dr. R. W. Gülch, Institute of Physiology II, University of Tübingen, D-7400 Tübingen (F. R. G.)

Local myocardial and global ventricular function compared during positive inotropic medication*

P. P. Lunkenheimer [1], A. Lunkenheimer [2], W. F. Whimster [5], G. Edel [3], N. Stroh [6], and H. Van Aken [4]

[1] Department of Experimental Thoraco-Vascular Surgery, [2] Department of Pediatric Cardiology, [3] Department of Morbid Anatomy, and [4] Department of Anesthesiology and Operative Care, University Hospital, Münster (F. R. G.), [5] Department of Morbid Anatomy, Kings College School of Medicine, London (England), and [6] Fraunhofer Institute für Verfahrenstechnik und Membrantechnologie, Stuttgart (F. R. G.)

Summary

The assessment of the pharmacological efficiency of cardiotonic drugs interferes with the complex force generation within the spatially netted myocardial meshwork. By multifocal local force and distance measurements we distinguished " afterloaded" from " unloading" force types, which essentially differ in their transient behaviour during changes in ventricular shape. Histologically we found the " afterloaded" force type in oblique fibre populations whereas the " unloading" force curve is generated in surface parallel fibres. Amrinon reduces pre- and afterload, thus inducing ventricular shrinkage. The resulting rearrangement of the intramural force pattern modifies the transmission of fibre tension to ventricular ejection in a way that contractility indices, derived from left ventricular pressure, become inapplicable. However, direct intracoronary drug injection, monitored by segmental force and distance measurements within the irrigated myocardial area, characterizes Amrinon as a potent positive inotropic drug.

Key words: Spatial netting of myocardial meshwork, unloading and afterloaded types of intramyocardial force generation, dualistic organization of ventricular function

Introduction

Which forces induce ventricular dilatation in myocardial insufficiency, in cardiomyopathy and in myocardial fibrosis? There are several well known concepts, such as Harvey's ventricular filling pressure (10), Brücke's spreading potency of the coronary arteries (7), Donder's intrathoracic sucking (8) and the passive elastic restoring forces recently re-examined by Rushmer (17) all of which have serious flaws as recent experiments on the empty beating heart have confirmed (21). Brachet (1814) (6) on the other hand put forward the idea of two myocardial fibre populations, one parallel to the surface and one radial (" fibres rayonnantes"). The surface-parallel fibres would produce ventricular constriction during systole whereas the radial fibres would actively diminish the wall thickness and produce active ventricular dilatation during diastole. Consequently Brachet postulated that the myocardial activation would be biphasic. Although no biphasic myocardial activation and no directly radial transmural fibres have been demonstrated, Brachet's concept led us to our present working hypothesis of a dualistic organization for ventricular function.

* Supported by Deutsche Forschungsgemeinschaft and by the Ministery of Research and Health NRW

Working hypothesis

We do not refer to radial fibres, but to oblique transmural fibres (Fig. 1) which take a variable course through the ventricular wall (19). Their angulation with respect to the epicardial surface continually changes with the length of their pathway. Some are curved

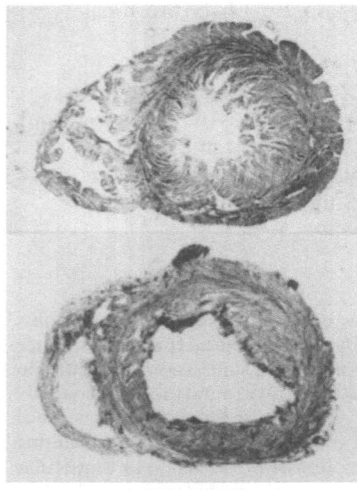

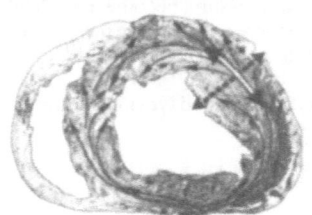

Fig. 1. Surface parallel and oblique transmural fibre orientation in the dog (upper) and calf heart (middle and lower) shown in the histological (upper) and macroscopical cross section after transcoronary air perfusion during formalin fixation. In the lower section the resulting main two force vectors are outlined: the tangential vector acts in ventricular constricting direction, the transmural one impedes wall thickening and thus acts in the direction of ventricular dilatation.

from the midwall to the epicardium and others from the midwall to the endocardium, thus giving a pennate pattern in cross section. Functionally this myocardial architecture produces tangential (ventricular constriction) forces and a complex force vector which is variably orientated transmurally. The transmural force vector has the effect of thinning the ventricle wall and thus promoting ventricular dilatation.

Thus, during systolic ventricular constriction, in response to wall thickening, the tension in the oblique transmural component of the heart muscle increases, whereas – according to Laplace's law (2, 16, 18, 20) – forces in the surface parallel component will decrease as the ventricular cross section decreases. This effect could be further elucidated by examining the myocardium during positively inotropic stimulation for which Amrinone was considered to be the best drug, since it also diminished ventricular pre- and afterload (1, 4, 5).

We therefore set out to assess the dualistic force pattern within the myocardial network, a method developed by our selves (11, 13, 15).

Methods

Twenty-seven anaesthetized mongrel dogs weighing 30–60 kg were used.

I. In each needle force probes, 1.1 mm thick and 9 mm long (Fig. 2), were implanted in the left ventricular wall parallel to the epicardial surface, one into the superficial fibres, and another into the midwall.

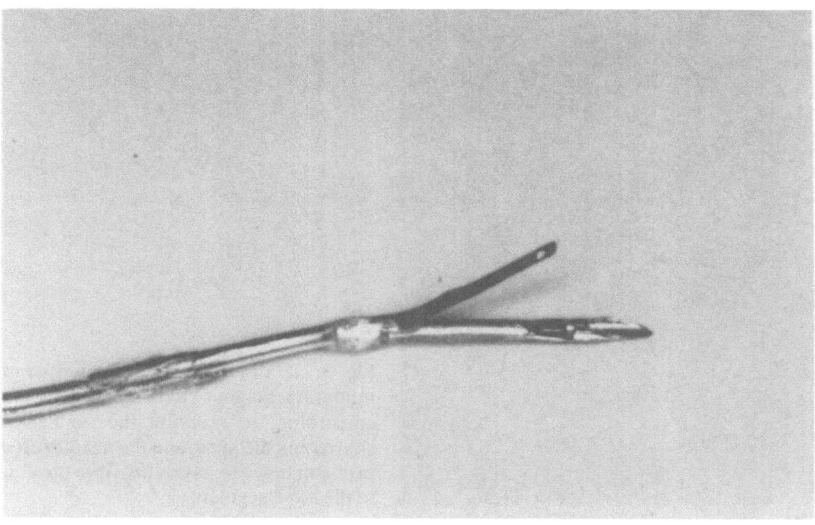

Fig. 2. The needle force probe, 1.1 mm thick, 9 mm long, for intramyocardial implantation at any site and in any depth of the ventricular wall, consists of the point of a hypodermic needle with a lateral window near the tip of the probe. An inner flexural bar is exposed by the window to the myocardial fibres which slip into the window during implantation. The lateral compression force of the surrounding myocardial meshwork acts on the flexural bar. Its deviation is sensed by strain gauges incorporated inside the needle lumen.

II. Hall-effect sensors in axial orientation to the fibres were implanted near the force probes (Fig. 3) to measure the shortening distance of the segment in which forces were assessed. In another preparation ventricular diameter was measured instead of segment lenght.

III. We clamped the measured segment in any position to make arbitrary measurements of the isometric constriction of the segment either shortened, stretched or afterloaded (free contraction) (Fig. 4).

Positive inotropic stimulation

We stimulated the heart with the positive inotropic drug Amrinone (i. v. bolus 2 mg/kg/b. w.). In the 27 dogs, we then compared the cardiodynamic data with classic cardiocirculatory data such as left ventricular pressure $\pm$ dp/dt, pulmonary artery pressure, cardiac output and heart rate.

Histology

A transmural block of tissue was taken at the site of the force probe and sectioned histologically to show the orientation of the myocardium around the probe for comparison with the probe signal (Fig. 5).

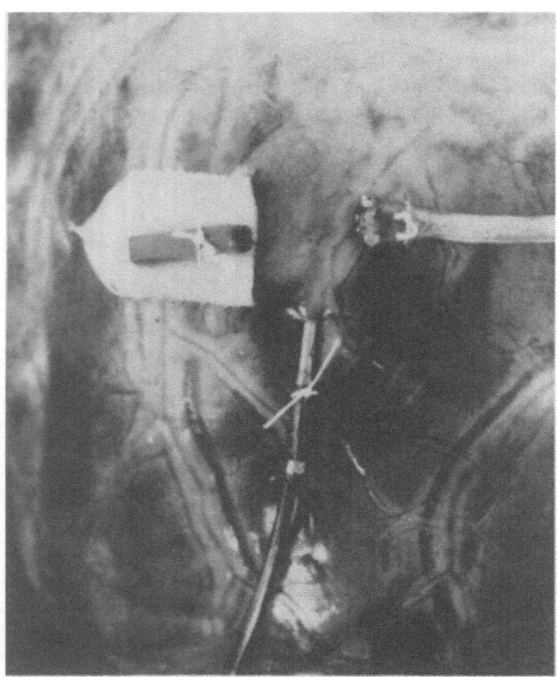

Fig. 3. Hall-effect Sensor (right) and miniature magnet (left) sutured to the epicardium to measure the segmental shortening distance, and the needle force probe in place to assess the fibre tension in the same segment.

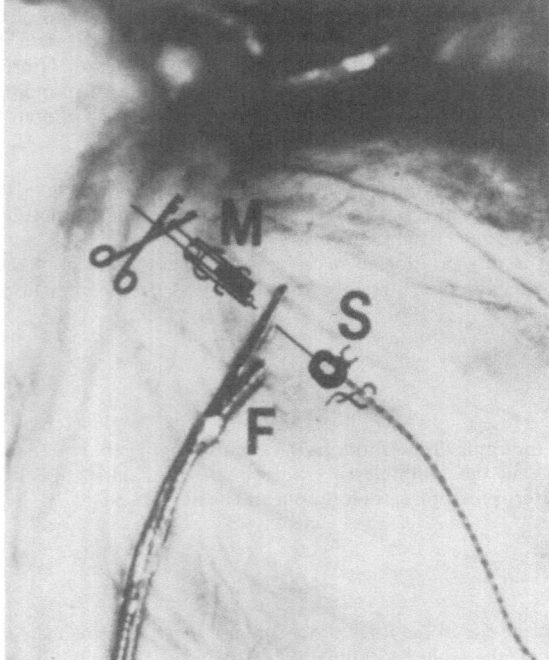

Fig. 4. Segmental clamp technique: S = Hall-effect Sensor; M = Miniature magnet; F = Force probe: Magnet and Hall-Sensor are bridged by a rigid wire which freely glides during the physiological contraction, but which can be clamped to induce isometric contraction.

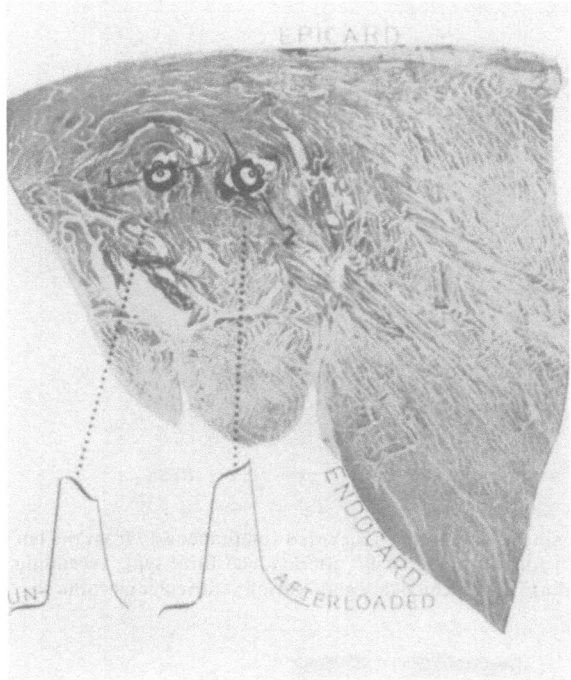

Fig. 5. Transmural histological cut through the left ventricular wall showing two implantation areas of force probes near the middle layer. Area 1 is located between surface parallel fibres which produce an "unloading" force signal. Area 2 corresponds to the oblique fibre population which engenders the "afterloaded" force signal.

Results

I. Dualism in cardiodynamics

Two types of force signal are generated within the intact ventricular myocardium (Fig. 6): The " afterloaded" type we confirmed histologically were in these areas where the force probes were coupled to oblique transmural fibre strands. The " unloading" force signal was measured when surface parallel fibres, confirmed histologically were loaded on the probe. The incidence of the " unloading" type of signal in an optional series of ca. 1,000 implantations in any area of the left ventricular wall was almost ten times that of the " afterloaded" type.

Haemodynamic manipulations going along with changes in ventricular diameter induce opposite changes in the two types of signal: in response to ventricular narrowing the unloading force signal decreases in amplitude whereas the afterloaded force increases in response to the increase in wall thickness. When left ventricular afterload was raised by blocking the descending aorta with a balloon catheter we regularly found a substantial increase in the unloading signal whereas the afterloaded type did not change, or its rise was poor because wall thickness decreased with left ventricular dilatation (Fig. 7).

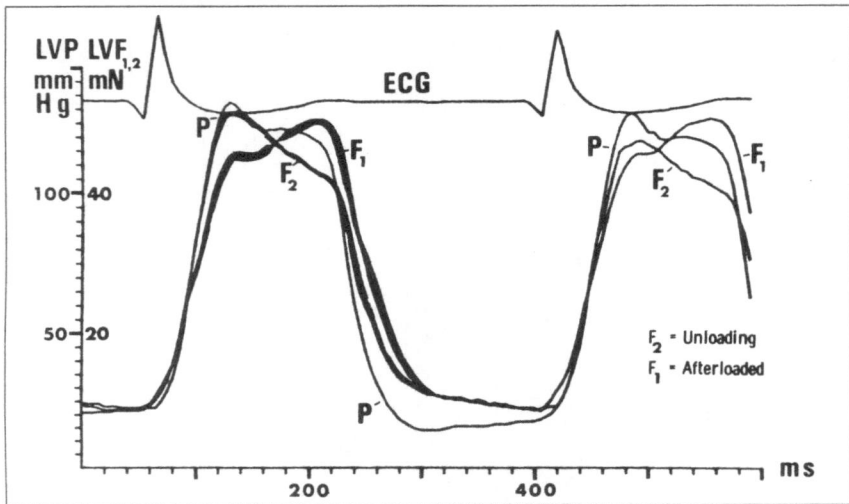

Fig. 6. ECG, LVP (P) and two local force singals (F $_1$ + F $_2$) recorded simultaneously from the left ventricular myocardium of a dog heart. F $_1$ follows the typical " afterloaded" force type, ascending during the ejection period. F $_2$ is an " unloading" curve which descends during ventricular ejection.

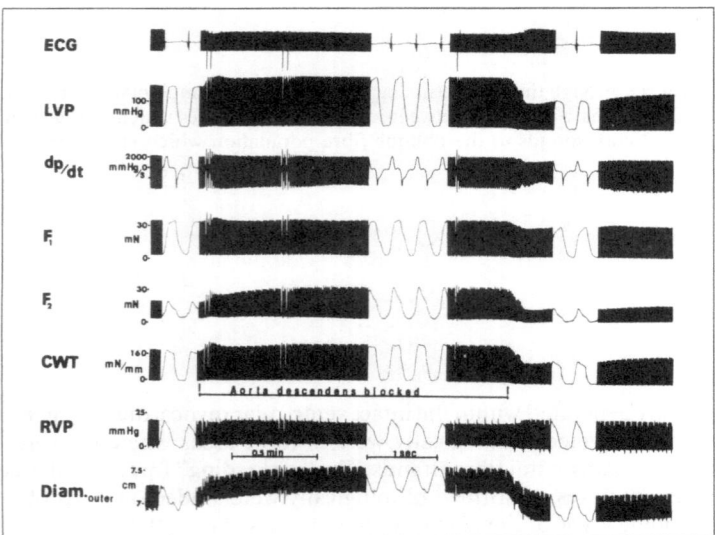

Fig. 7. Haemo- and cardiodynamic changes following an acute occulusion of the descending aorta near the aortic arch: the increase in afterload induces left ventricular dilatation (diam. outer = outer left ventricular diameter). Left ventricular pressure (LVP) and calculated wall tension (CWT) parallel one another. Myocardial fibre tension in the superficial fibres (F $_1$) follows the " afterloaded" type of force generation. Since ventricular dilatation induces thinning of a ventricular wall the increase in afterloaded force in the oblique transmural fibres is small. Some deeper fibres (F $_2$), following the " unloading" type of force generation (surface parallel fibres) show a marked increase in tension corresponding to the growing ventricular diameter.

II. Positive inotropic stimulation

a) Amrinone substantially reduces peripheral vascular resistance and increases venous capacitance. As a result left ventricular pre- and afterload decrease and hence the ventricular diameter decreases (Fig. 8). The wall thickness increases. In accordance with the working

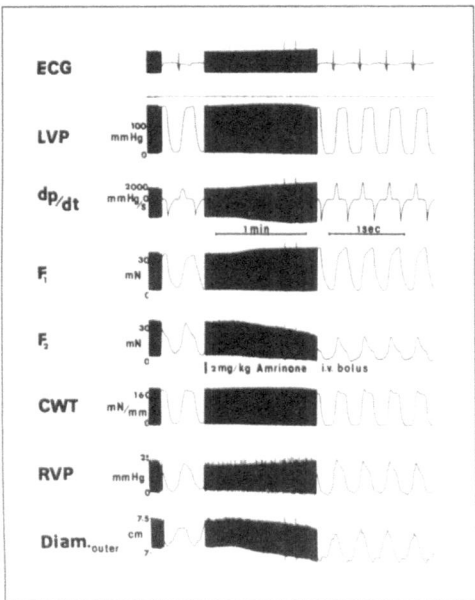

Fig. 8. Haemo- and cardiodynamic changes following a 2 mg/kg i. v. injection of Amrinone. The abrupt fall in ventricular diameter goes along with an increase in wall thickness. Hence the " afterloaded" force type (F_1) shows an increase in systolic force maxima, whereas the "unloading" force type markedly decreases. This complex rearrangement in the intramural force pattern is not reflected in the continuously calculated wall tension (CWT) (according to Laplace) nor can it be deduced from LVP.

hypothesis the left ventricular pressure, calculated wall tension, and the measured unloading force type decrease (Fig. 9). However, the afterloaded force signal increases *pari passu* with the wall thickness as the ventricular diameter decreases (Fig. 10). It is only paralleled by an increase in dp/dt max. and in cardiac output (Fig. 11).

b) When given directly into a branch of the coronary artery Amrinone significantly increased local forces both in the afterloaded and in the unloading types of signal (Fig. 12). Similarly the shortening distance in the perfused segment was drastically augmented. However, to get a response in left ventricular global function, a wall segment as extended as that which was perfused by the whole left circumflex artery had to be included in the inotropic medication.

c) The segment clamp technique revealed that Amrinone was able to shift the working diagram of a quasi-isolated myocardial segment from any control state to the left (Fig. 13). The end-diastolic local force was reduced in any state of control preload. Systolic local force maxima substantially increased. In the afterloaded contraction the shortening distance increased against an increase in peak force.

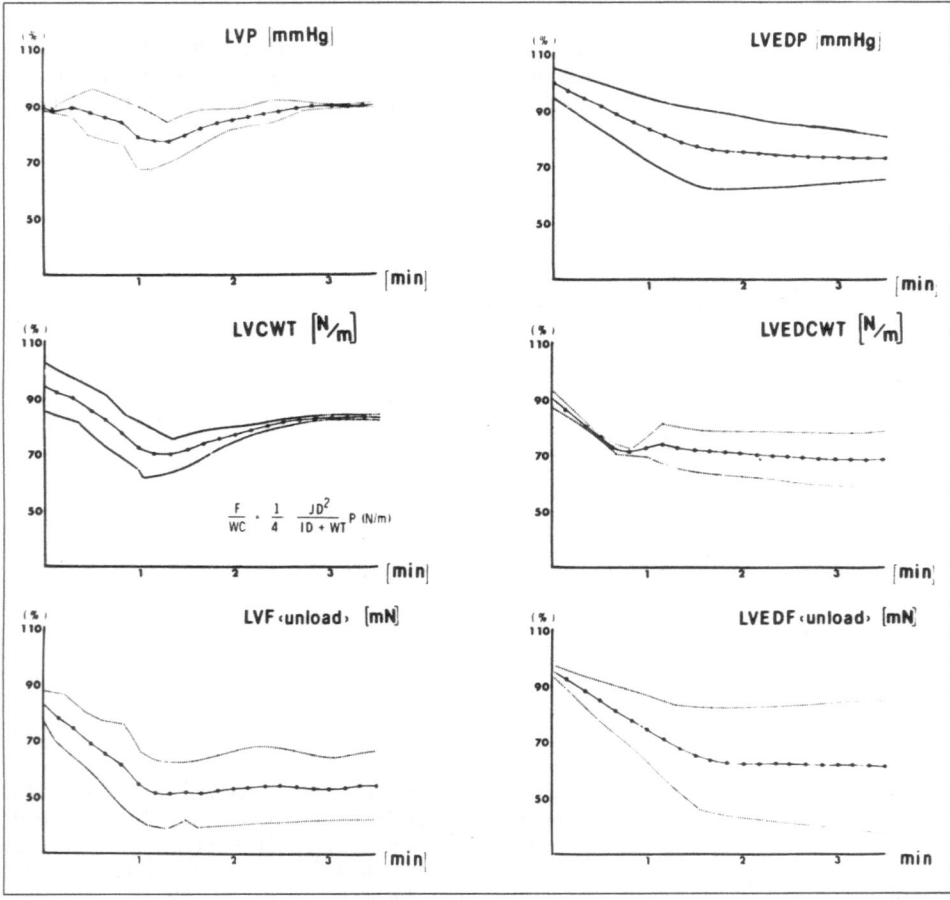

Fig. 9. Mean changes in left ventricular (end-diastolic) pressure LVP, LVEDP) in left ventricular calculated (end-diastolic) wall tension (LVCWT, LVEDCWT) and in left ventricular local " unloading" type forces following 2 mg/kg i. v. Amrinone. (———) Mean of 27 injections, (———) standard deviation.

Discussion

Haemodynamic data are likely to mask the positive inotropic effect of Amrinone except for the regularly reported increase in dp/dt max (1–5):

In the clinical situation we found an increase in cardiac output of up to 45 %. The left ventricular pressure was almost unchanged. The response in heart rate was variable. In view of the dramatic reduction in peripheral vascular resistance (afterload) and in central blood volume (preload), an increase in cardiac output gave little evidence of a positive inotropic intervention.

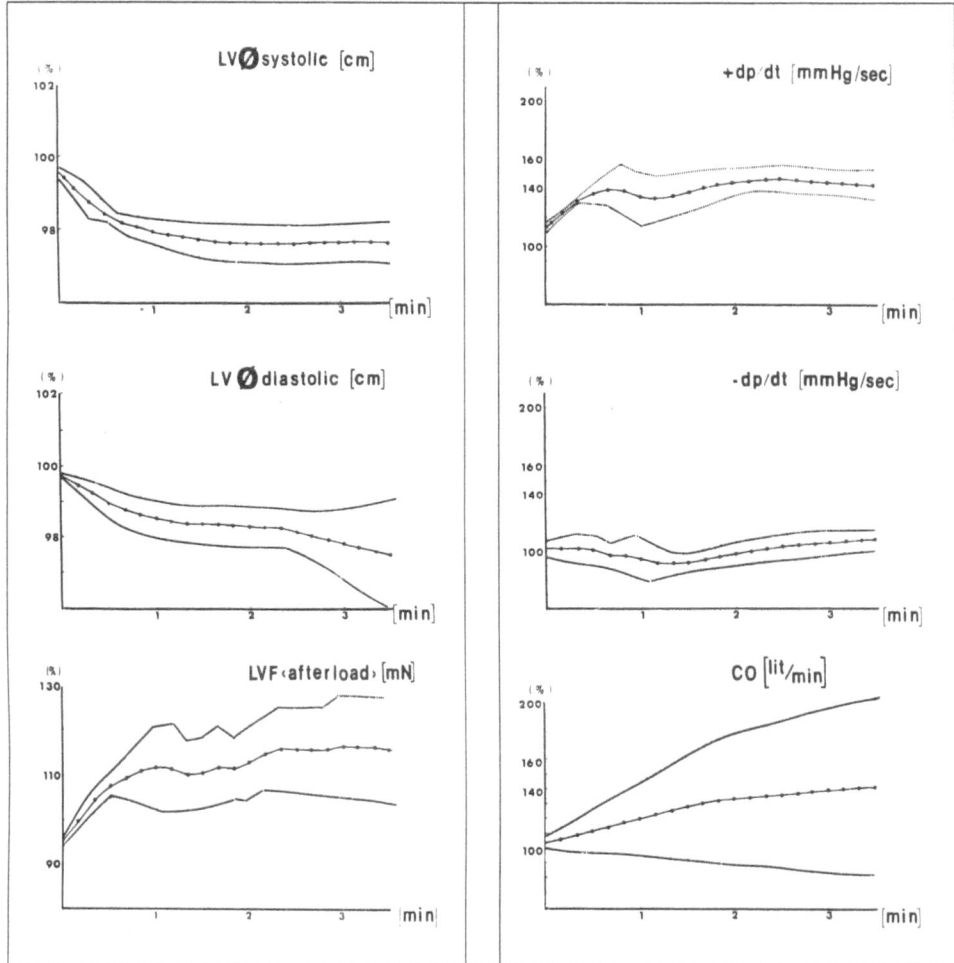

Fig. 10. Mean changes in left ventricular systolic and diastolic outer diameter (LVØ systolic, LVØ diastolic) and in the " afterloaded" type of local myocardial forces following 2 mg/kg i. v. Amrinone.

Fig. 11. Mean changes in left ventricular maximal pressure rise (+ dp/dt) and fall (− dp/dt) and in cardiac output (CO) following 2 mg/kg i. v. Amrinone.

Multifocal force measurements confirmed consistent inhomogeneities in intramural fibre tension. Local patterns were essentially modulated by changes in ventricular dimension. The unloading and the afterloaded types of force signal responded to changes in ventricular cross section in opposite directions.

The behaviour of the unloading type of force is in accordance with Laplace's law but the afterloaded force component defies the approved geometrical valuations (9, 16, 18, 20). This apparent dualism in myocardial force generations has to be kept in mind when inotropic

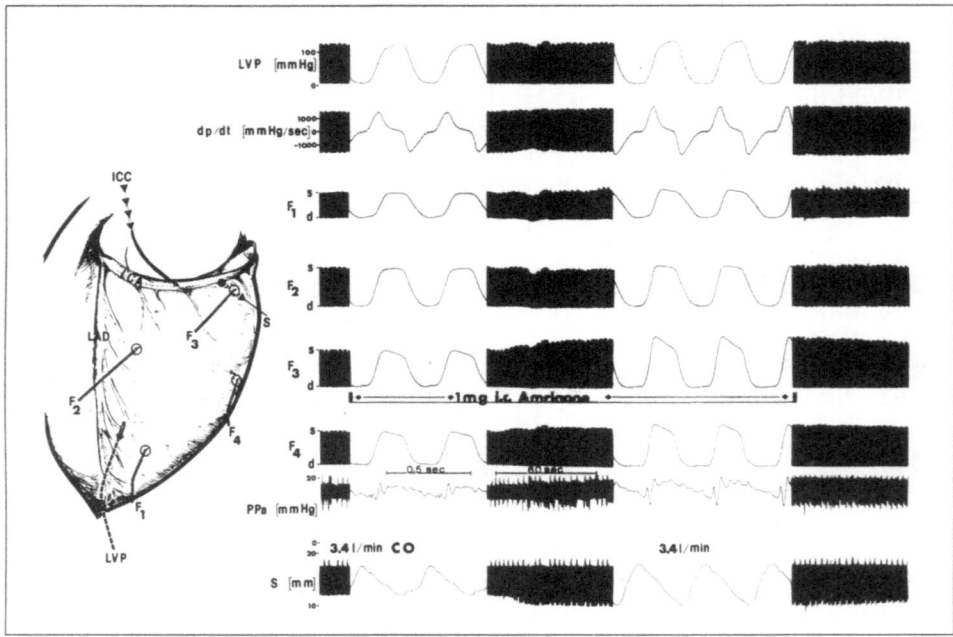

Fig. 12. Haemo- and cardiodynamic changes following an intracoronary injection of 1 mg Amrinone as a bolus. The drawing indicates the implantation areas of force probes (F_1 – F_4) and of the Hall-effect Sensor to measure segmental shortening (S). Following the injection of the drug into the distal circumflex artery local forces in F_3 and F_4 increase together with an increase in shortening amplitude (S). Forces in the non irrigated areas (F_1, F_2) are not influenced.

interventions are validated by any type of cardiodynamic measuring assembly whether it measures local forces (14), segment length or "intramyocardial pressure" (12).

Local dynamics, measured during segmental medication via isolated coronary perfusion, undeniably confirm the potent positive inotropic effect of Amrinone. This experimental protocol further determines the contribution of segmental function to global ventricular performance. Even substantial changes in segmental inotropy were not transmitted to the global ventricular function if the involved areas was essentially smaller than the territory which was perfused by the circumflex artery.

The segment clamp technique finally helped to range the actual myocardial function within the dimensions of the Frank-Straub-Starling mechanism e. g. in terms of the autoregulatory limits. Amrinone achieved a shift in the working diagram to the left (i. e. to a lowered preload). Positive inotropy of Amrinone emerged from an increase in isometric and afterloaded force maxima and an increase in segmental shortening distance starting from a reduced end-diastolic length.

However, the segment clamp technique also outlined the limitations of any procedure for measuring local myocardial dynamics: the spatial netting of the myocardial meshwork

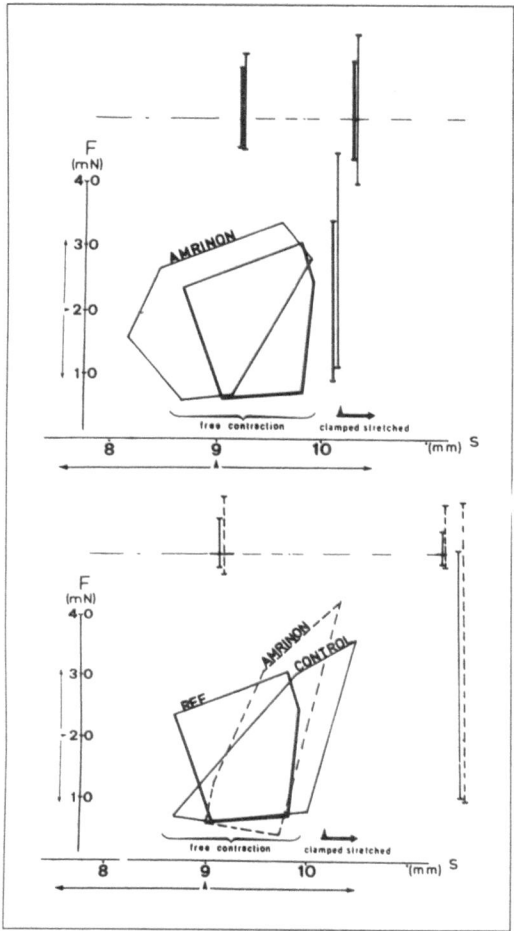

Fig. 13. Working diagrams of two dog hearts before (control) and after 2 mg/kg Amrinone i. v. Local force data (mN) are plotted against the distance of segmental shortening (mm). In the lower recording the control diagram of the first dog serves as a reference.
The graphs further show changes in max. isometric force generation (right columns) when the segment was clamped in stretched position, and dp/dt max. during free contraction and in a clamped and stretched position before and after Amrinone administration (bars above the working diagrams).

allows no access to a morphologically defined straight fibre band. Even the smallest separable segment is unpredictably influenced especially in its shortening distance by the diverging force trajectories of neighbouring interdigitations.

Conclusion

We conclude that global function cannot be validated from local dynamics. Similarly the rough ventricular dynamics observed by echocardiography or by ventricular angiography give no reliable insight into the intramural force patterns in any layer.

However, local measuring procedures which detect intramyocardial forces or shortening distances are helpful:
a) in quantifying inotropic drug effects,
b) in detecting local disturbances in the contractile state, for example in coronary surgery and
c) to monitor long-term changes in contractility in experiments which supposedly involve myocardial metabolism.

Amrinone has been shown to be a potent positive inotropic drug which also reduces ventricular pre- and afterload. Because of the complex interference of ventricular shape with local myocardial mechanical activity, global ventricular and even local functional indicators (force, shortening distance) are unreliable unless the mean ventricular size is kept constant during the pharmacological intervention. This experimental condition is perfectly guaranteed during intracoronary medication when measurements are done on the " quasi in situ isolated" myocardial segment. Our poorly invasive cardiodynamic measuring assembly is prepared for clinical application especially during coronary surgery when intracoronary medication is a matter of routine.

References

1. Alous; AA, -dobreck HP (1983) Amrihoue. In: Scriebine A (ed) New Drug Annual: Cardiovascular Drugs. Raven Press, New York, pp 259–276
2. Baker JF, Chalecki BW, Benziger, DP, O'Melia PE, Clemans SD, Edelson J (1982) Metabolism of Amrinone in Animals. Drug Metab Dispos 10: 168–172
3. Beek OG (1982) A Small Animal Model for Monitoring Inotropic Responses to Cardiotonic Agents. J Pharmacol Methods 7: 321–329
4. Benotti JR, Grossman W, Braunwald E, Carabello BA (1980) Effects of Amrinone on Myocardial Energy Metabolism and Hemodynamics in Patients with Severe Congestive Heart Failure Due to Coronary Artery Disease. Circulation 62: 28–34
5. Benotti JR, Grossman W, Braunwald E, Davolos DD, Alousi AA (1978) Hemodynamic Assessment of Amrinone. The New Engl J Med 25, 1373–1377
6. Brachet JL (1813) Sur la cause du mouvement de dilatation du coeur. Dissertation (18), (Imprimerie di Didot Jeune) Paris
7. Brücke E (1881) Physiologie des Kreislaufs, der Ernährung, der Absonderung, der Respiration und der Bewegungserscheinungen. " Vorlesungen über Physiologie" 1. Wilh Braumüller, Wien, pp 134–194
8. Donders FC (1853) Beiträge zum Mechanismus der Respiration und Circulation im gesunden und kranken Zustande. Z f Rationelle Med 3: 287–319
9. Falsetti HL, Mates RE, Grant C, Greene DG, Bunnel JL (1970) Left ventricular wall stress calculated from one-plane cineangiography. Circ Res 26: 71–83
10. Harvey W (1628) Exercitatio anatomica de motu cordis et sanguinis in animalibus. IV. Frankfurt
11. Lunkenheimer PP, Graham G, Stroh N, Welham K, Scharsich M (1976) Assessment of local force in myocardium disproving the distinctness of contractility parameters derived from left ventricular pressure. Eur Surg Res 8 (Suppl): 104–105
12. Lunkenheimer PP, Kirk Ed, Lunkenheimer A, Sonnenblick EdH (1981) Kritische Analyse zur Möglichkeit einer intramyokardialen Druckmessung. Zbl Vet Med A 28: 673–691
13. Lunkenheimer A, Lunkenheimer PP, Stroh N, Drüen B, Konermann Chr, Dittrich H (1983) Catheter tip force measurement: A new approach to the monitoring of myocardial function during cardiac surgery and during the postoperative period. Z Kardiol 72: 471–478

14. Lunkenheimer PP, Lunkenheimer A, Stroh N, Köhler F, Welham K, Graham G, Kirk Ed, Sonnenblick EdH, Kröller J (1982) Vergleich klassischer und neuer methodischer Zugänge zum intramyokardialen Kraftverteilungsmuster. Review Zbl Vet Med A 29: 557–601

15. Lunkenheimer PP, Stroh N, Scharsich M, Koubenec J, Schmuziger M, Achatz R, Dittrich H, Welham K, Graham G (1977) Continuous assessment of myocardial force during heart surgery. Curr Top Crit Care Med 3: 28–38

16. Mirsky I, Krayenbühl, HP (1981) The role of wall-stress in the assessment of ventricular function. Herz 6: 288–299

17. Rushmer RF, Crystal DK, Wagner C (1953) The functional anatomy of ventricular contraction. Circ Res 1: 162–170

18. Sandler H, Dodge, HT (1963) Left ventricular tension and stress in man. Circ Res 13: 91–104

19. Torrent-Guasp F (1980) La estructuracion macroscopica del miocardio ventricular. Rev Esp Cardiol 33: 265–287

20. Woods RN (1892) A few applications of a physical theorem to membranes in the human body in a state of tension. J Anal Physiol 26: 362–370

21. Yellin Ed L, Yoran Ch, Sonnenblick EOH, Frater RWM (1979) The relation between left ventricular relaxation and early diastolic filling in the intact dog heart. 5 th Workshop on the contractile behaviour of the heart, Antwerp (Abstr.)

Authors' address:

Prof. Dr. P. P. Lunkenheimer, Experimentelle Thorax-, Herz- und Gefäßchirurgie, Chirurgische Universitätsklinik, Jungeblodtplatz 1, D-4400 Münster (F. R. G.)

On the role of optimization in the cardiovascular system

T. Kenner

Physiologisches Institut der Universität Graz (Austria)

Summary

This essay discusses in a very simple manner several aspects of the meaning of optimization in general and, particularly, the role of optimization in relation to the work and action of the heart. Starting out with historical considerations the role of the properties of the heart as a pump, its relation to the arterial system, the problem of pulsatility and blood pressure and the role of time intervals and coronary perfusion is discussed. Mathematical methods permit the calculation of the time course of the cardiac ejection which, under certain constraints, minimizes the energy consumption of the heart. The saving of energy by this optimization compared with a nonoptimal ejection pattern is rather small – in the order of a few percent. It is therefore interesting and important to discuss the physiological meaning of small variations of the cost-effect function. It seems that unexplained phenomena like synchronization of heart beat and respiration have something to do with an optimization process. The most important conclusion is that any optimization has to be seen as a process related to the functioning of the organism as a whole.

Key words: optimization, cost function, heart, arterial system

Introduction: The meaning of the term optimization

There are two main questions: What does optimization mean? What should be optimized?

The word "optimize" implies that some function should be organized as advantageously as possible. Usually this means a compromise between several functions or variables. Mathematically this compromise can be calculated as an extremum of a certain function – the so-called optimization criteron – of the functions or variables mentioned above (6, 12).

The second question is related to the problem of which function can be used in a particular case as an optimization criterion and whether an effect-cost relation should be maximized or a cost function minimized. Depending on the kind of function it is termed a performance index on one hand, or simply a cost function on the other hand. In the following we will mainly discuss cost functions. Such an optimization criterion can include everything which is functionally related to the system under consideration. If we use the heart action as an example, the effect of optimization may primarily consist of providing a large minute volume. The cost in this case corresponds to the necessary energy consumption.

If an engineer designs an instrument, certain cost-effect constraints may be given beforehand. In the case of a biological system the possibly existing optimization criteria of nature have to be found by trail and error. Usually we have to start from conjectures, which in most cases can be reasonably explained, but often may or may not agree with the actual intentions of nature.

For these reasons there are some advantages to starting the trial for biological optimization with the assumption of very simple and basic optimization criteria. However, one always has to consider that possibly in reality more functions or variables may actually play a role than have been assumed. For example the following variables may play a role in the cost function: power, energy consumption, blood pressure, force, tension, material properties, and time.

Among other features this list shows that, if we discuss the optimization of the heart action, the latter may not be discussed as an isolated property but always has to be considered in the functional relation and connection with the system as a whole. This means that we have to consider at least the arterial and the venous part of the circulation.

A historical note on Broemser's theory of optimal matching

The first considerations of the question of optimization of the heart action are due to Ph. Broemser (1). In 1935 he used a simple model of the heart and the arterial system to examine the relation between the duration of the systole, the properties of the arterial windkessel and the cardiac output. As model of the heart Broemser used a pressure pump with a small internal impedance. Since the input impedance of the arterial windkessel is frequency dependent oscillations appear in the arterial and ventricular pressure during the ejection time. Due to the small internal impedance of the pump these pressure oscillations have a very marked influence on the cardiac ejection. Using this model Broemser found a maximum of the stroke volume if the duration of the systole is half the period of the auto-oscillation of the arterial windkessel. A minimum of the stroke volume was found if the duration of the systole equals the auto-oscillation period of the arterial windkessel. Under this condition ejection takes place during the first part of the systole. In the second half of the systole the positive oscillation of the aortic pressure impedes the ejection of further volume from the ventricle.

Broemser's assumptions about the properties of the heart were unrealistic. However they pointed to two interesting aspects: 1. The importance of the internal impedance of the heart. 2. The role of the aortic input impedance and its relation to the action of the heart.

The internal impedance of the pump

Broemser was not aware of the importance of the internal impedance of the heart. We now can say that 1) the higher the internal impedance of a pump the better it is suited as a flow pump and 2) a pump with a low internal impedance is unsuitable as a ventricular pump because it would be extremely sensitive to pressure variations of the aortic windkessel. It can be shown by a simple calculation that a pump is able to deliver a maximum of power to an external load resistance if the value of the internal impedance is equal to the value of the load resistance. This behaviour is actually realized in the cardiovascular system as can easily be shown experimentally. The internal impedance of the left ventricle can be measured by observing the decrease of stroke volume due to certain increases of the aortic pressure (4).

The minimum of the input impedance of the arterial windkessel

Whoever calculates the frequency dependence of the aortic input impedance from flow and pressure measurements will sooner or later come to the conclusion that the power which the left ventricle expends for the delivery of a given cardiac output should have a minimum at a certain frequency (14).

There is an interesting indirect argument for the importance of the relation between heart rate and the properties and geometry of the arterial system – the rules of the biological similarity, which in short express the following: the larger an organism, the lower is the working frequency of its different systems. Between the time period and length dimension of an organism a linear relationship exists. This implies that the heart rate can be matched to the characteristic frequencies of the arterial impedance in small as well as in large animals, because the heart rate is always proportional to the characteristic frequencies of the aortic impedance (4).

Pulsatility and blood pressure

As a rule of thumb for the calculation of the power expended by the ventricle we can state:

$$L = p.CO$$

where p is the mean arterial pressure and CO is the cardiac output. Therefore the expended power could be reduced by lowering the arterial pressure. Such a reduction can be made during anesthesia in recumbent patients; – it is certainly not possible during normal conditions.

The power expenditure of each ventricle consists of two parts: a mean or DC-component L_{DC} and a pulsatile component L_{PL}:

$$L = L_{DC} + L_{PL}$$

The latter part can be reduced somewhat by certain optimization manoenvres as will be shown later. Of course L_{PL} depends on stroke volume and heart rate. It is interesting to note that basically mean arterial pressure has about the same value in all warm blooded animals. Furthermore, the normal circulation is always driven with a pulsatile pump. A reduction to zero of L_{PL} by reduction of the pusatile power by application of continuous pumps is possible only under artificial conditions, e. g. by nonpulsatile working heart assist devices.

Both the reduction of arterial pressure and non-pulsatile perfusion would most probably lead to problems related to the control of the circulation. A condition of instability could appear during variations of the body position – which in human beings generates large variations of arterial and venous pressures even under normal conditions.

Blood pressure and coronary circulation

Coronary flow belongs to those functions which must be considered with respect to an optimization of the pulsatile heart action. The coronary perfusion depends 1) on the arterial pressure during diastole and 2) on the relative duration of the diastolic period in relation to the total period of one heart action. A shortening of the systole and corresponding lengthening of diastole is advantageous for coronary flow. On the other hand the stroke work increases at the same time because of the higher ventricular pressure peak generated during a short systole. The optimization consists here in the finding of a compromise with respect to the relation of diastole and systole (4).

Time course of ejection during systole

In order to discuss the principle of the following considerations we assume that the heart contracts with a certain frequency and ejects a certain stroke volume in a given ejection time S. Under such a condition one can examine the influence of the time course of the ejection flow q(t) on the energy expenditure of the ventricle. We have to assume a cost function which should be minimized by the optimization procedure. The most simple cost function equals the external stroke work of the ventricle (10):

$$J = \int_0^S p(t) \cdot q(t) dt$$

$p(t)$ is the time course of the aortic pressure.

For the calculation of the optimal time course of ejection an algorithm called the calculus of variations is applied. There are other numerical methods like dynamic programming which can be applied to problems of optimal time functions. The calculation leads to a time course of ejection flow which very much resembles the typical physiological central aortic flow contour: a triangular pattern with a steep upstroke and a somewhat slower descending slope which has a small notch in the later part of systole.

It is possible to extend the cost function and try the effect of additional terms. Hämäläinen introduced an additional term which "penalizes" fast changes of the ejection flow (3). The influence of the ventricular power expenditure can be adjusted by a constant factor a:

$$J = \int_0^S (q^2(t) + a \cdot p(t) \cdot q(t)) dt$$

Neither this type of cost function nor other variations seem to greatly improve the results. Another possible addition consists for example in the introduction of additional pressure dependent terms which penalize pressure or rate of pressure increase. – The word "penalize" in this context means that the process related to the particular term markedly increases the energy expenditure and thus should by reduced as much as possible as a result of the optimization.

On the meaning of the calculation of optimal functions

Calculations such as those reported above permit conclusions on the validity of cost functions used in the calculation. With respect to central aortic flow it seems that the expended stroke work is the most important component of the cost function.

Gain by optimization

If one calculates the energy per stroke which can be saved by an optimization procedure like that described above, the results often appear somewhat disappointing. It turns out that even under the worst nonoptimal control condition only a few percent of energy expenditure can be saved by optimization. However, it seems important from such a calculation to conclude that the organism uses even small advantages.

Regulation, stability and synchronization

In connection with the fact that the organism uses even small benefits it seems interesting in comparison with the above discussion to present cost functions which are applied to examine regulatory processes. In this case one tries to examine in which way the minimization of the variation of a state variable (e. g. blood pressure Δ_P) and certain control variables (like vasoconstrictor tonus etc., ΔU_1 ΔU_2) has effects on transients after the equilibrium of the system is disturbed. An example of such a cost function is given by the following equation (8):

$$J = \int_{t1}^{t2} ((\Delta_p)^2 + (\Delta U_1)^2 + (\Delta U_2)^2 \ldots \ldots)dt$$

One main consequence of optimal control functions of this kind is the avoidance of instabilities of the system, which means that a new equilibrium is attempted as fast as possible within time t_1 to t_2 and without much oscillation.

We have examined problems of stability in the circulation and the question of under which conditions oscillations may be generated (5). Here we just mention the components which from the action of the heart may favour instabilities: a complex interaction of frequency effects due to baroreceptor refelexes and to frequency potentiation.

In the context of these considerations of interaction of different systems it seems interesting to mention the synchronization of certain functions of these systems. Particularly it seems interesting to mention the synchronization between heart action and respiration which particularly can be observed during sleep (7). Such a synchronization seems to be connected with the use of certain natural optimization strategies. Here again the organism seems to be able to use small advantages.

Optimization through variation of the intervals

Stroke volume and pressure amplitude increase nonlinearly with increasing duration of the preceding diastolic interval. The relation between interval and stroke volume depends on the increasing filling volume of the ventricle and on interval or frequency potentiation of the myocardium. Related to unit time of the preceding intervall duration of a certain heartbeat one can calculate the average cardiac output. It can thus be found that this relation has a distinct maximum at a certain filling interval. In other words, the two phenomena generate under each condition of the organism a certain optimal stroke interval (11).

Optimization of the energy consumption of the heart

This problem is related to the following questions: 1) which variables permit a full description of the contraction process of the ventricle? and 2) which variables determine the oxygen consumption of the heart? There are several possible ways to attack the problem which finally lead to similar conclusions. Basically in all pertinent studies on the subject the myocardial oxygen or energy consumption is related to a sum of mechanical phenomena. One fundamental magnitude of such a sum is the pressure-volume area which includes the region of isometric contractions related to a certain end-systolic elastance and representing the internal work of the ventricle. Due to reflex effects on sympathetic activity and due to frequency potentiation, changes in heart rate have a rather complex influence on contractility and on each component of the energy consumption. It turns out that in each possible condition of the system (rest or exercise) the estimated oxygen consumption has a minimum at a certain frequency (2, 13).

From these considerations the conclusion can be drawn that there is an optimal contractility in terms of maximization of the cardiac efficiency and contractility and a corresponding minimum of the oxygen consumption, both related to the heart rate.

Optimality in the whole organism

Finally, the relation between the oxygen consumption of the whole organism and the oxygen consumption of the two pumps – heart and lung – should be mentioned. Since with increasing overall oxygen consumption the cost of transport by heart and respiration increases progressively more than the transport capacity, the amount of oxygen delivered to the periphery of the organism as function of the cardiac output has been found to have a distinct maximum. The calculations of Pennock and Attinger (9) estimated that the maximum of the oxygen consuption occurs at values of the cardiac output which are rather high, even for a well trained athlete.

Therefore this optimization can rather be interpreted as an upper limit of an overall power expenditure.

Acknowledgement

This study was supported by the Austrian Research Fund.

References

1. Broemser PH (1935) Über die optimalen Beziehungen zwischen Herztätigkeit und physikalischen Konstanten des Gefäßsystems. Z Biol 96: 1–10
2. D'Argenio DZ (1979) Minimum Energy Expenditure as a Basis for Myocardial Regulation. Ph D Dissertation, University of Southern California
3. Hämäläinen RP, Hämäläinen J, Miekkala U (1982) Optimal Control Modelling of Ventricular Ejection – do the Endpoint Conditions Dominate the Performance Criteria? Proceedings International Federation for Information Processing, Ghent, Belgium
4. Kenner T (1979) Physical and Mathematical Modeling in Cardiovascular Systems. In: Hwang NHC, Gross Dr, Patel DJ (eds) Quantitative Cardiovascular Studies. Clinical Research Applications and Engineering Principles. Univ Park Press, Baltimore
5. Kenner T (1971) Dynamics and Control of Flow and Pressure in the Circulation. Kybernetik 9: 215–225
6. Kenner T (1977) Zur Frage der Optimierung in der Abstimmung zwischen Herztätigkeit und Kreislauf. In: Festschrift zum 65. Geburtstag von H Reichel, Hamburg
7. Kenner T, Pessenhofer H, Schwaberger G (1976) Method for the Analysis of the Entrainment between Heart Rate and Ventilation Rate. Pflügers Arch 363: 263–265
8. Ono K, Uozumi T, Yoshimoto C, Kenner T (1982) The optimal Cardiovascular Regulation ot the Arterial Blood Pressure. In: Kenner T, Busse R, Hinghofer-Szalkay H (eds) Cardiovascular System Dynamics: Models and Measurements. Plenum, London New York
9. Pennock B, Attinger EO (1968) Optimization of the Oxygen Transport System. Biophysical J 8: 879–896
10. Pfeiffer KP, Kenner T (1982) The optimal Strategy of Cardiac Ejection. In: Kenner T, Busse R, Hinghofer-Szalkay H (eds) Cardiovascular System Dynamics: Models and Measurements. Plenum Press, London New York
11. Pfeiffer KP, Kenner T, Schaefer J (1984) Application of Statistical Methods for the Analysis of Interval related Cardiac Performance Variations during Cardiac Arrhythmia in Man. Cardiovasc Res 18: 80–98
12. Rosen R (1967) Optimality Principles in Biology. Butterworths, London
13. Suga H (1979) Minimal Oxygen consumption and optimal Contractility of the Heart: Theoretical Approach to Principle of Physiological Control of Contractility. Bull Math Biol 41: 139–150
14. Wetterer E, Kenner T (1968) Dynamik des Arterienpulses. Springer-Verlag, Berlin Heidelberg New York

Authors' address:

Prof. Dr. Thomas Kenner, Physiologisches Institut der Universität Graz, Harrachgasse 21, A-8010 Graz (Austria)

III. Cardiac energetics

Some problems of cardiac energetics

M. Siess, K. Stieler, J. Leuchtner and U. Delabar

Department of Pharmacology, Faculty of Theoretical Medicine University of Tübingen (F.R.G.)

Summary

Special problems of the aerobic metabolism in the cardiac muscle cell as an energy producing and energy consuming system are discussed and demonstrated with some experimental results using superfused resting and working guinea-pig atria as an energetic model:

1. Influence on resting O_2 uptake:
   a) Free fatty acids (FFA) increase the O_2 uptake rate to $\sim 20\%$ compared with glucose oxidation. This can be explained as a compensating effect due to the 9.7 % lower combustion value for 1 mol O_2 of C_{16}-FFA and the 10.7 % lower P/O-ratio related to glucose oxidation.
   b) K^+-depolarization increases the O_2 uptake
      b.1. between 15 and 65 mmol/l KCl from 110 to 200 % without activation of the actomyosin system. This effect is Ca^{++} dependent and is not observed in Ca^{++} free solution and can be inhibited completely by nifedipine. The enhanced O_2 uptake rate due to K^+-depolarization is not connected with an improved state of the energy quotient (ATP/ADP + AMP) indicating a lowering of the energy coupling,
      b.2. between 100 and 250 mmol/l KCl
          from 220 to $\sim 350\%$, not influenced by nifedipine and
          connected with activation of the actomyosin system at low Na^+ and/or high external Ca^{++} (contracture).
2. Stretching of resting atria up to 10 mN tension does not increase the O_2 uptake rate. The 'Feng' effect could not be confirmed.
3. a) The 'Frank-Starling' effect can be observed between 2.5 and 10 mN preload with increase of contractile work/beat connected with an enhancement of O_2 uptake rate to a lower percentage. At the maximum of the 'Frank-Starling' effect the highest efficiency of contractile work can be observed. With increasing beat rate this maximum is shifted to a lower preload.
   b) The *auxotonic contractile work* measured by a calibrated spring blade allows the calculation of the 'internal work' and the 'external contractile work'/beat in mm·mN. The total energy of the activated actomyosin system (total work) is stored by the displacement of the spring blade due to the constant of the spring blade, the preload (tension) and the afterload (force).
   The 'internal work' will be transformed into ATP dependent heat and force equal to the preload tension. The same ATP dependent energy from O_2 uptake is transformed at the same beat rate and the same preload a) with the *isometric type* of auxotonic contraction into high force and very low internal and low external work, b) with the *isotonic type* into a 6–8 fold higher 'internal work' and a considerably higher external work and lower force. The 'Fenn' effect can be explained by these findings. The efficiency of the contractile work related to the O_2 uptake depends therefore on the external conditions, which allow the sliding filament system to shorten or not. A general view of the cardiac energetics with the different sources of heat delivery during energy production and energy consumption is demonstrated.

Dedicated to Professor R. Jacob on the occasion of his 60th birthday

4. Differences in the economy of external cardiac work on the cellular level are reported:
   a) An increase of cardiac work/hour to the same degreee needs more O_2, if the contractile work is enhanced by chronotropy than by inotropy.
   b) The efficiency of cardiac work increases more by positive inotropy than by positive chronotropy and vice versa.
   c) The same cardiac work/beat of 1 mm·mN needs more picomol O_2 (resting O_2 uptake/hour subtracted) i) at a higher heart rate ii) with increasing degree of contractile work/beat.
   d) Similar observations could also be made with cumulative combinations of β-adrenergic stimulation, β-blockade and cardiac glycoside effects changing performance, O_2 uptake and efficiency in a difference degree. The efficiency of external contractile work therefore also depends on the various onsets of actions and the degree of activity of cardiotonic and cardiodepressive agents.

Key words: resting O_2 uptake: K^+ and FFA, Feng effect – O_2 uptake, Fenn effect – O_2 uptake, Frank-Starling mechanism, auxotonic contractile work, beat rate and O_2 uptake

I. Introduction

The problems of cardiac energetics can be studied from different points of view: We can determine 1) the aerobic energy production by measuring the O_2 uptake, 2) the energy consumption with the parameter of cardiac contractile work, 3) the heat delivered by 1) and 2), and 4) the cytoplasmatic phosphorylation potential. However, it has not yet been possible to calculate an exact total balance account of cardiac energetics and its regulations because we cannot measure all these parameters simultaneously under the same conditions.

We have studied the *aerobic energy production* (Fig. 1./I) measuring the O_2 uptake with a very sensitive method simultaneously with the $^{14}CO_2$ production rate of ^{14}C-labelled carbo-

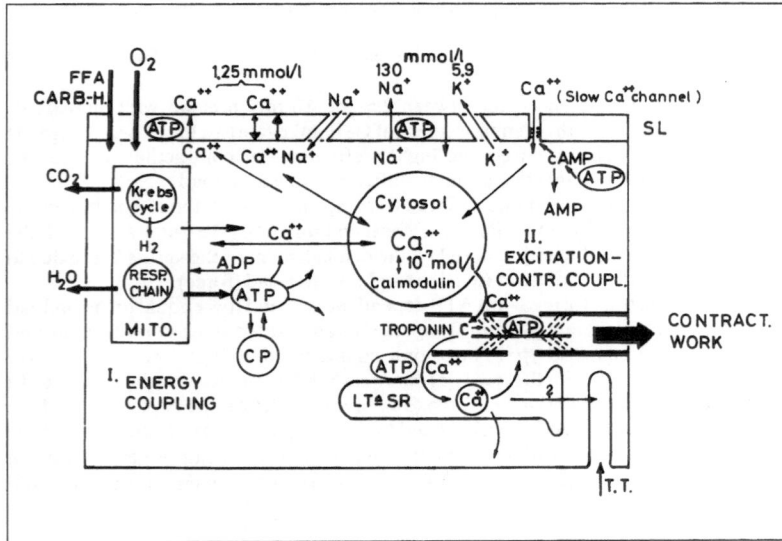

Fig. 1. Scheme of the cardiac muscle cell as an energy producing and consuming system ([22], modified).

hydrates or FFA and the *auxotonic contractile* work with a calibrated spring blade as the most important parameter of the *energy consumption* (Fig. 1./II) in isolated guinea-pig atria at rest and work. First we would like to point out some problems of cardiac energy production and energy consumption in connection with the efficiency of cardiac contractile work.

A) Energy production

The main source of aerobic energy production is the biological oxidation of carbohydrates and free fatty acids (FFA) in the respiratory chain located in the mitochondria, producing in the Krebs cycle CO_2 and in the respiratory chain H_2O and ATP together in the various energy coupling steps (1), (Fig. 1). Energy from ATP can be stored in creatine phosphate (CP) by the creatine kinase reaction and in cardiac muscle has about a doubled concentration related to ATP. The *efficiency* of this energy coupling step depends 1. on the substrate, 2. on the P/O-quotient and 3. on the caloric hydrolysis value of ATP and shows a wide range of variation (Table 1).

Table 1. Caloric value of 1 mol O_2 at combustion and biological oxidation of 1 mol glucose. The efficiency of the biological oxidation depends on the P/O-ratio and the caloric value of ATP hydrolysis, beside the free energy change of the substrate.

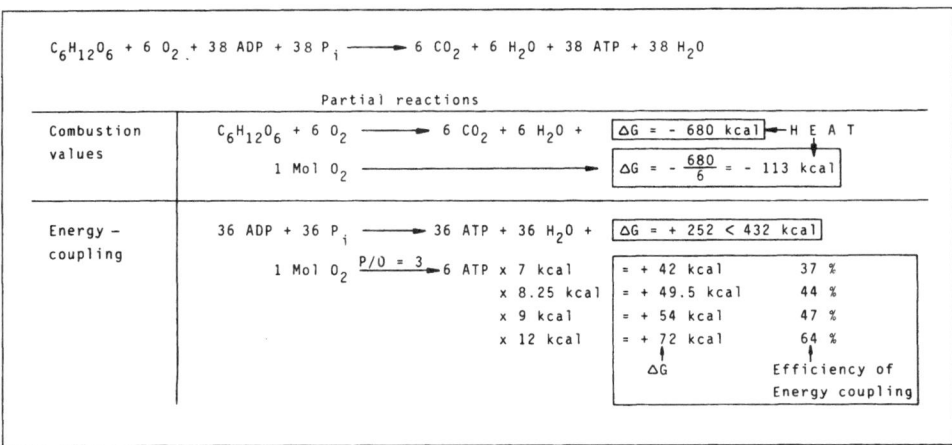

A 1) and 2) Substrate and P/O quotient:

The combustion value of 1 mol O_2 oxidizing *glucose* to CO_2 and H_2O has a ΔG free energy change of -113 kcal. During biological oxidation of glucose in the energy coupling steps 1 mol O_2 produces 6 mol ATP at a P/O quotient of 3.0 and if we add the yield of 2 ATP during the steps of aerobic glycolysis 1 mol O_2 produces a total of 6.33 mol ATP during glucose oxidation (1, 11, 12).

The combustion value of *palmitate* shows for 1 mol O_2 only a ΔG free energy change of -102 kcal (-9.7% compared with glucose). The energy coupling during biological oxidation of palmitic acid with a P/O quotient of only 5.65 for 1 mol O_2 is 10.7% less than the yield in ATP during oxidation of glucose. This lower yield of energy can be compensated however by a higher oxidation rate of FFA connected with an increase of O_2 uptake (12, 18, 19, 20, 21, 22).

A 3) Caloric value of ATP hydrolysis:

The efficiency of energy production however is not only dependent on the P/O ratio but also on the changing caloric hydrolysis value of 1 mol ATP split to ADP + P_i in a wide range from 7.0 to 12 and 14 kcal ($\times$ 4.18 $\triangleq$ KJ). Lehninger (1965) calculated this value to 9.0 kcal (12). At standard conditions of 25°C and pH 7.0 this value is assumed today in textbooks to amount 8.25 kcal (11).

Recently the 'affinity value' (A) for ATP hydrolysis has been calculated by various equations (editorial 6) measuring intracellular concentrations of ATP, ADP, AMP, P_i, CP (creatine phosphate), C (creatine) and the creatine kinase activity (CK) using a ΔG for 1 mol ATP hydrolysis of 7.30 kcal observed at 37°C and 1 mmol/l Mg^{++}. The *calculated* 'affinity values' (A) of 1 mol ATP hydrolysis may change in vivo between 9 and 14 kcal dependent on the "cytosolic phosphorylation potential' at normoxic and anoxic conditions (5, 6, 8, 10). The ΔG free energy change for 1 mol creatine phosphate (CP) amounts to 10.3 kcal at standard conditions (11). There are observations that the free energy change of the caloric hydrolysis value of ATP can also be different in various cell compartments dependent on the intracellular pH, temperature, electrolytes and pO_2. The ATP molecule usually exists in several charged forms that complex with cations dependent on the pH (6). This could be responsible for an early hypoxic failure of the heart at a time when considerable reserves of ATP and CP are available. Also it would explain that at special experimental conditions the heart can contract quite well with low reserves of creatine phosphate when ATP is present. Therefore the caloric ATP hydrolysis value shows a wide range of efficiency between 37 and 75% and we can assume that the normal values in vivo in cardiac muscle at aerobic conditions would range between 45 and 60%. However, we have to consider that all these calculations are very rough and give only approximative values. Therefore, the heat lost during energy production will also change in a corresponding range in the mean values between 55 to 40%. Because this heat is produced during energy production we would call this metabolic heat (H I.)

To summarize:

The efficiency of the energy produced by 1 mol O_2 during biological oxidation and transferred into high energy phosphates (ATP, CP) depends on 1) the combustion value of the substrate, 2) the P/O quotient, 3) the caloric value of ATP hydrolysis.

This efficiency ranges between $\sim$ 34 and 75%, at physiological in vivo conditions between $\sim$ 45 and 60%. The rest is lost as 'metabolic' heat (H I.).

B) Cardiac energy consumption

In Fig. 1 are demonstrated some important *ATP consuming* biochemical reactions in the various electrolyte fluxes through the membranes and as most important energy requiring factor the excitation contraction coupling system (II).

1. Resting state:
   The maintenance of the *resting metabolism* requires a relatively constant amount of O_2 uptake for steady state conditions of the resting potential and other basic metabolic ATP dependent biochemical reactions for synthesis and degradation.
2. Contraction:
   The transfer from the resting state of the cardiac muscle cell into the *activated state* starts with the action potential resulting in the contraction of the sliding filaments of the actomyosin system. This is induced by increase of the intracellular free calcium from 10^{-7} to $\sim 10^{-5}$ mmol/l. But Ca^{++} activates not only the actomyosin system, but also the mitochondrial function as one regulator of the O_2 uptake (13, 19, 22, 23). According to the increased energy need more ATP is produced in the energy coupling step corresponding together with more 'metabolic heat'. During activation of the actomyosin system by

splitting ATP in the crossbridge reactions to ADP, energy will be transferred into contractile work and also in this way additional 'ATP dependent heat' will be liberated during the other ATP consuming steps at excitation contraction coupling and relaxation. The amount will be depend on the *external* conditions of contractions: The preload, the afterload and the isotonic, auxotonic or isometric type of contraction. These external conditions will relieve or inhibit the shortening of the sliding filament system during activation.

By the measurement of the *auxotonic* contractile work/beat with a calibrated spring blade we can calculate the 'external' work together with the 'internal' and 'total' work/ beat in mm · mN and by multiplication with the beat rate the *'total work'*/hour as most important *parameters of cardiac energy consumption*. Because the amount of the 'internal' work (mm · mN) is transferred during contraction only into additional heat and force (equal to the preload tension) we can calculate changes of the *ratio of external contractile work* and the ATP dependent heat of the *internal work* important for the efficiency of energy consumption during excitation contraction coupling.

3. Efficiency of contractile work:

As mentioned above we can determine in this way changes of the efficiency of the 'external contractile work' in relation to the measured O_2 consumption. For the total determination of the balance of the produced and the consumed energy it would be necessary to measure the delivered heat during both phases. This however is technically impossible in our studies.

However, we can assume that around 50% of heat is developed during energy production as metabolic heat (H I). The ATP dependent ana- and catabolic biochemical reactions (ACBR) will compete with the high energy phosphates used for the contraction cycle: an unknown smaller amount of heat (H II a) will be lost by ATP hydrolysis at ACBR and a considerably higher amount (H II b) during ATP hydrolysis at the contraction cycle dependent on the developed force (afterload). H II b will be different in degree between *isometric* and *isotonic* contraction. At *auxotonic* contraction the *internal work* can be measured as mechanical energy loaded in the spring blade. This energy will be transferred in force ($\triangleq$ preload) and heat (H III). The 'external' auxotonic contractile work can also be measured. Therefore the efficiency of the external and the total contractile work can be related to the O_2 consumption and the efficiency can be calculated. By this method we can also observe the change of the ratio between internal and external work (see results section 3 b_1 and b_2).

4. Relaxation:

The cytosolic free Ca^{++} has to be restored for relaxation to inactivate the actomyosin system (see Fig. 1) 1) by the ATP dependent Ca^{++} uptake in the sarcoplasmatic reticulum (SR), 2) by the Ca^{++} efflux through the sarcolemma (SL): here the Na^+/K^+ and the Ca^{++} ATPase as well as the electrogenic H^+/Na^+ and Ca^{++}/Na^+ exchange are important, 3) by Ca^{++} uptake in mitochondria regulated by the proton potential of the respiratory chain (13).

C) Regulation of energy production by energy consumption

1. The mitochondrial function measured as O_2 uptake is controlled in the cell 1) by the ATP/ADP quotient (1) and as measure of the total cellular energy supply the mentioned 'cytosolic phosphorylation potential' (6), 2) the availability of reducing substrates which determine the $NAD^+/NADH$ quotient, (6, 7), 3) the cellular O_2 concentration depending on O_2 pressure, 4) the rate of oxidation of cytochrome c by the activity of the cytochrome

oxidase (6), 5) the pH, 6) the temperature, 7) Ca^{++} fluxes through the membranes (13, 19, 22), and 8) K^+ depolarization (13, 19, 22, 23).

2. Determinants of O_2 uptake:

We would like to present in this volume on 'controversial issues in cardiac pathophysiology' some results from our studies concerning the points mentioned in the following disposition of the determinants of O_2 uptake and the efficiency of contractile work:

Determinants of cardiac O_2 uptake and the efficiency of contractile cardiac work.
1. Resting O_2 consumption $\rightarrow$ (a) FFA oxidation, b) K^+ depolarization
2. Resting tension $\rightarrow$ 'Feng' effect
3. Auxotonic contractile $\rightarrow$ (a) 'Frank Starling' effect
     work/beat
        ↙ ↘
     Isometric   Isotonic $\rightarrow$ (b) 'Fenn' effect
     type   type

4. Beat rate (frequency)

The methods in detail (20, 22) and most of the results mentioned here in this disposition are published elsewhere (2, 17–23) and therefore will only be touched on briefly. However, we would like to point out in this chapter some special findings of interest, because they could perhaps give explanations of controversial results in problems on cardiac energetics especially in the factors influencing the efficiency of cardiac contractile work, the question of internal and external work and the connection to the delivery of heat.

II. Results and Discussion

II. 1. Resting O_2 consumption:

If the environmental conditions (temperature, pH, K^+ concentration and substrates of biological oxidation) are not altered the resting O_2 consumption remains constantly during 4 hours and more with a weak tendency to decline during 6 to 10 hours.

1. a) Influence of free fatty acids (FFA)

Short and long chain FFA are preferentially oxidized and inhibit external glucose oxidation as well as oxidation of endogenous glycogen (18–22). Addition of C_6, C_8, C_{10} FFA in a range of 0.5 to 0.1 mmol/l increases the resting O_2 consumption very quickly to around 20%, whereas the inhibition of the oxidation rate of carbohydrates and the substitution by oxidation of FFA is a process lasting some hours until a new steady state is reached. Therefore direct effects on FFA on the cardiac mitochondrial activity have also been assumed (19, 22). It could be observed that even in beating atria FFA suddenly increase the O_2 consumption in low concentrations without changing the contractile work/beat thus diminishing the efficiency of cardiac work. The 11% lower combustion value of 1 mol O_2 for palmitate compared with glucose together with a 10% lower P/O quotient would explain the observed $\sim 20\%$ increase of O_2 uptakes as a compensative effect to obtain the same amount of energy gained with glucose by a correspondent higher rate of O_2 uptake.

1. b) K^+-depolarization (Table 2)

Increase of external *Ca++ concentrations* from 0 to 7.5 mmol/l in *resting* atria does not influence the *resting O_2 consumption*. During rest the sarcolemma seems to be a barrier for external Ca^{++}.

However, increase of *external K^+* enhances the resting O_2 consumption starting with 10 mmol/l K^+ very sensitively in a non linear function to a high degree from 10% to 250% (19, 22, 23).

Table 2. Calculated resting potential (RP), increase of resting O$_2$ uptake and diastolic tension (DT = 5 mN preload) during K$^+$ depolarization with increasing KCl concentrations added to K. H.-solution (5.9 mmol/l K$^+$; see text) (19).

K$^+$	5,9	+	10	20	30	60	100	150	200	MMOL/L
RP	-83		-57	-45	-36	-20	-7	+3	+10	MV
O$_2$	100 %		108	130	180	200	220	250	350	%
DT	5		5	5	5	5	5*<	5*<	5*<	MN

RP = CALCULATED RESTING POTENTIAL MV

O$_2$ = RESTING O$_2$ CONSUMPTION IN K.H.SOLUTION + 15 MMOL/L GLUCOSE, 30°C 100 %

DT = DIASTOLIC TENSION 500 MP (= 5 MN)

DT*= INCREASED DIASTOLIC TENSION (CONTRACTURE) OBSERVED WITH HIGH EXTERNAL
      CA^{++} (7.5 MMOL/L) OR LOW NA$^+$ (25 MMOL/L)

From Table 2 it can be observed that with a concentration of 60 mmol/l KCl which lowers the calculated resting potential from − 83 mV to − 36 mV, the resting O$_2$ uptake is doubled without any activation of the actomyosin system, the diastolic tension of 5 mN remaining constant. This effect is Ca^{++} dependent: 1) inhibition by K$^+$ depolarization in Ca^{++} free medium and increase by adding of higher external Ca^{++} concentrations or epinephrine 10^{-6} mol/l during depolarization. 2) Blockade of the slow Ca^{++} channels by nifidepine (10^{-6} mol/l) before or directly after K$^+$ depolarization (10–60 mmol/l KCl) completely inhibits the K$^+$ induced increase of O$_2$ uptake. 3) Epinephrine (10^{-6} mol/l) or high external Ca^{++} does not influence the resting O$_2$ consumption without depolarization.

Higher concentrations of KCl above 100 mmol/l up to 250 mmol/l increase the resting O$_2$ uptake around 3.5 fold now raising the diastolic tension by low external Na$^+$ and/or high Ca^{++}. Here blockade of the slow Ca^{++} channels with nifedipine no longer has any inhibiting effect. With these concentrations the mitochondrial activity decreases as sign of detrimental effects and the developed contracture is irreversible. The increased O$_2$ uptake between 15.9 and 65.9 mmol/l KCl is not correlated with a higher energy state quotient (ATP/ADP + AMP) and also inhibits NAD- and adenine nucleotide-synthesis from precursors (2). The increased resting O$_2$ uptake due to K$^+$ depolarization is therefore not connected with a correlating yield of high energy phosphates. Even in anoxia, low concentrations of KCl decrease the anoxic lowered energy state quotient to detrimental values. Concentrations above 15 mmol/l external KCl in cardioplegic solutions can therefore not be recommended.

II. 2. Resting tension and O$_2$ consumption ('Stretch' or 'Feng' effect):
'When a resting isolated muscle is stretched its metabolic rate increases'. The effect (known as the 'stretch' or 'Feng' effect [3], 1932) has also been observed in cardiac muscle preparations (review in [14]). Several authors (14) have attributed the 'Feng' effect in papillary muscles to the existence of an anoxic inside zone, the extent of which would be diminished by the stretch of the muscle because it cannot be seen in preparations thinner than the critical wall thickness for penetration of O$_2$. We have investigated this problem in resting left atria of guinea-pigs, increasing the diastolic tension from 0 to 15 mN. In former investigations (17) by measuring the aerobic glycogen containing zone stained with the PAS reaction in isolated atria of guinea-pigs in histological slices, we could observe that this aerobic zone shows an exactly marked red stained band of 250–300 μm, each from outside and inside, whereas unstained anerobic inside zones change according to the wall thickness between 0 and 150

μm. This can be demonstrated only in atria with 300 mg of guinea-pigs, weighing 300 to 500 g. In isolated left atria (25–75 mg) of guinea-pigs with a weight between 150 and 200 g the critical wall thickness for O_2 can be neglected. We have never seen changes in O_2 consumption with our very sensitive method. There is no increase of resting O_2 consumption during stretch. Stretching the parallel and serial elastic elements in isolated resting atria is therefore not connected with any activation of the sliding filament system leading to a higher energy need connected with an augmented ATP turnover and an increased O_2 consumption. The question of whether there are differences between papillary and atrial muscle is open. Because other authors (14) have seen obviously with thin papillary muscle preparations no stretch effect on the O_2 consumption either, we assume that the 'Feng' effect was a misinterpretation.

II. 3. Auxotonic contractile work/beat and O_2 consumption:

3. a) 'Frank-Starling' mechanism

Whereas increased diastolic tension has no effect on the resting O_2 consumption, an increased tension in beating atria enhances the contractile work/beat in accordance with the Frank-Starling mechanism together with the O_2 consumption. We have studied this in several groups of experiments all showing the same results (18, 19, 21, 22). In one spontaneously beating atrium (120 bpm) (Fig. 2) with increasing preload from 1.5 to 10.0 mN the work/beat

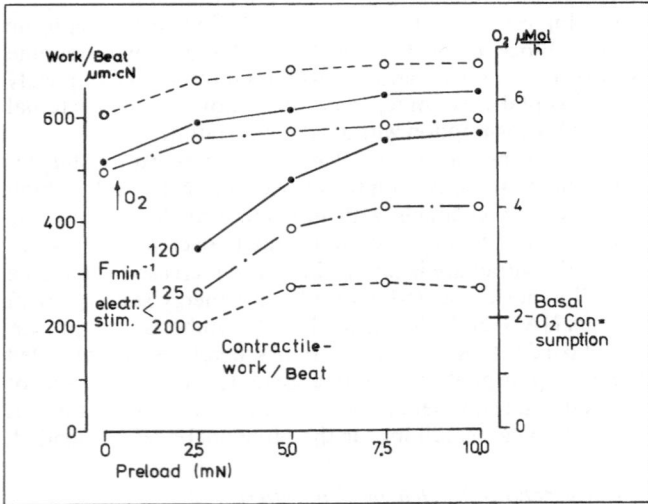

Fig. 2. 'Frank-Starling' effect and O_2 consumption at 120 (•——•) 125, (O–·–O) 200 O----O) bpm and increasing preload (0 <2.5 <10 mN). Spontaneously beating guinea-pig atrium 30°C (19). Upper panel: O_2 uptake, lower panel: work/beat (19).

increases with a maximum in the range between 7.5 and 10.0 mN. The O_2 consumption (upper part of the figure) increases to a lower degree than the work. Electric stimulation with 125 beats/min in the same atrium demonstrates the same effect.

The contractile work/beat is lowered, however with increase of the pacing to 200 beat/min and the maximum of the 'Frank-Starling' is here shifted to 5 mN. Also, according to the higher beat rate the O_2 consumption is enhanced and reaches the maximum at an earlier stage of 5 mN preload. We can summarize these results:

a) The maximum of 'Frank-Starling' is connected with the highest efficiency of cardiac work/beat.

b) The maximum of 'Frank-Starling' is shifted with increasing beat rate from 120 to 200 beats/min to a lower preload.

c) The same cardiac work/beat of 1 mm·mN measured at the maximum efficiency of 'Frank-Starling' needs around +40% more picomol O_2 with a beat rate of 200 bpm than was measured with 120 bpm (resting O_2 consumption subtracted). Therefore the 'Frank-Starling' effect as a higher beat rate has a lower efficiency.

3. b) Comparison of energy production, energy consumption and efficiency between the 'isometric' and the 'isotonic' type of *auxotonic contractile work/beat* and its possible connection with the 'Fenn'-effect

3. b) 1. The auxotonic contraction measured by displacement of a calibrated spring blade

At rest the diastolic tension is caused by stretching the parallel and serial elastic components in the cardiac muscle by the preload. In Fig. 3 the calibrated spring blade (10 mN/

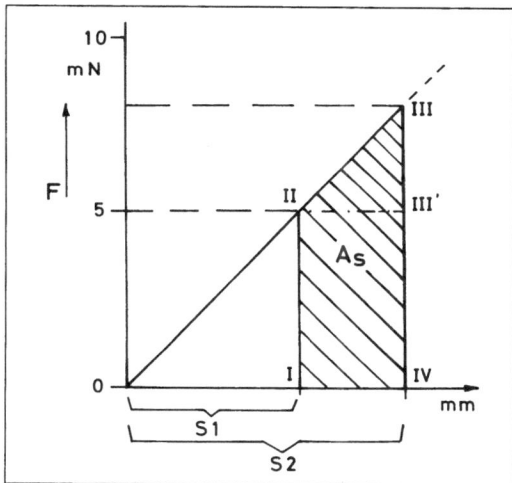

Fig. 3. Calculation of 'internal work' (0 – I – II) and 'external contractile work' (I – II – III – IV) loaded as mechanical energy in the spring blade during atrial auxotonic contraction at 5 mN preload ([22], modified).

1 mm) is moved by stretching the left atrium with 5 mN preload in position II and displacement of the spring blade (S 1) in position I. At electric stimulation (0.1 ms, 0.3–2.0 mA, 15% above threshold) the sliding filaments in the actomyosin system are activated and force will be developed in direction I–II in Fig. 2 counteracting the 'tension' of the elastic elements. Contraction starts, when the energy stored in the spring blade by the preload and shown in the white triangle (0 – I – II) in Fig. 3 is overcome by the activation of the actomyosin system and the developed force of the cross-bridge reactions in the actomyosin system exceeds the force of 5 mN. This required energy measured in mm·mN·10^{-2} can be considered as 'internal' work (2) and will be delivered for the most part as heat of the 'internal' work (H III) and 5 mN force due to the splitting of ATP to ADP. When the 'internal' force exceeds the tension of the preload (II = 5 mN) the sliding filaments will move and the spring blade is auxotonically displaced from position II to position III. This hatched area I – II – III – IV corresponds in mm·mN·10^{-2} to the *'external'* contractile work. Visible on the chart is only the 'contractile amplitude' with the energy of the triangle II – III – III'.

The white triangle and hatched area together (0 – IV – III), represent the 'total energy' stored in the displaced spring blade during activation and contraction and transferred 1) into heat of the 'internal work' and 5 mN force and 2) to external contractile work.

After inactivation the stored energy of the spring blade is unloaded and the blade moves to position I/II corresponding to the *tension* of the elastic elements and the lengthening due to the preload.

In Fig. 4 is demonstrated that according to the formula for the calculation of the auxotonic work/beat a Ca^{++} induced positive inotropic effect measured as force (F) in mN does not

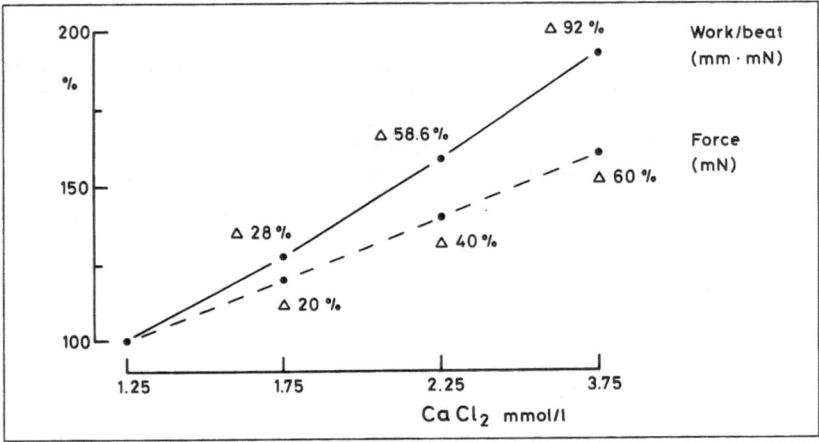

Fig. 4. Calculated external contractile work/beat (mm·mN) and developed force (mN) at atrial auxotonic contraction increased by positive inotropic action due to $CaCl_2$, presented in percent.

parallel the percentage of the increased auxotonic external contractile work/beat, calculated in mm·mN. The higher the increase in force the higher is the difference between the increasing contraction work/beat (mm·mN) and the force (mN) dependent also on the constant of the spring blade, the afterload and the preload.

3. b) 2. The energy balance of isometric and isotonic types of auxotonic contraction

If we stretch with the same preload of 5 mN the resting atrium from L_0 to L_{5mN} to the same length with spring blades of different constants it can be shown in Fig. 5 that the displace-

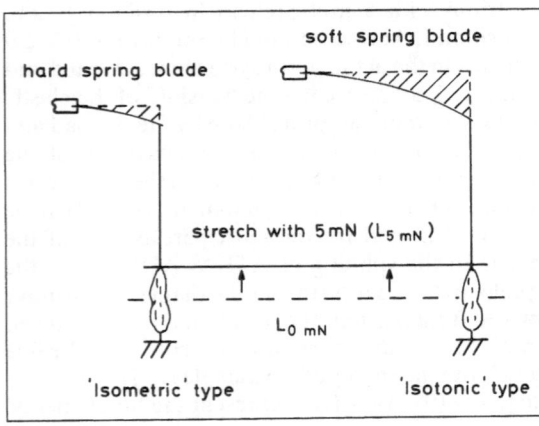

Fig. 5. Scheme demonstrating the difference of loaded energy between a 'hard' and a 'soft' spring blade stretched with the same preload of 5 mN. The mechanical energy loaded in the hard spring blade is considerably lower than in the soft blade (hatched areas). This energy has to be overcome as 'internal work' during activation before contraction occurs.

ment of the 'hard' spring blade is less than that of the 'soft' one. The hatched area in this figure shows that the energy loaded in the spring blade by stretch of the 'isometric' type is considerably lower than that of the more 'isotonic' type. We have tested with the same spontaneously beating atrium (Fig. 6) the change of the auxotonic contractile work/beat and

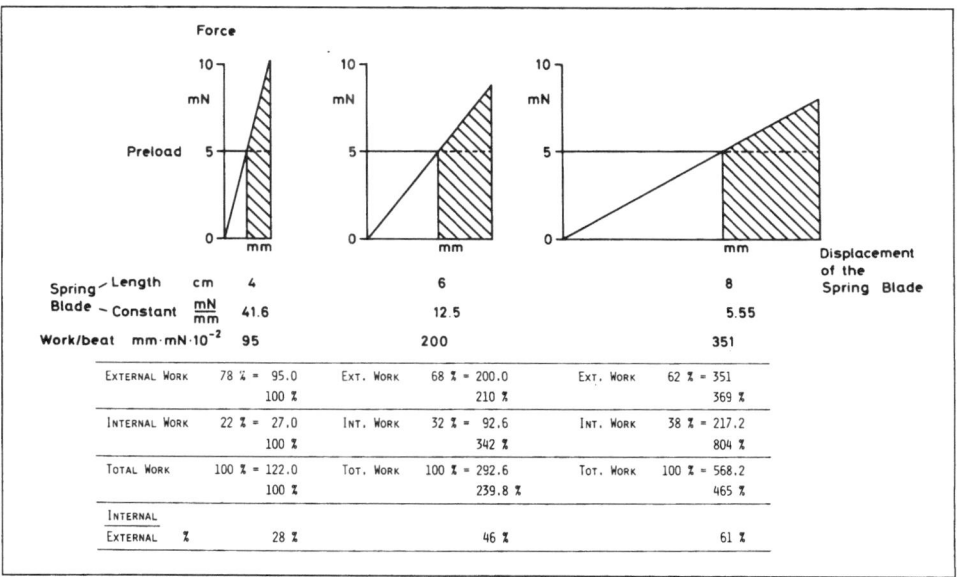

Fig. 6. Graph and calculation of external, internal and total work/beat of the same atrium during auxotonic contraction moving spring blades with different constants (41.6 > 5.55 mN/mm).
With the hard 'isometric' type a high force (mN) and a low 'internal work' can be observed compared with the soft 'isotonic' type of spring blade. The ratio of the 'internal' to the 'external' contractile work/beat increases with the softness of the spring blade.

per hour by switching with the same preload of 5 mN the hardness of the same spring blade in three steps from the more 'isometric' hard type to the more 'isotonic' soft one. It can be clearly demonstrated that the white triangle, which presents the energy of the 'internal work' increases with 5 mN preload around 8 fold from 27 to 217 mm $\cdot$ mN $\cdot 10^{-2}$. Auxotonic contractions measured with the hard spring blade (isometric type) develop a considerably higher force as afterload and a lower 'external' contractile work compared with the values of the soft one (isotonic type). The external work increases 3.69 fold from 95 to 351 mm $\cdot$ mN $\cdot 10^{-2}$. Therefore the quotient of internal/external work is shifted from 28 % at the hard (isometric) type to 61 % at the soft (isotonic) type (Fig. 6).

Figure 7 demonstrates that in this experiment, in spite of the increasing external work and the total work at the *same spontaneous beat rate no change in O$_2$ uptake occurs*. Therefore the efficiency of the external contractile work increases considerably from the 'isometric' type of auxotonic contraction to the more 'isotonic' type and we can assume that the efficiency would be even higher at a solely isotonic contractile work and an afterload of 5 mN. This means that cardiac work against a high afterload, for example a high blood pressure, will be connected with a considerably lower efficiency of contractile work if we compare the whole

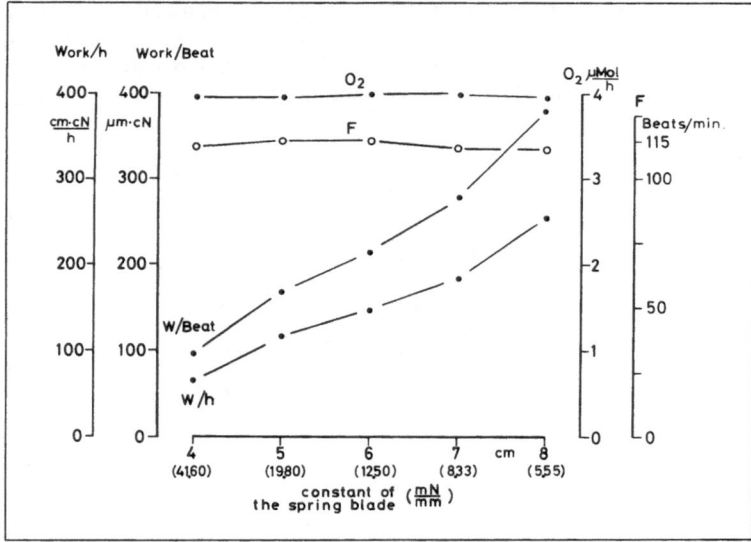

Fig. 7. Values of atrial performance (external contractile work per beat and per hour and spontaneous beat rate) compared with O_2 consumption demonstrated in the experiment of Fig. 6.

The O_2 consumption remains unchanged, whereas the external contractile work increases at auxotonic contraction moving the soft spring blade (19) resulting in a considerably improved efficiency of external contractile work.

heart with our model. This experiment demonstrates that at the *same preload* with the same lengthening of the sarcomeres and the *same beat rate the O_2 uptake remains constant. The efficiency of external cardiac work therefore depends only on the external conditions which allow the sliding filaments to contract or not.*

In Table 3 we give a general view of this experiment on the energetics considering energy production, energy consumption and the efficiency of energy coupling as well as the efficiency of contractile work. The data of Table 1 and Figs. 6 and 7 are rounded to give a better understanding of the important points. We assume here that the caloric hydrolysis value of ATP remains unchanged.

At rest the O_2 uptake is assumed to be 100%. From the energy of this O_2 uptake about 50% will be transferred in ATP in the energy coupling step for the ATP requiring ana- and catabolic biochemical reactions at rest and 50% is lost as 'metabolic' heat. *At work* the O_2 uptake increases from 100% to 400% with a 4 fold increase of the ATP production rate (200%). In the following estimation we have not subtracted the resting O_2 consumption (50%) because according to our observations at a higher frequency the resting O_2 consumption increases and after standstill needs about 30 min to decrease to the initial value as a sign of an O_2 debt.

Only the energy stored in high energy phosphates can be used for the auxotonic contractile work and the other ATP dependent anabolic or catabolic biochemical reactions. The isometric and the isotonic type of auxotonic contractile work/beat have the same energy supply of 200% in ATP stored energy. Both differ however around 4 fold in external and total work.

We can assume that in the *isometric type* therefore around 40% of 200% produced ATP will be transferred in internal and external contractile work. The remaining 160% will be

Table 3. Energy balance and distribution of the produced energy in *work* (activation of actomyosin system) and *heat*, calculated from data of Figs. 6 and 7 and Table 1). Observe the 6-fold higher 'internal work' at isotonic type of contraction compared with the isometric type, delivered as heat and 5 mN force (= preload): 'Fenn' effect? (see text).

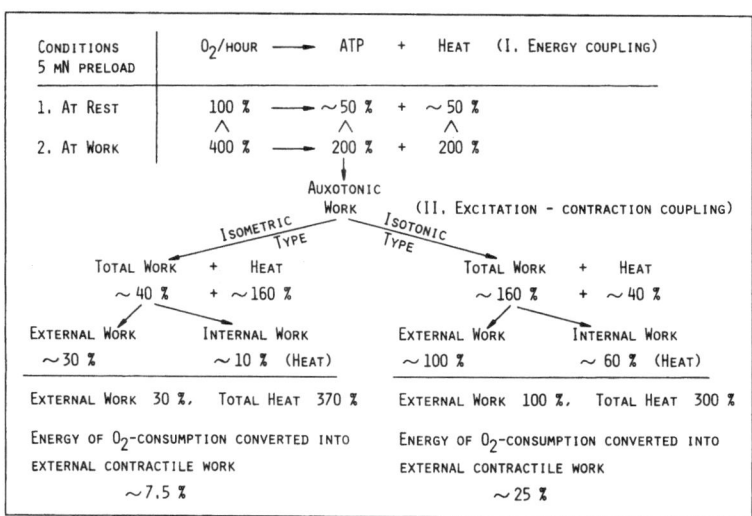

transferred mostly in heat by the resistance of the hard spring blade against contraction of the activated sliding filament system, leading to an increased force as afterload which will deliver additional ATP dependent heat (H II b). An unknown amount of energy will however be used for ana- or catabolic ATP dependent biochemical reactions with an unknown amount of heat (H II a). From the 'total work' 30 % of the energy is transferred into 'external' work and only 10 % of the energy used for the 'internal' work and transferred into heat H III + 5 mN force. As total balance of the isometric type of contraction it is shown that from 400 % energy of the O₂ consumption only 30 % is transferred into external auxotonic work with an 'efficiency' of 7.5 % and 40 % into the total work with an efficiency of 10 %. Around 370 % of the supplied energy may be transferred into heat with the exception of a small part used for ATP dependent ana- and catabolic biochemical reactions. This may even be lowered by competition with the high energy need during the activated state compared with the normal resting state conditions of ~ 50 % and result in the mentioned O₂ debt at rest after a high beat rate.

At the *isotonic type* of contraction with the same amount of 200 % energy stored in high energy phosphates, 160 % is used for the total work and only 40 % lost as heat (H II b) or used for ATP dependent reactions. The energy used for the *external contractile work* however amounts here to 100 % and 60 % is transferred into heat and 5 mN force for the internal work (H III). In comparison to the isometric type here the internal work at the isotonic type of contraction *delivers around 6 fold more heat* than the isometric type with the same preload conditions. From the energy production of 400 % O₂ consumption is 100 % transferred into external contractile work with a calculated 'efficiency' of 25 % and 160 % into the 'total work' with 40 % 'efficiency' ~ 300 % delivered as heat with the exception of the small amount of ATP dependent ACB reactions.

These values of the 'efficiency' are here not related to the real efficiency calculated from the measured work in cm · cN/hour and the energy gain by O₂ uptake in μmol/h. They represent only the calculated distribution values of the produced energy in percent converted in external and total work which also includes the ATP dependent heat of the internal work. In this calculation we do not include the loss of mechanical energy by friction and by hydrostatic pressure of the system as well as the variable directions of myofibrils in the preparation changing the vector 'force'. The real efficiency is therefore lower.

3. b) 3. These calculations however, clearly show that we have to expect more *total heat* production during the isometric type of contraction observation of heat production during tetanus and isometric exercise.

As we can see in Table 3, the total calculated heat has several sources mentioned above in the introduction:

3. 1. 200% heat from 400% energy of the O_2 is lost during the energy coupling in the phase of energy production ('metabolic' heat) during biological oxidation of substrates (H I).

3. 2. Heat will be delivered to around 50% at resting state conditions by ACBR (H II a). Heat is also developed during the excitation contraction coupling in the most energy consuming step of contraction correlated to the developed force as afterload (H II b). Here in the isometric type with 160% the H II b value is higher than in the isotonic type (40%) and corresponds with the different force (afterload). During activation of the ATP consuming crossbridge reactions the contraction of the sliding filament system is aggravated by the hardness of the spring blade. Therefore more heat H II b and more force will be developed compared with the isotonic type, where more ATP is transferred into external contractile work and less in heat H II b.

3. 3. Heat of the 'internal work' and the 'Fenn' effect (H III)

There seems to be a discrepancy here to the *'Fenn' effect,* where it has been shown by measuring the heat production that the delivered heat is higher at 'shortening' during isotonic contraction than at isometric contraction. However, if we consider that the 'internal work' is 6 fold higher in the isotonic type of auxotonic contraction than in the isometric type, and the internal work is transferred only into force and heat, this would explain with our calculation the observed 'Fenn' effect (4, 7, 15, 16). The measurements of heat in muscle preparations are completely different from our measurements of O_2 consumption comparing this value with the auxotonic work of contraction differentiated in external and internal work. Therefore it seems difficult to compare the different sources of delivered heat of our theoretical estimation with the classification terms 'shortening heat', 'activation heat' and 'tension determined heat' introduced by heat measurement.

The origin finding of 'Fenn' (4) at the frog sartorius with a thermopile was that less heat is liberated in the isometric contraction than in any of those where shortening is allowed. He found that in afterloaded tetanic contraction of brief duration more energy was liberated in isotonic than in isometric contraction. Mommaerts (15) tried to propose a new definition of this effect: 'A muscle doing work mobilizes, over and above that needed for activation and the maintenance of tension energy accounting for the work and for the dissipation of energy accompanying the work process'. Both definitions are also in agreement with our findings.

All methods used so far do not include a total and exact balance of energy production and energy consumption. Also it is very difficult to make conclusions of the efficiency of cardiac work by measuring heat and contractile work, because as we have seen, the sources of heat are different.

Only the measurement of O_2 consumption together with the delivered heat and the contractile work would allow to calculate the total balance. From the technical point of view this is not impossible but very difficult and connected with many sources of experimental errors.

3. b) 4. *To summarize:*

4. 1. The advantage of the registration of cardiac contractile work at auxotonic type of

contraction is the exact measurement of 'internal' and 'external' work in $mm \cdot mN$ dependent on preload and afterload. Since the internal work is measured in mechanical loaded energy the developed heat of internal work can be calculated by the mechanical heat equivalent (1 kcal $= 427$ mkg). Together with the external contractile work the total energy connected with the ATP dependent reactions of the actomyosin system can be measured in the loaded energy of the spring blade.

4. 2. From Table 3 we can assume that the same amount ATP is consumed in the crossbridge reaction at the same preload lengthening the sarcomeres to the same degree.

At the *isotonic type* of auxotonic contraction the same amount of ATP will be consumed as observed at the *isometric* contraction. The distribution of energy however is different: Here, less energy will be transferred into force and heat H II b, but a considerably higher part into the heat of the internal work H III (Fenn effect) and into external mechanical work by shortening of the sliding filament system due to the low afterload. The efficiency of the external contractile work related to the O_2 uptake therefore increases.

II. 4. Beat rate and cardiac O_2 uptake:

It is well known from whole heart preparations as well as from isolated cardiac muscle preparations that the O_2 consumption increases with the beat rate according to the multiplication effect of the contraction cycles. The controls of mitochondrial activity and the O_2 uptake have been mentioned before. There are differences in the economy of cardiac work on the cellular level (18–22):

a) An increase of cardiac work/hour to the same degree needs more O_2 if the contractile work is enhanced by chronotropy than by inotropy.

b) The efficiency of cardiac work increases more by positive inotropy than by positive chronotropy and 'vice versa', because changes in O_2 consumption are more expressed by the same change in percent by chronotropy than by inotropy.

c) The same cardiac work/beat of $1 \; mm \cdot mN$ needs more picomol O_2 (resting O_2 uptake/ hour subtracted)

 i) at a higher heart rate

 ii) at a higher degree of contractile work/beat as was observed with adrenergic stimulation at a constant beat rate.

These observations could also be made with cumulative combinations of β-adrenergic stimulation, β-blockade and cardiac glycoside effects changing the performance and O_2 uptake. The efficiency of external contractile work obviously depends on the various onsets of actions of cardiotonic and cardiodepressive agents (19, 22) as was shown recently by differences in heat production in a similar way (9).

Acknowledgements

These investigations have been partly supported by the DFG (Si 103) and the Dr. Karl Kuhn Foundation.

We appreciate gratefully the skilful technical assistance of Mrs A. Weible performing experiments and completing tables, figures and photographs and the excellent help of Mrs. G. Koschmieder for typing and revising the manuscript.

References

1. Chance B, Williams GR (1956) Respiratory enzymes in oxidation phosphorylation. J Biol Chem 217: 409–427
2. Delabar U, Stieler K, Reich I, Zeitler K, Weible A, Siess M (1984) Uncoupling effects in the respiratory chain due to K+ depolarization in resting left atria of guinea-pigs and anoxic myocardial salvage. In: IUPHAR 9th International Congress of Pharmacology, London. Abstracts, 1764 P

3. Feng TP (1932) The effect of length on the resting metabolism of muscle. J Physiol (Lond) 74: 441–454

4. Fenn WO (1923) A quantitative comparison between the energy liberated and the work performed by the isolated sartorius muscle of the frog. J Physiol (Lond) 58: 175–203

5. Fiolet, JWT, Baartscheer A, Schumacher CA, Coronel R, Ter Welle HF (1984) The change of free energy of ATP hydrolysis during global ischemia and anoxia in the rat heart. J Mol Cell Cardiol 16: 1023–1036

6. Gibbs CL (1985) The cytoplasmatic phosphorylation potential. Its possible role in the control of myocardial respiration and cardiac contractility. J Mol Cell Cardiol 17: 727–731

7. Gibbs CL, Chapman JB (1979) Cardiac energetics. In: Handbook of Physiology: The cardiovascular system I. Am Physiol Soc, Washington DC, pp 775–804

8. Giesen J, Kammermeier H (1980) Relationship of phosphorylation potential and oxygen consumption in isolated perfused rat hearts. J Mol Cell Cardiol 12: 891–907

9. Holubarsch Ch, Hasenfuß A, Blancherd E, Alpert NR, Mulieri LA, Just H (1985) Effects of positive inotropic substances on cardiac energetics. Abstracts, 8th Congress of the European Section, International Society for Heart Research, Stockholm, 1985

10. Kammermeier H, Schmid P, Jüngling E (1983) Free energy change of ATP hydrolysis: a causal factor of early hypoxic failure of the myocardium? J Mol Cell Cardiol 14: 267–277

11. Karlson P (1980) Lehrbuch der Biochemie. Thieme Inc, Stuttgart New York, pp 86–88

12. Lehninger AC (1965) The mitochondrion. Molecular basis of structure and function. WA Benjamin, Inc, New York Amsterdam, pp 106–131

13. McCormack JG, Denton RM (1986) Ca^{2+} ions as a link between functional demands and mitochondrial metabolism in the heart. In: Rupp H (ed) Regulation of Heart Function. Basic Concepts and Clinical Applications. Thieme Inc, New York, pp 186–200

14. Loiselle DS (1982) Stretch induced increase in resting metabolism of isolated papillary muscle. Biophys J 38: 185–194

15. Mommaerts WFHM (1970) What is the 'Fenn' effect? Muscle is a regulatory engine, the energy output of which is governed by the load. Naturwissenschaften 57: 326–330

16. Rall JA (1982) Sense and nonsense about the 'Fenn' effect. Am J Physiol 242 (Heart Circ, Physiol 11): H1–H6

17. Schmid W, Siess M (1956) Über Grenzbedingungen von Zelleben und spezifischer Zellfunktion am isolierten Muskel. Pflügers Arch Gesamte Physiologie 263: 492–510

18. Siess M (1977) Influences on the efficiency of cardiac work. Basic Res Cardiol 72: 299–305

19. Siess M (1983) Influences on the mitochondrial function of cardiac tissue. In: Sono KH, Nagano M (eds) 2nd Congress of the working group: 'Cardiac structure and metabolism'. Tokyo, pp 1–42

20. Siess M, Keller HJ, Scharre E, Geisler J, Müller G (1970) The continuous and simultaneous measurement of O_2 consumption rate of decarboxylation of ^{14}C substrates and the performance of spontaneous beating isolated heart atria of guinea-pigs. J Mol Cell Cardiol 1: 261–289

21. Siess M, Mensing HJ, Stieler K (1976) Investigations about the determinants of the myocardial oxygen consumption. In: Knoll J, Szekeres L, Papp JGY (eds). Akadémiai kiadó, Pergamon Press, Kiadó, Budapest, pp 65–73

22. Siess M, Stieler K (1984) Methods for studying mitochondrial function in superfused cardiac muscle preparations. In: Dhalla NS (ed) Methods in studying cardiac membranes. Vol 1. CRC Press Inc, Boca Raton, FL 33431/USA, pp 87–109

23. Stieler J, Reich I, Stiess M (1984) Mitochondrial function and activation of the actomyosin system during K+ depolarization of resting left guinea-pig atria in dependence of Ca++ and nifedipine. In: IUPHAR, 9th International Congress of Pharmacology, London, Abstracts 848 P

Authors' address:

M. Siess, Department of Pharmacology Faculty of Theoretical Medicine University of Tübingen, Wilhelmstraße 56, D-7400 Tübingen (F.R.G.)

Myothermal economy of rat myocardium, Chronic adaptation versus acute inotropism

Ch. Holubarsch[+], G. Hasenfuss[+], E. Blanchard[*], N. R. Alpert[*], L. A. Mulieri[*], and H. Just[+]

[+]Department of Cardiology, Medizinische Universitätsklinik III, Freiburg (F. R. G.) and
[*]Department of Physiology & Biophysics, University of Vermont, Burlington, Vermont (U. S. A.)

Summary

By means of rapid planar Hill type antimony-bismuth thermopiles the initial heat liberated by papillary muscles was measured synchronously with developed tension for control (C), pressure-overload (GOP), and hypothyrotic (PTU) rat myocardium (chronic experiments) and after application of 10^{-6} M isoproterenol or 200 10^{-6} M UDCG-115. Economy of force production was analyzed by the ratio of initial heat versus developed tension-time integral. This ratio was found to be reduced by 34% in GOP and by 43% in PTU myocardium (P <0.01, respectively) indicating increased economy of force production. In contrast, isoproterenol increased initial heat versus tension-time integral by 70% (P<0.01) indicating reduced economy of force production. No change in this ratio was found for UDCG-115. The presented data indicates that long and short term modulation of myocardial energetic costs of force generation is possible. The basic mechanisms for these myocardial alterations are discussed.

Key words: myothermal economy, pressure overload, hypothyroidism, catecholamines, positive inotropic drugs, initial heat

Introduction

Myocardial failure is an unresolved problem in cardiology. There is a lack of convincing parameters which indicate failure on the level of the myocardium. Recently, it has been hypothesized that physiological and pathological types of cardiac hypertrophy are due to the increase and decrease in ATPase activity, respectively (24, 25). By means of myothermal studies (2, 14) it is possible to define the economy of force development and to acquire more information about the performance of myocardium in addition to mechanical and biochemical parameters (ATPase activity, myosin isoenzymes, mechanical "V_{max}" (1, 2, 3, 7, 16, 18, 23, 24, 26).

Furthermore, in addition to chronic structural changes of the sarcoplasmic reticulum and contractile proteins, the acute influence of catecholamines may modulate the chemomechanical transduction efficiency (myocardial economy) on the level of activation processes as well as the contractile apparatus. The knowledge of inotropic influences and energetic consequences is important for the clinical treatment of heart failure. Therefore, chronic and acute changes of myocardial economy of force generation were investigated using highly sensitive thermopiles (21).

Methods

Animals

The rats used in these experiments were Wistar Kyoto males at an age of 10 weeks. The rats were made hypothyrotic by treatment with propylthiouracil (PTU) which was added to the drinking water in a concentration of 0.8 mg/ml over a period of three weeks. Renal hypertension (one clip, two kidneys according to Goldblatt (GOP)) was induced at an age of five weeks so that arterial blood pressure was 220 mm Hg on the average compared to 120 mm Hg in the control animals. The left ventricular-to-body-weight-ratio was 3.40 ± 0.32 mg/g in hypertensive and 2.14 ± 0.10 mg/g in control rats (15).

Instruments and preparations

Rapid thermopiles were used to separate between initial heat and recovery heat (2, 21). Initial heat is calculated as illustrated in Figure 1. In the present paper recovery heat is not discussed.

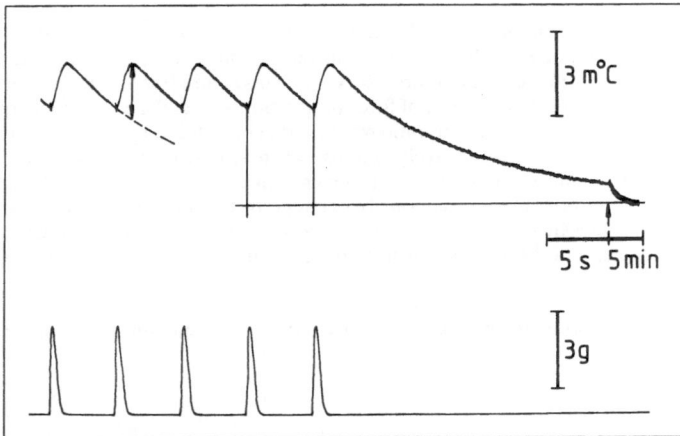

Fig. 1. A typical record of the temperature signal (upper trace) and the isometric tension (lower trace) is shown. Note that temperature increases rapidly when the contraction starts, and decreases slowly ("cool-off") when the contraction is finished. Initial heat is the temperature difference (arrow) between the peak of the oscillating signal and the extrapolated cool-off curve (dotted line) multiplied by the heat capacity of the system. The dotted line is obtained from the cool-off curve after stimulation was stopped (right part of the figure). Total heat can be analyzed from the area between the oscillating temperature signal and the temperature baseline during a twitch interval (unbroken line).

The hearts were removed from the thorax after ether anesthesia. After repetitive exsanguinations the left ventricle was opened along the septum interventriculare. The thinnest papillary muscle was chosen, and its connections with the free wall were cut carefully. On both ends of the muscle, silk loops were attached by means of silk ligatures. The silk loops served for mounting the muscle between the force transducer and a fixed glass hook and contained thin platinum wires for stimulation. The muscle was then pulled against the central hot junctions using a permanent tether applied to the lower silk loop.

Experimental protocol

After mounting the muscle, it was surrounded by Krebs Ringer solution. The muscle length was left unchanged somewhat below optimum length during a two hour equilibration period. The muscle preparation was paced with a 2 ms square wave 10% suprathreshold stimulus every 5 seconds. Thereafter the muscle was stretched by 0.1 mm steps until no further increase or very little decrease in developed force was observed (13).

Krebs Ringer solution was drained and the muscle was surrounded by temperature-equilibrated (21°C) moisturized gas (95% O_2 and 5% CO_2). Under steady state conditions, temperature and force records were taken for several twitches. The stimulation was stopped and a cool-off curve after activity was obtained for analysis of initial and total activity-related heat (Fig. 1). Thereafter the muscle was heated physically by means of infrared diodes (21), and cool-off curves after infrared-heating were obtained.

Myothermal analysis

Initial heat was calculated from the distance between the peak of the oscillating temperature signal and the extrapolation of the cool-off curve to the previous temperature records (Fig. 1, arrow). This temperature change multiplied by the thermal capacity of the muscle and the pile is the initial heat. Thermal capacity was calculated from the cool-off curves after infrared-heating and the heat loss coefficient (17). As a measure of economy of force development, initial heat was related to the developed tension-time integral.

Pharmacological interventions

After data was obtained under control conditions, the muscle was submerged in normal Krebs Ringer solution (resting heat rate). Isoproterenol was then added at a concentration of 10^{-6} M/l. After an equilibration period of at least 10 minutes, data was obtained under steady state conditions as described above. Thereafter, the solution was exchanged three times at ten minute intervals, and a one hour period was allowed for washout of isoproterenol. UDCG 115 was applied in a concentration of 200 10^{-6} M/l. The recording procedure was then repeated as described above. In half of the experiments UDCG-115 was administered before isoproterenol.

Results

Chronic experiments

Typical isometric contractions of hypothyrotic (PTU) and pressure-overloaded myocardium (GOP) are shown in Figure 2 (upper diagram). Contraction and relaxation phases are significantly prolonged in PTU myocardium, whereas peak developed tension is decreased by 24% (6.11 ± 1.75 g mm^{-2} in control versus 4.64 ± 0.89 g mm^{-2}; n = 10; P <0.05) (14). Peak developed tension was found to be 5.83 ± 0.89 g mm^{-2} in GOP and 5.88 ± 1.61 g mm^{-2} in controls (N.S.; n = 6). Contraction time was slightly but not significantly increased (Fig. 2).

The relation of initial heat to tension-time integral was decreased from 6.76 ± 1.28 ucal/g cm s to 3.85 ± 0.45 ucal/g cm s in the PTU myocardium (n = 10; P <0.01), and from 7.24 ± 1.48 ucal/g cm s to 4.60 ± 1.77 ucal/g cm s in GOP myocardium (P <0.01; n = 6; Fig. 2).

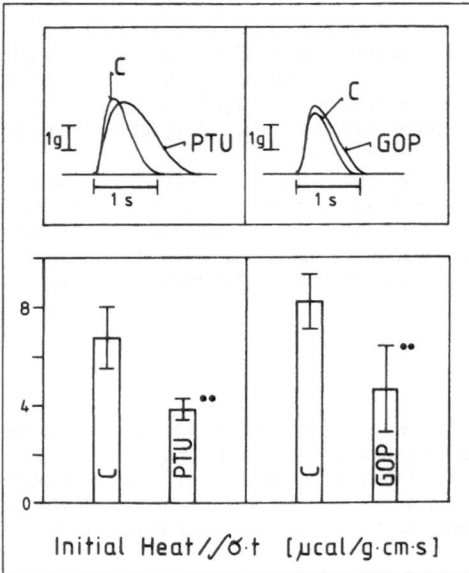

Fig. 2. Upper diagram: Isometric twitch contraction of hypothyrotic (PTU, left), hypertrophied (GOP, right), and control myocardium (C, left and right). Note that the PTU myocardium exhibits a prolonged contraction time.

Lower diagram: Initial heat related to the tension-time integral as an inverse measure of economy of force production for control (C), hypothyrotic (PTU), and hypertrophied (GOP) rat myocardium. A significant decrease of this ratio was found for PTU (N = 10; P <0.01) and GOP myocardium (n = 6; P <0.01).

Acute inotropic interventions

Isoproterenol decreases the contraction time drastically so that time to peak tension and relaxation time are decreased by 28.0 ± 1.8% and 39.5 ± 5.0%, respectively (n = 6; P <0.01, respectively). These changes are obvious in 2.5 mM as well as in 0.625 mM calcium. The 28% increase in peak developed tension is only observed in 0.625 mM calcium (Figure 3).

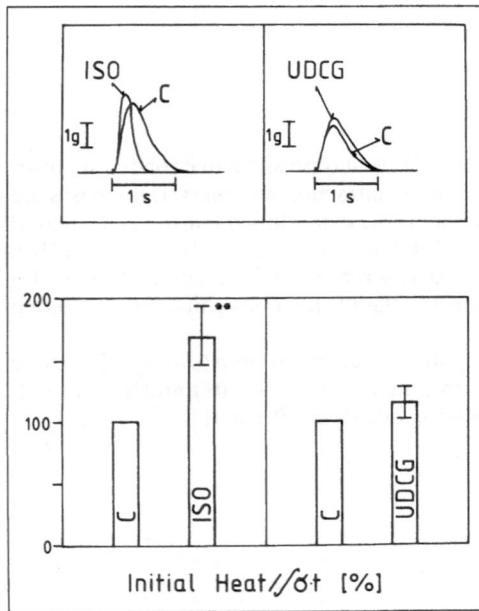

Fig. 3. Upper diagram: Isometric twitch contraction under isoproterenol (ISO, 16^{-6} M/l), UDCG-115 (UDCG, 200 10^{-6} M/l), and control conditions. Note the obvious reduction of contraction time due to isoproterenol.

Lower diagram: Initial heat related to the tension-time integral as an inverse measure of economy of force production for control (C), isoproterenol (ISO), and UDCG-115 (UDCG). A significant increase of this ratio was found for isoproterenol (n = 6; P <0.01), but not for UDCG-115 (n = 6; N. S.).

UDCG 115 does not change the contraction time significantly, however, in two preparations aftercontractions were observed. UDCG 115 increased peak developed tension by 34.1 ± 11.7% at a calcium concentration of 0.625 mM (P < 0.01).

Whereas no significant change in the initial heat versus tension-time integral ratio is found for UDCG 115 (Fig. 3, lower right diagram), isoproterenol increases this ratio significantly by 70% (Fig. 3, left lower diagram; p < 0.01; n = 6).

Discussion

Data presentation

In the present paper, the ratio of initial heat to tension-time integral is given. We think that this ratio is the best index of economy of myocardial force production for the following reasons: 1) The tension-time integral is preferred in contrast to peak developed tension (4, 9), because the tension-time integral covers the whole period of activation including all instantaneous tension values. By choosing this parameter different rates of activation and inactivation are taken into account (see also appendix). 2) Initial heat includes energy-dependent processes due to activation and inactivation ("calcium cycling") and the chemomechanical process on the level of the contractile proteins ("cross-bridge cycling"). 3) Initial heat reflects only the ATP splitting, whereas recovery heat (ATP production) is not taken into account.

Chronic structural changes

As shown by Hoh et al. (11) and Rupp (23), hypothyrosis and pressure overload lead to myosin isoenzyme shifts from V1 towards V3 in rat myocardium. In addition to the reduction of maximum unloaded shortening velocity (7, 16) and the decrease of the ATPase-activity (1, 27), the present paper demonstrates that the shift in myosin insoenzyme pattern is also associated with a significant decrease in initial heat per tension-time integral for both preparations, i. e., economy of moycardial force production is increased. This important result was also found by Loiselle et al. (19) for the hypothyrotic rat myocardium, whereas Coughlin and Gibbs (6) did not find any change in myocardial economy of force production in pressure overload myocardium. However, the pressure overload in their aortic coarctation model was much lower than in the GOP rats. Therefore, the degree of cardiac hypertrophy was low in their coarctation model and high in the GOP rats.

As stated above, these energetic changes may be due to mechanisms of either activation or cross-bridge cycling. Previous data suggests that the increased economy of myocardial force production is primarily due to a decrease in tension-dependent heat (12, 14). Therefore, chronic changes of economy of force production occur due to hypothyrosis and pressure-overload on the level of cross-bridges. Because energy is preserved during force development and maintenance in these preparations, the reduced shortening velocity and decreased myosin ATPase activity per se cannot be taken as parameters which indicate impaired contractility. Additionally, a reduction in mechanical and biochemical parameters should not be interpreted as being pathological or even detrimental (24, 25). The improved economy of force production indicates adaptational processes on the molecular level including the membrane system (activation) and contractile proteins (chemomechanical transduction). In the hypothyrotic rat, the slow myocardium is adapted for slow work (low cardiac output), whereas in the hypertensive rat, the slow myocardium is adapted for increased wall stress.

Acute pharmacological interventions

The influences of isoproterenol and UDCG on cardiac energetics are presented as the ratio of initial heat versus developed tension-time integral. The reasons for this procedure are discussed in the section of data presentation as well as in the appendix. Isoproterenol clearly increases the energy demand of myocardium for a unit of developed tension-time integral. Again, is the 70% increase in initial heat versus tension-time integral due to changes in activation heat or tension-dependent heat or both? Preliminary experiments in which a new method was applied for separation between tension-dependent and tension-independent heat (BDM [5]) give evidence that both tension-dependent and tension-independent heat are increased by about 70% (when related to the tension-time integral) due to isoproterenol. Therefore, it seems that the decreased economy of force production has to be attributed not only to an increased speed and number of calcium turnover (4, 9), but also to an alteration of cross-bridge cycling mechanisms. The later conclusion was not drawn by Gibbs (9) when relating total activity-related heat versus peak developed tension. However, in a later paper from this group (4) it was shown that both the slope and the intercept of the plot of total activity-related heat versus tension-time integral are increased significantly in the same manner as discussed here.

Furthermore, in preliminary reports, Hoh and Rosmanith (12) and Winegrad (26) gave evidence that catecholamines modulate the speed and therefore the chemomechanical transduction of the cross-bridges in rat myocardium. These authors thereby support our conclusion drawn from the presented data, i. e., isoproterenol decreases the economy of force production in rat myocardium.

In contrast to isoproterenol, the novel nonglycoside non-catecholamine UDCG-115 does not change the economy of force production. Preliminary unpublished data from our group do not even show a significant increase in activation heat as was shown for oubain (10). In light of the data from Rüegg and Pfitzer (22), UDCG 115 seems to act by increasing the sensitivity of the contractile proteins to calcium ions. Our data supports this hypothesis, because neither an increase in activation heat nor a decrease in economy of force generation on the level of cross-bridges was found. In contrast to catecholamines (or other substances increasing the cyclic AMP concentration), which speed up the cross-bridge cycling, and digitalis, which increases the calcium release into the cells, UDCG-115 seems neither to increase the cycling rate of the cross-bridges and thereby the tension-dependent heat per tension-time integral nor to enhance the calcium release in to the cell and thereby activation heat.

Appendix

It was clearly shown in tetanic contraction experiments that in V3 myocardium (hypothyrotic rat; guinea-pig; cat) the ratio of heat versus tension-time integral is lowered by a factor of about two compared to V1 myocardium (normal young rat) (8, 14). The same energetic differences between V1 and V3 myocardium were shown for single twitches in normal and hypothyrotic rat myocardium (14, 19). However, Loiselle and Gibbs (20) did not find species differences between rat and cat (guinea-pig) with respect to chemomechanical transduction efficiency of the cross-bridges for single twitches when plotting total activity-related heat versus peak developed tension. These results would imply that species differences are obvious only in tetanic, but not in single twitches. This seems unlikely because structural changes of myosin are involved in these energetic differences. However, when relating initial heat or total activity-related heat to the tension-time integral, species differences become evident also for single twitches of V3 rabbit myocardium (6.0 ucal/g cm s total heat versus tension-time integral and 2.9 ucal/g cm s initial heat versus tension-time integral [3]) and V1 rat myocardium (11.0 ucal/g cm s total activity-related heat versus tension-time integral and 6.8 ucal/g cm s initial heat versus tension-time integral [14]). This is an additional argument which supports the use of initial heat versus tension-time integral ratio.

References

1. Alpert NR, Mulieri LA (1977) The partitioning of altered mechanics in hypertrophied heart muscle between the sarcoplasmic reticulum and the contractile apparatus by means of myothermal measurements. Basic Res Cardiol 72: 153–159
2. Alpert NR, Mulieri LA (1982) The functional significance of altered tension dependent heat in thyrotoxic myocardial hypertrophy. Basic Res Cardiol 75: 153–159
3. Alpert NR, Mulieri LA (1984) The inhomogeneity and appropriateness of the myocardial response to stress. Hypertension 6 (Suppl III): 50–57
4. Barclay JK, Gibbs CL, Loiselle DS (1979) Stress as an index of metabolic cost in papillary muscle in the cat. Basic Res Cardiol 54: 594–603
5. Blanchard EM, Mulieri LA, Alpert NR (1984) The effect of 2,3-Butenedione monoxime (BDM) on the relation between initial heat and mechanical output and on the activity of the contractile apparatus of rat papillary muscle. Conference of Muscle Energetics, Burlington, Vermont
6. Coughlin P, Gibbs CL (1981) Cardiac energetics in short and long term hypertrophy induced by aortic coarctation. Cardiovasc Res 15: 623–631
7. Ebrecht G, Rupp H, Jacob R (1982) Alterations of mechanical parameters in chemically skinned preparations of rat myocardium as a function of isoenzyme pattern of myosin. Basic Res Cardiol 77: 220–234
8. Gibbs C, Loiselle D (1978) The energy output of tetanized cardiac muscle: species differences. Pflügers Arch 373: 31–38
9. Gibbs CL (1967) Role of catecholamines in heat production in the myocardium. Circ Res 21 (Suppl III): 223–230
10. Gibbs CL, Gibson WR (1969) Effect of oubain on the energy output of rabbit cardiac muscle. Circ Res 24: 951
11. Hoh, JFY, McGath PA, Hale PT (1977) Electrophoretic analysis of multiple forms of rat cardiac myosin: effects of hypophysectomy and thyroxine replacement. J Mol Cell Cardiol 10: 1053–1076
12. Hoh JFY, Rosmanith HG (1983) Crossbridge dynamics in rat papillary muscles containing V1 and V3 isomyosins: effects of adrenaline. J Mol Cell Cardiol 15 (Suppl 2): 65
13. Holubarsch Ch, Alpert NR, Goulette R, Mulieri LA (1982) Heat production during hypoxic contracture of rat myocardium. Circ Res 51: 777–786
14. Holubarsch Ch, Goulette RP, Mulieri LA, Alpert NR (1985) The economy of isometric force development, myosin isoenzyme pattern and myofibrillar ATPase activity in normal and hypothyroid rat myocardium. Circ Res 56: 78–86
15. Holubarsch Ch, Goulette RP, Mulieri LA, Alpert NR (1983) Heat liberation in experimentally induced tetanic contractions of myocardium from normal and Goldblatt rats. In: Jacob R (ed) Cardiac Adaptation of Hemodynamic Overload, Training and Stress. Steinkopff Verlag, Darmstadt, pp 158–166
16. Jacob R, Ebrecht G, Holubarsch Ch, Medugorac I (1980) Elastic and contractile properties of the myocardium in experimental cardiac hypertrophy in the rat. Methodological and pathophysiological considerations. Basic Res Cardiol 75: 253–261
17. Kretzschmar KMM, Wilkie DR (1972) A new method for absolute heat measurements, utilizing the Peltier effect. J Physiol (Lond) 224: 18p–20p
18. Litten RZ, Martin BJ, Low RB, Alpert NR (1982) Altered myosin isoenzyme pattern from pressure-overload and thyrotoxic hypertrophied rabbit hearts. Circ Res 50: 856–864
19. Loiselle DS, Wendt IR, Hoh JFY (1982) Energetic consequences of thyroid-modulated shifts in ventricular isomyosin distribution in the rat. J Muscle Res Cell Motil 3: 5–23

20. Loiselle DS, Gibbs CL (1979) Species differences in cardiac energetics. Am J Physiol 237: H90–H98
21. Mulieri LA, Luhr G, Trefry J, Alpert NR (1977) Metal-film thermopiles for use with rabbit right ventricular papillary muscles. Am J Physiol 233: C136–C156
22. Rüegg JC, Pfitzer G (1984) Myokardkontraktilität und Phosphorylierung der kontraktilen Proteine. In: Keul J, H-H Dickhuth (eds) Herzinsuffizienz. Pathophysiologie, Klinik und Therapie. Perimed Fachbuch-Verlagsgesellschaft, Erlangen, pp 53–56
23. Rupp H (1982) Polymorphic myosin as the common determinant of myofibrillar ATPase in different hemodynamic and thyroid states. Basic Res Cardiol 77: 34–46
24. Scheuer J, Malhotra A, Hirsch C, Capasso J (1982) Physiologic cardiac hypertrophy corrects contractile protein abnormalities associated with pathologic hypertrophy of rats. J Clin Invest 70: 1300–1305
25. Wikman-Coffelt J, Parmley WW, Mason DT (1979) The cardiac hypertrophy process. Analyses of factors determining pathological versus physiological development. Circ Res 45: 697–707
26. Winegrad S, Weisberg A, Lin LE, McClellan G (1986) Adrenergic regulation of myosin adenosine Friphosphatase activity. Circ Res 58: 83–95
27. Yasaki Y, Raben MS (1975) Effect of the thyroid state on the enzymatic characteristics of cardiac myosin. A difference in behavior of rat and rabbit cardiac myosin. Circ Res 36: 208–215

Authors' address:

Doz. Dr. Ch. Holubarsch, Medizinische Universitätsklinik, Department of Cardiology, Hugstetter Straße 55, D-7800 Freiburg (F.R.G.)

The influence of myosin isoenzyme pattern on increase in myocardial oxygen consumption induced by catecholamines

G. Kissling and H. Rupp

Physiologisches Institut II, Universität Tübingen (F.R.G.)

Summary

Investigations were performed in a modified heart-lung preparation of the rat in situ to ascertain to what extent the myosin isoenzyme pattern affects the catecholamine-induced increase in myocardial oxygen consumption. Accordingly, the myocardial oxygen consumption was measured in young Wistar rats with mostly VM-1 myosin and older spontaneously hypertensive rats with mostly VM-3 myosin, both under control conditions and after 0.05 mg/kg orciprenaline. In the controls (73.7 ± 3.35 % VM-1) the oxygen consumption related to TTI increased from 0.098 ± 0.003 to 0.129 ± 0.004 μM O$_2$/g · beat under orciprenaline ($+32\%$, p <0.005). In the SHR (27.8 ± 0.58 % VM-1) there was no significant increase in O$_2$-consumption related to TTI (control conditions 0.093 ± 0.003; orciprenaline 0.095 ± 0.004 μM O$_2$/g · beat; $+2\%$, n. s.). Our investigations demonstrate that the degree of catecholamine-induced increase in myocardial O$_2$-consumption depends on the isoenzyme pattern of myosin.

Key words: myocardial oxygen consumption, isoenzyme pattern of myosin, catecholamine, tension-time index

In the myocardium of the rat, 3 types of isoenzymes of myosin with different ATPase-activity can be distinguished by electrophoresis (3, 5, 13). The percentage proportion of the various isoenzymes can change under hemodynamic and hormonal influences (3, 14). Variations in isoenzyme pattern of myosin influence the mechanics as well as the energetics of the heart. A redistribution towards VM-3, the isoenzyme with the lowest ATPase-activity, leads to a reduction in myocardial oxygen consumption (9, 10). Also the isoenzyme pattern of myosin influences the degree of the positive inotropic action of catecholamines (17, 18): the greater the proportion of VM-3, the less is the positive inotropic effect. According to the investigations of Hoh and Rossmanith (4) this diminished sensitivity to catecholamines is due to limited increase in the rate of cross-bridge cycling. This limitation in the rate of cross-bridge cycling means less increase in ATP splitting under the action of catecholamines when VM-3 is predominant. Since the resynthesis of ATP is basically an aerobic process, also the increase in myocardial oxygen consumption under the effect of catecholamines must be less under predominance of VM-3.

The aim of the present study was to establish possible correlations between the isoenzyme pattern of myosin and the increase in myocardial O$_2$-consumption induced by catecholamines. Thus, the latter was measured in young Wistar rats with mainly VM-1 myosin and older spontaneously hypertensive rats (SHR) with mainly VM-3 myosin under control conditions and under the activity of orciprenaline.

Supported by the Deutsche Forschungsgemeinschaft

Methods

The investigations were performed on 12 week-old Wistar rats and on 21 week-old spontaneously hypertensive rats (SHR/Kisslegg of the Aoki-Okamoto strain; Ivanovas, Kisslegg, F.R.G.). The modified heart-lung preparation in situ has been described in previous publications (7–10). Thus we only give a brief description here including some improvements made on the original set-up.

After opening the chest under urethane anesthesia (1.2–1.5 g/kg b. w.) the animals were ventilated with air using a respirator (Schuler; Braun-Melsungen, F.R.G.). An electromagnetic flow probe was placed around the pulmonary artery trunk. The left ventricle was pierced at the apex with a steel cannula for pressure measurement. The right ventricle was pierced with a second cannula for pressure measurement and slow blood infusions (0.075–0.1 ml/min). Subsequently the superior and the inferior venae cavae were ligated and also the ascending aorta immediately above the aortic valves. The ligatures cut off the entire systemic circulation with the exception of coronary circulation, pulmonary circulation

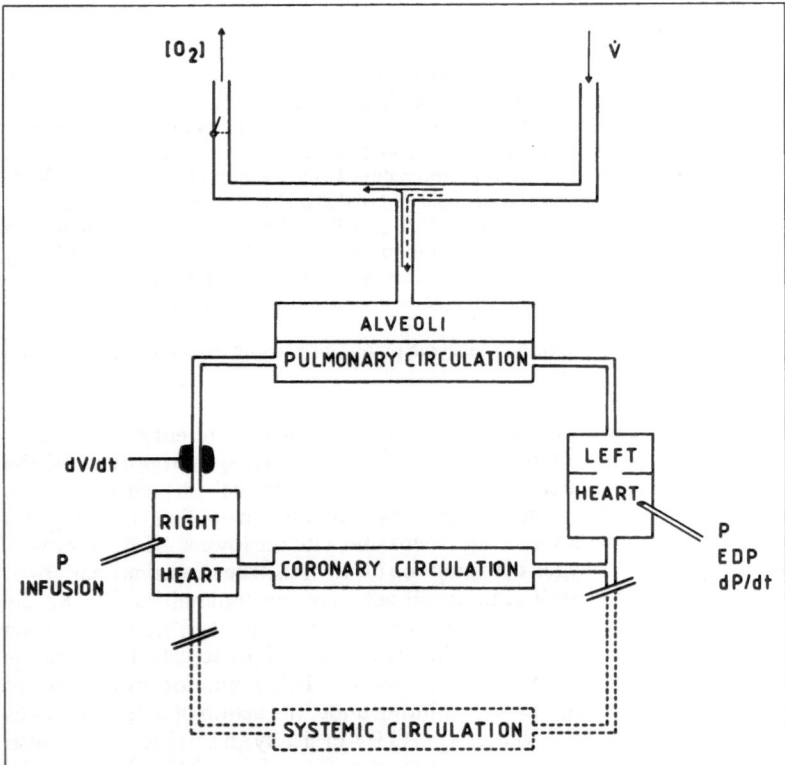

Fig. 1. Schematic presentation of experimental procedure. After clamping the aorta ascendens and venae cavae, ejected blood from the left ventricle is directed over the coronary circulation to the right ventricle. The pulmonary circulation remains intact. Under steady state conditions the flow in the arteria pulmonalis measured by electromagnetic flow probe corresponds to coronary perfusion. Left ventricular pressure is continuously registered over a cannula. Circulating blood volume is variable either by slow blood infusions or blood letting over a second cannula pierced into the right ventricle.

The flow of the respirator is measured using a spirometer. The duration of inspiration can be adjusted over the outlet valve. Oxygen concentration at the outlet valve is continuously measured. The O_2-consumption of the preparation can be ascertained from the flow of the respirator and from the O_2-concentration gradient between inlet- and outlet-valve.

remaining intact (Fig. 1). The left and right ventricular output are equal under steady state conditions, allowing for indirect measurement of left ventricular stroke volume over pulmonary flow.

The following parameters were recorded on a Hellige 7-channel recorder: left ventricular pressure amplitude (P_{LV}), left ventricular end-diastolic pressure (EDP), first derivative of left ventricular pressure (dP/dt), right ventricular pressure (P_{RV}), and pulmonary flow (dV/dt).

At the end of each experiment the atrioventricular border of the still beating heart was ligated and end-diastolic pressure-volume relationships were recorded as relaxation curves (6). The end-diastolic pressure-volume relationships were used to determine the respective end-diastolic volume from the measured end-diastolic pressure of each beat.

Blood volume in each animal was varied either by blood letting or by slow blood infusions. Thus, O_2 consumption could be measured at different mechanical activity of the heart, both under control conditions as well as under the effect of 0.05 mg/kg orciprenaline.

Left ventricular wall stress was calculated assuming a thick-walled sphere, using the formula (15)

$$\sigma = \frac{P}{[(V + W) \cdot V^{2/3}] - 1}$$

(P = ventricular pressure; V = internal ventricular volume; W = wall volume; whereby myocardial specific weight is set to 1 g/cm^3).

In order to calculate the maximum rate of tension development (dσ/dt), P was substituted by dP/dt$_{max}$ and V by end-diastolic ventricular volume. This is justifiable since the maximum value of dP/dt is reached before the onset of ejection. However, peak tension is reached during the ejection period when the ventricular volume is smaller than the end-diastolic volume. Since in our preparation the left ventricle operates against elevated afterload, the ejection fraction is only about 10%. In calculating the peak tension (σ) and tension time index (TTI) we assumed an averaged ventricular volume that is smaller than the end-diastolic volume by half the stroke volume ($\overline{V} = Vd - \frac{Vs}{2}$). To calculate σ the peak pressure was measured and to calculate the TTI the averaged pressure was determined planimetrically. The averaged wall tension was then calculated from this pressure-value and from the averaged ventricular volume. For comparison we also calculated, in different hearts, instantaneous wall tension by measuring simultaneously at intervals of 4 ms the pressure-volume values. Average wall tension derived from instantaneous measurements correlates very well with that calculated using the simplified formula (Fig. 2).

In contrast to our previous investigations (8–10) where the O_2-consumption of the modified heart-lung preparation was measured by determining cardiac output and the arterio-venous oxygen concentration difference, in the present studies the O_2-consumption was measured from the minute respiratory volume and the concentration of oxygen in inspired and expired gas volumes (Fig. 1). The advantage of the latter method is that arterial and venous blood samples need not be taken for each measurement, the number of which is limited by the small blood volume of approx. 1.5 ml/100 g b. w. in the model used (8). The respirator we are currently using pumps a continuous flow of air. The duration of the inspiration and expiration can be varied over a valve. Since the pump forwards a continuous flow also during expiration, the expired air by the animal is mixed with normal athmospheric air so that the oxygen concentration at the outlet valve is higher than that in the air expired by the animal. The oxygen concentration in the gas mixture at the outlet valve was measured using an oxygen analyzer (model S-3 A, Ametek, Pittsburgh, U.S.A.). This apparatus gives measurements with a reproducible accuracy of 0.01 vol% O_2. The output of the respirator was constantly registered using a spirometer (approx. 100 ml/min). The O_2-consumption of the modified heart-lung preparation could then be calculated from the output of the respirator and from the oxygen concentration gradient in the outlet and inlet air. Despite constant output of the pump, the ventilation of the animal could be regulated in such a way that, by varying the duration of inspiration, a pH of 7.2 could be maintained in the blood.

At the end of each experiment, the heart was excised, the left ventricle and ventricular septum was dissected, weighed and frozen in liquid nitrogen. The isoenzyme pattern of each individual heart was determined using polyacrylamide gel electrophoresis in the presence of sodium pyrophosphate (3, 13).

Statistical analysis of the data was performed using Student's t-test. Differences were considered to be significant when $p < 0.05$. When deviation is given, it represents standard error ($\overline{x} \pm s_{\overline{x}}$).

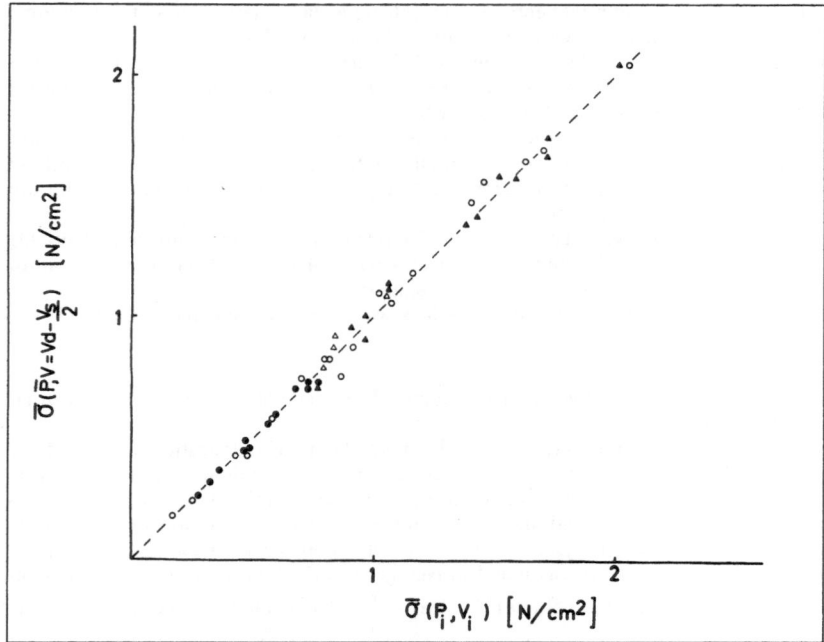

Fig. 2. Comparison of systolic wall stress values determined by different procedures. The values that were calculated from planimetrically determined mean pressure ($\overline{P}$) and from mean ventricular inner volume ($\overline{V} = V_d - \frac{V_s}{2}$) are plotted along the ordinate. The values calculated from instantaneous pressure and volume (P_i, V_i) – measured at intervals of 4 ms – are plotted along the abscissa. The values obtained by either procedure correspond very well also in chronically altered hearts.
Δ control animals $\bigcirc$ aorta coarctation
$\blacktriangle$ Goldblatt $\bullet$ spontaneous hypertension

Results

Body weight, left ventricular weight and the isoenzyme pattern of myosin of control (C) and spontaneously hypertensive rats (SH) are shown in Table 1. Although the body weight of SH is less than that of C by 10%, the left ventricular weight of SH is higher by 19%.

Table 1. Mean value and standard error ($\overline{x} \pm s_{\overline{x}}$) of body weight, left ventricular weight, left ventricular weight per 100 g body weight and proportion of the various isoenzymes of myosin.

	Body weight (g)	Left ventricular weight (mg)	Left ventr. w. 100 g b. w. (mg)	VM-1 (%)	VM-2 (%)	VM-3 (%)	α-chains (%)
Controls (n = 5)	352.0 ±12.51	761.8 ±16.45	217.2 ± 7.06	73.7 ±3.35	16.8 ±2.10	9.5 ±1.27	82.1 ±2.31
SH (n = 6)	317.5 ±10.55	903.8 ±37.84	284.8 ±7.93	27.8 ±0.58	29.1 ±0.46	43.1 ±0.95	42.4 ±0.74
p	<0.05	<0.01	<0.0005	<0.0005	<0.005	<0.0005	<0.0005

Left ventricular weight per 100 g body weight is thus higher in SH than in C by 31 %.

The percentage proportion of VM-1 – the isoenzyme of myosin with the highest ATPase-activity – is less in SH than in C by 45 %. The proportion of VM-3 in SH is higher by 34 %. The isoenzymes differ in the structure of their heavy chains of myosin (3). Both VM-1 and VM-3 are homodimers, with 2 α and 2 β chains respectively. VM-2 is a heterodimer, having 1 α and 1 β chain. Given the relative proportion of all three isoenzymes, the fraction of α and β chains can then be calculated. The proportion of α chains in SH is less than that in C by 40 %.

Prerequisite for the measurements of energetics is that the preparation be mechanically and energetically stable for a longer period of time. As Fig. 3 shows, our preparation fulfills this requirement. Three series of infusion, each lasting for 30 minutes, were done. Prior to each infusion, the volume of circulating blood was reduced by blood letting. Figure 3 shows the O_2-consumption per gram and beat as a function of various mechanical parameters.

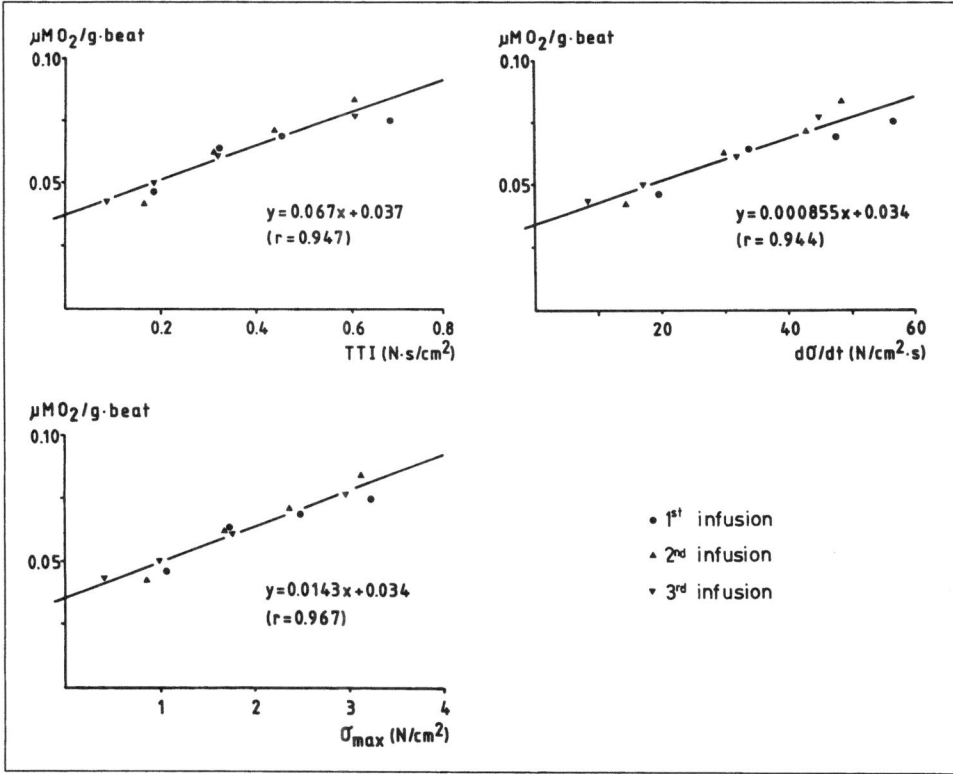

Fig. 3. The O_2-consumption per g and beat measured in a control animal at various end-diastolic volumes is plotted as a function of TTI, $d\sigma/dt$ and σ_{max}, respectively, giving a linear correlation in each case. The point of interception of the regression line on the ordinate corresponds to the O_2-consumption, independent of mechanical activity of the left ventricle. The slope gives a measure of O_2-consumption related to the respective mechanical parameters of the left ventricle. The values were measured during 3 successive infusions, each lasting about 30 minutes. After a period of 90 minutes (i. e. during the third infusion) the points still lie on the same regression line as during the first infusion. This proves that the preparations remain energetically stable even over a longer period of time.

During a period of 90 minutes the O_2-consumption of the preparation related to tension-time index (TTI), maximum rate of stress development ($d\sigma/dt$) and peak tension (σ), respectively, is constant. After ascertaining that our preparation remains mechanically and energetically stable for at least two hours, measurements of O_2-consumption were done by varying blood volume firstly under control conditions and finally after application of 0.05 mg orciprenaline/kg b. w. This procedure was performed for each individual animal, both for C and SH.

Table 2 shows various pressure values and the ejection fraction measured at an end-diastolic left ventricular pressure of 7 mm Hg, under control conditions and after application of orciprenaline, for both C and SH. Systolic peak pressure, the maximum rate of pressure rise and fall as well as the ejection fraction increase significantly under orciprenaline in both collectives. However, the pressure time integral increases significantly only in SH, remaining constant in C. The calculated wall tension parameters show similar alterations under orciprenaline (Table 3). The increase in TTI found in SH could, at least in part, be due to the moderate yet significant decrease in heart rate. For the same reason SH did not show a significant reduction in duration of systole under orciprenaline.

Table 2. Peak pressure (P_{max}), max. rate of pressure rise ($dP/dt_{max\ syst}$) and pressure fall ($dP/dt_{max\ diast}$), pressure time integral ($\int p \cdot t$) and ejection fraction, each measured at the end-diastolic pressure of 7 mm Hg both under control conditions and under orciprenaline (0.05 mg/kg). The values represent mean values and standard error ($\bar{x} \pm s_{\bar{x}}$).

	P_{max} (mm Hg)	$dP/dt_{max\ syst}$ (mm Hg/s)	$dP/dt_{max\ diast}$ (mm Hg/s)	$\int p \cdot t$ (mm Hg $\cdot$ s)	Ejection fraction (%)
Controls (n = 5)					
Control conditions	160 ± 9	3025 ± 214	1263 ± 136	29.25 ± 2.06	$7.5 \pm .0.7$
Orciprenaline	213 ± 9	4925 ± 368	2038 ± 126	30.50 ± 2.18	13.5 ± 1.1
p	<0.0005	<0.0025	<0.025	n. s.	<0.0005
SH (n = 6)					
Control conditions	163 ± 12	2550 ± 312	1313 ± 128	32.75 ± 1.89	5.6 ± 0.3
Orciprenaline	250 ± 9	4300 ± 334	1925 ± 217	45.50 ± 1.50	10.6 ± 0.7
p	<0.0025	<0.0005	<0.0125	<0.025	<0.0005

As depicted in Fig. 3 TTI, σ, and $d\sigma/dt$ have a linear correlation with O_2-consumption per gram and beat. This strictly linear correlation also holds under the application of orciprenaline. The results of a representative experiment on a control rat are shown in Fig. 4. The O_2-consumption of the preparation, independent of the mechanical activity of the left ventricle, determined by extrapolating the regression line to the point of intersection with the y-axis, increases under orciprenaline in all three correlations. However, the slope of the regression lines, which corresponds with the O_2-consumption per unit of mechanical parameter of the left ventricle is different for each correlation. Related to TTI, the increase in O_2-consumption per gram and beat is moderate although statistically significant under orciprenaline; while the O_2-consumption related to σ and $d\sigma/dt$ significantly decreases.

Also in spontaneously hypertensive rats a linear correlation was found between the O_2-consumption and the various mechanical parameters, both under control conditions and under orciprenaline.

The relative O_2-consumptions are depicted by the histograms in Fig. 5. In C the O_2-con-

Table 3. Peak tension (σ_{max}), maximal rate of tension development ($d\sigma/dt_{max\ syst}$) and relaxation ($d\sigma/dt_{max\ diast}$), tension time integral (TTI), heart rate and duration of systole, each measured at diastolic wall stress of 0.08 N/cm² both under control conditions and under orciprenaline. The mean values and standard error ($\bar{x} \pm s_{\bar{x}}$) are given.

	σ_{max} (N/cm²)	$d\sigma/dt_{max\ syst}$ (N/cm² · s)	$d\sigma/dt_{max\ diast}$ (N/cm² · s)	TTI (N · s/cm²)	Heart rate (min⁻¹)	Duration of systole (ms)
Controls (n = 5)						
Control conditions	1.775 ±0.095	34.250 ±2.780	13.900 ±1.100	0.320 ±.020	159 ±11	342 ±20
Orciprenaline	2.265 ±0.165	58.500 ±3.797	31.100 ±3.900	0.338 ±.029	158 ±6	256 ±7
p	<0.005	<0.005	<0.025	n. s.	n. s.	<0.005
SH (n = 6)						
Control conditions	1.850 ±0.155	29.500 ±3.617	15.400 ±1.600	0.385 ±0.032	146 ±8	354 ±17
Orciprenaline	2.775 ±0.085	46.750 ±2.983	24.400 ±2.200	0.545 ±0.030	127 ±5	320 ±16
p	<0.0025	<0.005	<0.0025	<0.0025	<0.05	n. s.

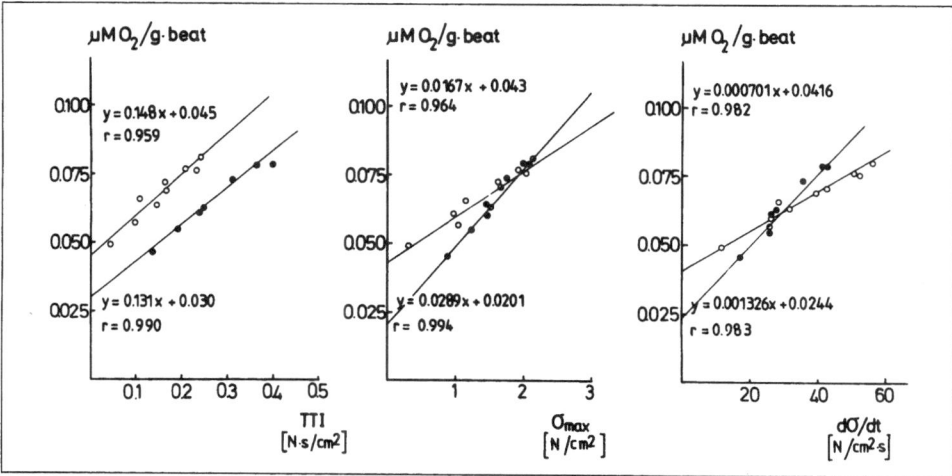

Fig. 4. Representative study performed on a control animal depicting O_2-consumption per g and beat related to tension time index (TTI), to peak tension (σ_{max}) and to maximum rate of tension development $d\sigma/dt$ under control conditions (●) and under orciprenaline (○), respectively. In both cases there is a close linear correlation between O_2-consumption and the respective mechanical parameter. All 3 diagrams show the increase in O_2-consumption independent of left ventricular mechanical activity under orciprenaline. Whereas the O_2-consumption related to TTI increases slightly but significantly, it decreases significantly when related to $d\sigma/dt$ and σ_{max}.

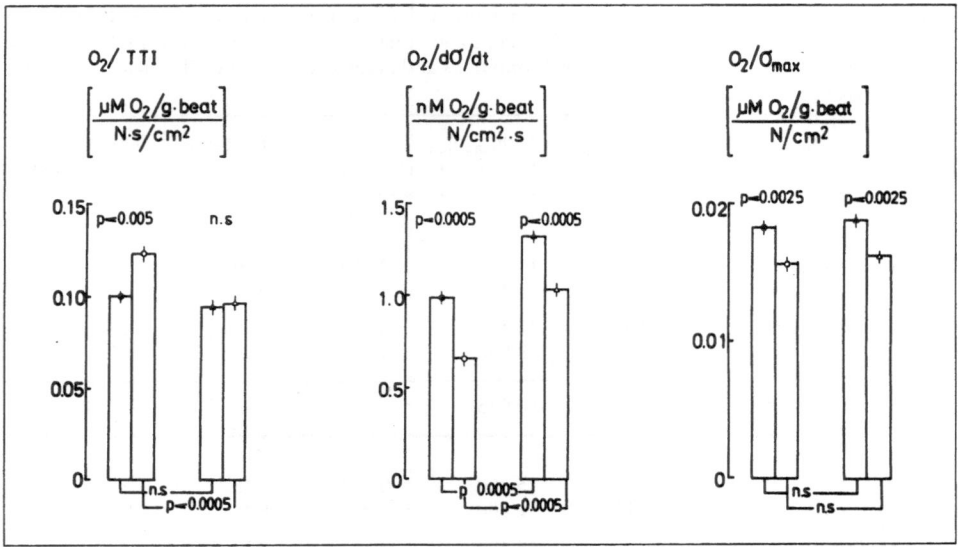

Fig. 5. Diagrammatic presentation of results derived from measurements on 5 control and 6 spontaneously hypertensive rats. For each animal the values of O_2-consumption related to the various mechanical parameters were plotted and the slope of each regression line was then calculated (for specific examples see Fig. 4). The histograms depict the mean slope of the various regression lines.

● controls: control conditions
○ controls: orciprenaline
▲ SHR: control conditions
△ SHR: orciprenaline

sumption related to TTI increased from 0.098 ± 0.003 to 0.129 ± 0.004 μM O_2/g $\cdot$ beat ($+32\%$, p < 0.005) under orciprenaline; in SH, however, there was no significant change in O_2-consumption related to TTI under orciprenaline (control conditions: 0.093 ± 0.003; orciprenaline: 0.095 ± 0.004 μM O_2/g $\cdot$ beat). In contrast, O_2-consumption related to $d\sigma/dt$ decreased under orciprenaline from 0.980 ± 0.036 to 0.648 ± 0.025 nM O_2/g $\cdot$ beat (-34%, p < 0.0005) in C and from 1.305 ± 0.053 to 1.017 ± 0.058 nM O_2/g $\cdot$ beat (-22%, p < 0.0005) in SH. Also the O_2-consumption related to σ decreased from 0.0183 ± 0.0007 to 0.0156 ± 0.0004 μM O_2/g $\cdot$ beat (-15%, p < 0.0025) in C and from 0.0189 ± 0.0007 to 0.0162 ± 0.0005 μM O_2/g $\cdot$ beat (-14%, p < 0.0025) in SH. The O_2-consumption independent of the left ventricular activity increased under orciprenaline from 0.018 ± 0.003 to 0.024 ± 0.003 μM O_2/g $\cdot$ beat ($+33\%$, p < 0.05) in C and from 0.016 ± 0.003 to 0.030 ± 0.004 μM O_2/g $\cdot$ beat ($+88\%$, p < 0.005) in SH.

Discussion

The myocardium, like all other animal cells, derives the energy it requires for processes of metabolism from ATP-splitting. Since the resynthesis of ATP is basically an aerobic process, the O_2-consumption can be taken as an index of ATP-splitting. Only in the metabolism of glucose, about 5% of the ATP is obtained anaerobically over glycolysis. In our previous studies, the heart-lung preparation we used derives 50% of its energy requirement from glucose (8). We can therefore assume that, in the present investigations, 97–98 % of the ATP is resynthetized aerobically. Strictly speaking, the respiratory equivalent of oxygen also should be taken into consideration since, from the standpoint of energetics, it is not altogether without bearing which substrate is burnt. When pure fat is metabolized, with 1 mol O_2 the amount of ATP resynthetized is about 7 % less than that obtained when the substrate burnt is pure carbohydrate. According to our previous studies on control rats and on Goldblatt rats (8) as well as on rats with aortic coarctation (unpublished results), about 80 % of the myocardial energy turnover is derived from carbohydrates and 20 % from fat. It is therefore unlikely that in the present experiments the respiratory equivalent for C and SH should differ from the above values. An alteration in respiratory equivalent under the effect of catecholamines cannot be ruled out but should be practically identical for both SH and C.

Since our measurements were performed after opening the chest, extrapulmonary oxygen uptake by diffusion from the air to the myocardium cannot be excluded. The portion of myocardium that is supplied by oxygen diffusion from the surface can be estimated from the extent of penetration. Assuming a spherical shape for the heart, the depth of penetration can be calculated using the formula

$$r_0 = \sqrt{6k \cdot \frac{P_0}{a}}$$

(r_0 = depth of penetration, k = O_2 diffusion conductance, P_0 = partial pressure of O_2 at the surface, a = O_2-consumption of the myocardium per unit volume).

By substituting the corresponding values in the formula, penetration depth of approx. 0.006 mm is calculated, thus rendering the portion of myocardium that is supplied by extrapulmonary O_2-intake to be about 3 %.

With our experimental procedure, however, only the O_2-consumption of the whole heart-lung preparation can be measured, i. e. our measurements include the active and the resting energy turnover of the whole heart and the turnover in the lungs. A linear correlation was found between O_2-consumption per gram and beat on the one hand and TTI, σ, and $d\sigma/dt$ on the other hand (Figs. 3 and 4). By extrapolating the regression line to the point of intersection on the ordinate, the O_2-consumption independent of the left ventricular activity can be ascertained. This value includes the resting O_2-consumption of the left ventricle as well as the total O_2-consumption of the other heart compartments and of the lungs. The slope of the regression line is a direct measure of the O_2-consumption per unit left ventricular mechanical parameter.

A linear correlation between the measured O_2-consumption and a specific mechanical parameter is often interpreted to the effect that the latter must be the limiting factor for the O_2-consumption (for literature see [2]). By our comparing the O_2-consumption before and after application of orciprenaline, we proved that this assumption need not always be correct (Figs. 4, 5). Although we did find before and after application of orciprenaline a linear correlation between the O_2-consumption on the one hand and TTI, σ, and $d\sigma/dt$ on the other, all three mechanical parameters cannot be limiting factors for O_2-consumption. This is because the O_2-consumption related to TTI increases under orciprenaline whereas O_2-consumption related to σ and $d\sigma/dt$, respectively decreases.

Linear correlations between these mechanical parameters and the O_2-consumption are then plausible when a linear correlation is also found among the three mechanical parameters. This is in fact true as can be seen from Fig. 6. Granted that only one of these mechanical parameters is the limiting factor for O_2-consumption then, inevitabily, the two other parameters must also show a linear correlation with O_2-consumption.

Which of the three mechanical parameters is, in the final analysis, decisive for O_2-consumption? To elucidate this problem, supplementary O_2-measurements under β-blockade were done. The relationships between the mechanical parameters under control conditions on the one hand and under β-stimulation (0.05 mg/kg orciprenaline) as well as under β-blockade (10 mg/kg atenolol) on the other hand are shown in Fig. 6. Assuming that the mechanical parameter plotted on one coordinate is the limiting factor for O_2-consumption

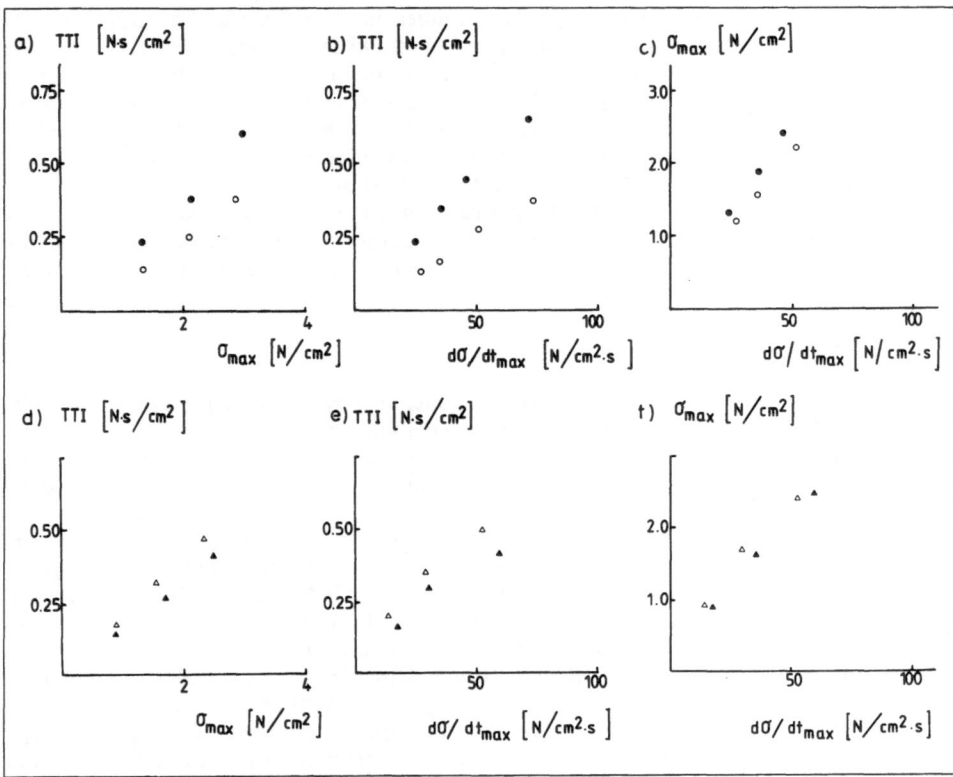

Fig. 6. The influence of orciprenaline (a–c) and atenolol (d–f) on the correlation between the individual mechanical parameters. Each symbol represents the mean value of at least 7 coordinates.
a–c: ● control conditions
     ○ orciprenaline
d–f: ▲ control conditions
     △ atenolol

then the second coordinate should reveal how the O_2-consumption related to the second parameter varies under orciprenaline and atenolol, respectively. The expected changes in O_2-consumption derived from the diagrams can be compared to the actually measured alterations shown schematically in Table 4.

Assuming firstly that σ is the mechanical parameter decisive for O_2-consumption, then the O_2-consumption per unit TTI should increase under orciprenaline (Fig. 6a) and the O_2-consumption per unit $d\sigma/dt$ should decrease (Fig. 6c). Table 4 verifies both statements. However, under atenolol, the O_2-consumption per unit TTI should decrease (Fig. 6d) and the O_2-consumption per unit $d\sigma/dt$ should slightly increase (Fig. 6f). The measured O_2-consumption per unit TTI, however, does not change under atenolol (Table 4).

Table 4. Qualitative change in O_2-consumption per gram and beat related to the specific mechanical parameter, measured under orciprenaline and under atenolol.

	$\Delta O_2/TTI$	$\Delta O_2/\sigma_{max}$	$\Delta O_2/d\sigma/dt_{max}$
Orciprenaline	$\uparrow$	$\downarrow$	$\downarrow$
Atenolol	$\rightarrow$	$\uparrow$	$\uparrow$

If, on the other hand, $d\sigma/dt$ is taken to be the limiting factor, then the O_2-consumption related to unit TTI (Fig. 6 b) as well as to unit σ (Fig. 6 c) should increase under orciprenaline.

In Table 4, however, the O_2-consumption increases when related to unit TTI and decreases when related to unit σ. Under atenolol, the O_2-consumption per unit TTI (Fig. 6 e) and per unit σ (Fig. 6 f) should decrease. According to Table 4, however, the O_2-consumption per unit TTI measured under atenolol does not change at all, even increasing when related to unit σ.

Finally, granted that TTI has the decisive effect on O_2-consumption, the O_2-consumption per unit σ (Fig. 6 a) as well as per unit $d\sigma/dt$ (Fig. 6 b) should decrease under orciprenaline. This is verified in Table 4. Conversely, under atenolol the O_2-consumption per unit σ (Fig. 6 d) and per unit $d\sigma/dt$ (Fig. 6 e) should increase. Table 4 again verifies this postulation.

Hence, TTI is the only parameter where the postulated changes in O_2-consumption based on the various correlations correspond to the actual values measured under orciprenaline and atenolol, respectively. On the strength of these considerations, we conclude that TTI is the limiting parameter for the O_2-consumption.

In agreement with our findings in control animals under orciprenaline, other researchers have also described displacements in the correlation between O_2-consumption and TTI due to acute alterations in contractility. For example, less O_2-consumption per unit TTI was found under hypothermia (11) whereas a greater consumption was found under paired stimulation (12) and also under epinephrine (16), compared to control conditions. Based upon this, it was concluded that TTI could not be the limiting parameter for O_2-consumption (2). In contrast to this concept, we have ground to believe that the cross-bridge kinetics can be directly influenced by alterations in contractility. Changes involving cross-bridge kinetics need not necessarily anual the close correlation found between O_2-consumption and TTI under control conditions. On the basis of our investigations we think that these correlations are merely displaced by acute changes in contractility and that TTI is the decisive mechanical parameter for O_2-consumption, also under positive inotropic effect of catecholamines. Interestingly, in SHR, the O_2-consumption related to unit TTI did not increase under orciprenaline. We postulate that the reason for this must lie in the state of isoenzymes pattern of myosin which in SHR, compared to C, is redistributed towards VM-3.

According to the investigations of Hoh and Rossmanith (4), the increase in rate of cross-bridge cycling in rat myocardium under the effect of catecholamines is less under predominancy of VM-3 than of VM-1. Given that per cross-bridge cycle 1 mole ATP is split, this would mean that under the influence of catecholamines the increase in amount of ATP required – and hence also the O_2-consumption – is less in a myocardium with a predominancy of VM-3 than in one containing mostly VM-1.

According to a working hypothesis of Alpert and Mulieri (1) the rate of cross-bridge cycling in myocardium increases under thyroxine. Concurrently, the period of time in which the cross-bridges are in the state of forcegeneration ("on-time") decreases overproportionally. This alteration in cross-bridge kinetics could explain the poor efficiency of the heart under these conditions. Assuming that the increase in rate of cross-bridge cycling under the influence of catecholamines is paralleled by a reduction in "on-time", then an impaired

114

efficiency should ensue. We were actually able to register in the controls with relatively high proportion of VM-1 an increase in O_2-consumption per unit TTI, under orciprenaline. Since VM-3 is predominant in SHR only a slight increase in rate of cross-bridge cycling can be expected under catecholamine. It can be supposed that the "on-time" of the cross-bridges decreases little and thus the efficiency also changes to a lesser degree than in C. In our measurements on SHR we actually found no significant change in O_2-consumption related to TII, under orciprenaline.

Our investigations have shown clearly that, under the effect of catecholamines, the O_2-consumption of the heart related to the mechanical activity does not increase to the same extent in SH as it does in C. The differences in the increase of myocardial O_2-consumption can be traced back to variations in the isoenzyme pattern of myosin.

References

1. Alpert NR, Mulieri LA (1980) The functional significance of altered tension dependent heat in thyrotoxic myocardial hypertrophy. Basic Res Cardiol 75: 179–184
2. Gibbs CL, Chapman JB (1979) Cardiac energetics. In: Berne RM (ed) Handbook of Physiology. Sect 2 Vol I, Amer Physiol Soc, Bethesda Maryland, 775–804
3. Hoh JFY, McGrath PA, Hale PT (1978) Electrophoretic analysis of multiple forms of rat cardiac myosin: Effects of hypophysectomy and thyroxine replacement. J Mol Cell Cardiol 10: 1053–1076
4. Hoh JFY, Rossmanith GH (1983) Crossbridge dynamics in rat papillary muscles containing V_1 and V_3 isomyosins: effect of adrenaline. J Mol Cell Cardiol 15 (Suppl 2): 65
5 Jacob R, Ebrecht G, Holubarsch Ch, Rupp H, Kissling G (1983) Mechanics and energetics in cardiac hypertrophy as related to the isoenzyme pattern of myosin. In: Alpert NR (ed) Perspectives in cardiovascular research. Vol 7, Myocardial hypertrophy and failure. Raven Press, New York, 553–569
6. Kissling G, Gassenmaier T, Wendt-Gallitelli MF, Jacob R (1977) Pressure-volume relations, elastic modulus and contractile behaviour of the hypertrophied left ventricle of rats with Goldblatt II hypertension. Pflügers Arch 369: 213–221
7. Kissling G, Ziegler Ch (1978) A new in situ heart preparation for measurement of oxygen consumption under isovolumic conditions. Pflügers Arch 373: R8
8. Kissling G (1980) Oxygen consumption and substrate uptake of the hypertrophied rat heart in situ. Basic Res Cardiol 75: 185–192
9. Kissling G, Rupp H, Malloy L, Jacob R (1982) Alterations in cardiac oxygen consumption under chronic pressure overload. Significance of the isoenzyme pattern of myosin. Basic Res Cardiol 77: 255–269
10. Kissling G, Malloy L, Rupp H (1983) Energetics of the rat heart in chronic pressure overload. In: Jacob R, Gülch RW, Kissling G (eds) Cardiac adaptation to hemodynamic overload, training and stress. Steinkopff Verlag, Darmstadt, 167–173
11. Monroe RG, Strang RH, La Farge CG, Levy J (1964) Ventricular performance, pressure-volume relationships, and O_2 consumption during hypothermia. Am J Physiol 206: 67–73
12. Ross J, Sonnenblick EH, Kaiser GA, Frommer PL, Braunwald E (1965) Electroaugmentation of ventricular performance and oxygen consumption by repetitive application of paired electrical stimuli. Circ Res 16: 332–342
13. Rupp H (1981) The adaptive changes in the isoenzyme pattern of myosin from hypertrophied rat myocardium as a result of pressure overload and physical training. Basic Res Cardiol 76: 79–88
14. Rupp H, Kissling G, Jacob R (1983) Hormonal and hemodynamic determinants of polymorphic myosin. In: Alpert NR (ed) Perspectives in cardiovascular research, Vol 7, Myocardial hypertrophy and failure. Raven Press, New York, 373–383
15. Sandler H, Dodge HT (1963) Left ventricular tension and stress in man. Circ Res 13: 91–104
16. Sonnenblick EH, Ross J, Covell JW, Kaiser GA, Braunwald E (1965) Velocity of contraction as a determinant of myocardial oxygen consumption. Am J Physiol 219: 1490–1495
17. Takeda N, Dominiak P, Türck D, Rupp H, Jacob R (1985) The influence of endurance training on

mechanical catecholamine responsiveness, β-adrenoceptor density and myosin isoenzyme pattern of rat ventricular myocardium. Basic Res Cardiol 80: 88–99

18. Winegrad S, McClellan G, Tucker M, Lin LE (1983) Cyclic AMP regulation of myosin isoenzymes in mammalian cardiac muscle. J Gen Physiol 81: 749–765

Authors' address:

Prof. Dr. G. Kissling, Physiologisches Institut II, Universität Tübingen, Gmelinstraße 5, D-7400 Tübingen (F.R.G.)

Function and energy-rich phosphate content of the hypertrophied ventricle after global ischemia and reperfusion

G. Fenchel, R. Storf, H.-E. Hoffmeister, and W. Heller

Department of Thoracic and Cardiovascular Surgery, Surgical Clinic, University of Tübingen (F.R.G.)

Summary

Using an isolated rat heart preparation (Langendorff perfusion, perfusion pressure 100 cm H_2O) the response of the hypertrophied heart (spontaneous hypertensive rats lv/bw ratio 3.6 ± 0.5) to global normothermic (30 min) and hypothermic (25°C, 120 min) ischemic and cardioplegic arrest and reperfusion (30 min) was examined and compared with normal hearts (Wistar rats lv/bw ratio 2.0 ± 0.3). St. Thomas solution and verapamil (2 mg/l Ringer solution) were used as cardioplegic agents.

Before ischemia hypertrophied hearts had a significantly higher pressure-rate product, a lower myocardial perfusion/g myocardium and a lower myocardial ATP and adenine nucleotide content.

Unmodified ischemia reduced myocardial function in the hypertrophied hearts to a greater degree than in normal hearts in both normo- and hypothermia. St. Thomas solution and verapamil protected significantly the myocardial function in the normal and hypertrophied heart after normothermic ischemia in a similar manner (60–70 % of the initial value). In the hypertrophied ventricle ATP decay and adenine nucleotide loss was greater in verapamil than in St. Thomas solution treated hearts. In hypothermic ischemia only St. Thomas solution protected left ventricular function and adenine nucleotide loss in both normal and hypertrophied hearts. Verapamil was ineffective in the normal ventricle and protected left ventricular function but not the ATP and adenine nucleotide decay in the hypertrophied heart.

Key words: myocardial ischemia, myocardial function, myocardial hypertrophy, myocardial metabolism, St. Thomas cardioplegia

Introduction

Myocardial hypertrophy leads, depending on the type and duration of the ventricular loading, to functional (5, 14, 17) and biochemical (38, 43) changes which reduce the reserve of the heart as well as change its reaction to any ischemic stress. In clinical practice the increased sensitivity of hypertrophied hearts to ischemic stress during open cardiac operations has been noted (10, 26) and thus the experiments by Sink (36) on rats and by Attarian (3, 4) on canine hearts have been confirmed.

Despite these facts the majority of experiments carried out to assess anti-ischemic protective methods have been performed on young and previously undamaged hearts. Experiments on hypertrophied hearts which could come close to clinical conditions are very rare and hardly lead to any definite conclusions (3, 11, 12, 23, 25, 30, 36).

The purpose of this work was to show the differences between the reactions of normal and hypertrophied hearts to ischaemia during normothermia and hypothermia (25°C); as well as to ascertain and examine the state of these hearts subsequent to reperfusion, and to assess how far these differences could be reduced or eliminated by using myocardial protecting agents such as St. Thomas solution or the calcium antagonist verapamil.

Material and methods

The experiments were performed on spontaneously hypertensive rats (SHR) aged 24 to 30 weeks and weighing 250–320 gm as well as on Wistar rats of the same age. The left ventricular/body ratio was significantly higher in SHR than in Wistar hearts ($3.6 \pm 0.5 \times 10^{-3}$ versus $2.0 \pm 0.3 \times 10^{-3}$ wet weight and $0.65 \pm 0.11 \times 10^{-3}$ versus $0.38 \pm 0.04 \times 10^{-3}$ dry weight respectively). The water content of the left ventricle and the right ventricular weight were not different between SHR and Wistar rats.

After cannulation of the aorta the hearts were perfused aerobically for a 15 minute period in a Langendorff apparatus at a perfusion pressure of 100 cm H_2O, followed by either a pure or cardioplegic cardiac arrest. Modified Krebs-Henseleit bicarbonate buffer gassed with carbogen (95% O_2 and 5% CO_2) was used as the perfusion solution.

To induce a pure ischemic cardiac arrest the perfusion to the heart was interrupted. For cardioplegic arrest the hearts were perfused after clamping the aortic cannula either by St. Thomas solution or verapamil solution (2 mg verapamil/liter Ringer's solution) at a speed of 3 ml/minute for 4 minutes. For hypothermic investigations the hearts were cooled after the 15 minute normothermic perfusion period by the perfusion medium to 25° C. The cardioplegic solutions were likewise perfused at a temperature of 25° C. After 30 minutes of normothermic ischemia or 120 minutes of hypothermic ischemia the hearts were reperfused at 37° C for 30 minutes. Coronary flow, the developed left ventricular pressure and dp/dt were measured before ischemia and after 30 minutes of reperfusion. The left ventricular pressure was measured using a fluid filled Latex ballon introduced into the left ventricle via the left atrium.

The heart rate was calculated from the left ventricular pressure curve. Because the hearts could not be paced at a constant rate, the pressure-rate product was used as a measure of the left ventricular function. The energy-rich phosphate levels were determined by the bioluminescence technique.

For statistical evaluation of the resulting experimental data multifactorial variance analysis was carried out, whereas the influence of independent variables – animal, temperature and mode of cardiac arrest on the variables pressure-rate product and energy-rich phosphates was analysed. For respective comparisons within groups the Scheffe procedure was employed. $P < 0.05$ was regarded as significant.

Results and discussion

Corresponding to the clinical conditions in which many patients in the compensated stage of left ventricular hypertrophy undergo open heart operations, animals which were not in heart failure but characterized by high degree of left ventricular hypertrophy were used in our experiments.

From the work of Bürger and Strauer (6, 7) and Mayr, Bürger and Strauer (24) it is concluded that hearts from spontaneously hypertensive rats up to the age of 40 weeks are not different from normal hearts of the same age with regard to left ventricular mechanics and myofibrillar ATPase activity. According to the definition of Wikman-Coffelt there is a "physiologic hypertrophy" in these animals (43).

Before ischemia, we found in hypertrophied hearts a significantly higher pressure-rate product, a decreased blood flow per g myocardium (SHR: 11.7 ± 1.5 ml/g/min, Wistar: 16.8 ± 3.9 ml/g/min) and a decreased ATP and adenine nucleotide content compared to normal hearts. Similar changes have been observed in hypertrophied hearts by other authors (1, 3, 4, 22, 30, 36).

For spontaneously hypertensive rats also a decreased growth of the capillaries during developing hypertrophy up to 7 months of age (39) and a decrease in reception and binding ability of the sarcoplasmatic reticulum for calcium ions in the presence of increased calcium-ATPase activity (20) was demonstrated.

The imbalance between energy production and its need during ischemia leads to a decrease in the important energy-rich phosphates, especially ATP, which are needed for the maintenance of normal cell functions. Dephosphorylization of adenine nucleotides through the monophosphate shunt leads to the loss of adenosine and inosine during reperfusion (29, 31, 40). After extended periods of ischemia the regeneration of ATP is thus limited because the rates of both "de novo synthesis" and "salvage pathway" of adenosine nucleotides are low (45). In several reports a close relationship between the content of myocardial energy-rich phosphates and the attainment of adequate left ventricular function after ischemia is postulated (31, 40, 42). Reduced ATP or adenine nucleotide content may not only be the cause of myocardial failure but appears to be an indicator of the damage to many myocardial structures (29, 40).

Apart from the loss of energy-rich phosphates during ischemia the excessive calcium inflow during reperfusion was connected to the irreversible damage of the myocardial cells (28, 34, 35). The increased level of calcium ions in the cytosol led to an uncoupling of the mitochondrial oxidative phosphorylization (41), activation of phospholipases accompanied by membrane damage (9), activation of the calcium ATPase resulting in diminution of the cellular energy reserve and decrease in intracellular pH (2) and to blocking of the sodium pump (37). In many experiments the favourable action of calcium antagonists on the myocardium during ischemia has been observed, where by the majority of investigators link the main action of these drugs to their negative inotropic effect (8, 18, 21, 27, 33, 42).

Apart from the mainly experimental tests with calcium antagonists, cold crystalloid hyperkalaemic solutions, in an optimal concentration of 15–35 mmol K^+/liter, are widely used to protect the myocardium under clinical conditions during open heart surgery (13, 15, 19, 32, 33). Hyperkalaemia leads, through depolarization of the cell membrane, to a rapid diastolic cardiac arrest and thus results in sparing cellular energy reserves (15, 19).

Our results indicate that the function of the hypertrophied heart is more damaged in normothermia as in hypothermia of 25° C by ischemia than the function of the normal heart. Normothermic ischemia is quite unfavourable for the hypertrophied ventricle because in our experiments more than half of the hypertrophied hearts developed left ventricular contracture during reperfusion (Fig. 1). This is in agreement with the clinical observation after normothermic ischemia reported by Cooley (10) and Najafi (26). Experimentally, Sink (36) and Attarian (4) have shown respectively in rats and dogs that after normothermic ischemia left ventricular contracture appeared earlier in hypertrophied hearts than in normal ones. Also Mundt and co-workers (25) stress that after ischemia the hypertrophied left ventricle is considerably depressed in comparison with the normal ventricle. According to them hypothermia and potassium cardioplegia were able to prevent these differences up to 75 minutes of ischemia.

Myocardial protection using St. Thomas solution gave favourable results in normothermia as well as in hypothermia. No differences were noticed in the decrease of the left ventricular function of normal and hypertrophied hearts. The corresponding fall in ATP or loss of adenine nucleotides during ischemic cardiac arrest modified by St. Thomas solution cardioplegia was the smallest and there were no differences between normal and hypertrophied hearts.

We postulate that through the rapid cardiac arrest after the start of ischemia only basal metabolism takes place which is not different for the hypertrophied and normal ventricles. However it cannot be ruled out that during prolonged ischemia there will be differences between normal and hypertrophied hearts. Coughlin and co-workers (11) induced cardiac arrest using potassium cardioplegia in hypertrophied and hypothermic canine hearts and they concluded that cardioplegia provided the same protection for normal and hypertrophied hearts. Ellis (12) on the other hand could not, under hypothermic conditions, obtain extra protection using potassium cardioplegia.

There is a different observation when verapamil solution is used as cardioplegic agent.

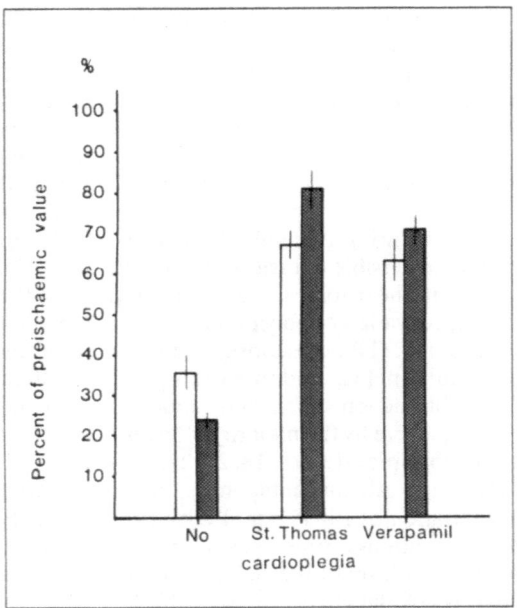

Fig. 1. Pressure-rate-product after normothermic ischemia (30 min) and reperfusion (30 min).
White bars: normal ventricle; dark bars: hypertrophied ventricle. No cardioplegia: normal hearts n = 9, hypertrophied hearts n = 11 – seven out of eleven hearts developed left ventricular contracture – St. Thomas solution: normal hearts n = 14, hypertrophied hearts n = 10; verapamil: normal hearts n = 12, hypertrophied hearts n = 11; ($\bar{x}$, ± SEM).

With regard to normothermic ischemia in normal hearts our results demonstrate, similar to other investigations (18, 21, 27, 33, 42), that verapamil cardioplegia gives good myocardial protection as does St. Thomas cardioplegia, considering the decrease in left ventricular function and the fall in ATP content and loss of adenine nucleotides (Fig. 1). On the other hand in hypertrophied hearts after normothermic ischemia there was a greater fall in ATP content and greater loss of adenine nucleotides following the use of verapamil than of St. Thomas solution for myocardial protection (Fig. 1). Despite the significant lower ATP and adenine nucleotide content after normothermic cardioplegic arrest of hypertrophied hearts with verapamil the left ventricular function is however maintained and not different to the hypertrophied hearts which are protected by St. Thomas solution.

As already shown by Yamamoto (44) and Hearse (18) in hypothermia of 25°C verapamil does not protect the normal heart more effectively than pure ischemic arrest. Hearse argued that by some mechanism common to both hypothermia and verapamil, the anti-ischemic and negative inotropic effects of verapamil are rendered redundant under conditions of hypothermia. In hypothermia verapamil is not significantly more effective than pure ischemic arrest in preventing ATP and adenine nucleotide loss from hypertrophied left ventricle, however left ventricular function is better maintained after verapamil than after ischemic arrest (Fig. 2). The cause of this discrepancy between ATP and adenine nucleotide content and the function of the hypertrophied hearts after verapamil cardioplegia, which was observed in our investigation in normo- and hypothermia is not clear. Possibly the disturbed calcium homeostasis is favourably influenced by verapamil.

Table 1. Myocardial high energy phosphate content (normal ventricle) before and after normothermic ischemia (30 min) and reperfusion (30 min).
Control: n = 9; no cardioplegia: n = 4; St. Thomas: n = 5; verapamil: n = 4; ($\bar{x}$, ± SEM)

	Control	Cardioplegia Nil	St. Thomas	Verapamil
ATP $\frac{nMol}{mg\ Protein}$	36.9 ± 1.6	6.1 ± 1.4	22.3 ± 1.7	21.3 ± 1.5
ADP $\frac{nMol}{mg\ Protein}$	6.4 ± 0.9	4.3 ± 0.4	4.4 ± 0.4	5.7 ± 0.8
AMP $\frac{nMol}{mg\ Protein}$	3.5 ± 0.8	6.3 ± 1.4	2.5 ± 1.0	2.2 ± 0.6
$\sum$ AN $\frac{nMol}{mg\ Protein}$	46.8 ± 2.1	16.5 ± 2.5	29.2 ± 2.1	29.2 ± 2.6
Energy charge	0.86 ± 0.02	0.50 ± 0.07	0.84 ± 0.03	0.83 ± 0.02
ATP/ADP	7.0 ± 1.2	1.4 ± 0.3	5.2 ± 0.08	4.0 ± 0.5

Table 2. Myocardial high energy phosphate content (hypertrophied ventricle) before and after normothermic ischemia (30 min) and reperfusion (30 min).
Control: n = 4; no cardioplegia: n = 4; St. Thomas: n = 4; verapamil: n = 4; ($\bar{x}$, ± SEM)

	Control	Cardioplegia Nil	St. Thomas	Verapamil
ATP $\frac{nMol}{mg\ Protein}$	$30.6\ \pm 1.5$	$3.1\ \pm 0.8$	$20.8\ \pm 1.0$	$13.1\ \pm 1.2$
ADP $\frac{nMol}{mg\ Protein}$	$4.7\ \pm 0.5$	$3.2\ \pm 0.4$	$4.3\ \pm 0.5$	$3.8\ \pm 0.3$
AMP $\frac{nMol}{mg\ Protein}$	$1.6\ \pm 0.5$	$5.0\ \pm 0.4$	$1.9\ \pm 0.2$	$2.5\ \pm 0.2$
$\sum$ AN $\frac{nMol}{mg\ Protein}$	$35.9\ \pm 1.5$	$11.3\ \pm 0.7$	$27.0\ \pm 0.8$	$19.4\ \pm 1.4$
Energy charge	0.89 ± 0.02	0.41 ± 0.06	0.85 ± 0.02	0.77 ± 0.01
ATP/ADP	$6.8\ \pm 0.8$	0.94 ± 0.14	$5.2\ \pm 1.0$	$3.5\ \pm 0.4$

Table 3. Myocardial high energy phosphate content (normal ventricle) before hypothermic ischemia (25°C, 120 min) and after reperfusion (30 min). Control: n = 9; no cardioplegia: n = 6; St. Thomas: n = 6; verapamil: n = 8; ($\bar{x}$, ± SEM)

	Control	Cardioplegia Nil	St. Thomas	Verapamil
ATP $\frac{nMol}{mg\ Protein}$	$36.9\ \pm 1.6$	$6.1\ \pm 0.8$	$15.4\ \pm 1.8$	$7.9\ \pm 0.7$
ADP $\frac{nMol}{mg\ Protein}$	$6.4\ \pm 0.9$	$3.2\ \pm 0.5$	$3.7\ \pm 0.3$	$3.6\ \pm 0.3$
AMP $\frac{nMol}{mg\ Protein}$	$3.5\ \pm 0.8$	$2.1\ \pm 0.2$	$1.0\ \pm 0.2$	$1.5\ \pm 0.3$
$\sum$ AN $\frac{nMol}{mg\ Protein}$	$46.8\ \pm 2.1$	$11.4\ \pm 1.4$	$20.1\ \pm 0.4$	$13.0\ \pm 0.9$
Energy charge	0.86 ± 0.02	0.67 ± 0.02	0.85 ± 0.03	0.74 ± 0.02
ATP/ADP	$7.0\ \pm 1.2$	$2.0\ \pm 0.09$	$4.3\ \pm 0.07$	$2.3\ \pm 0.2$

Table 4. Myocardial high energy phosphate content (hypertrophied ventricle) before hypothermic ischemia (25°C, 120 min) and after reperfusion (30 min). Control: n = 4; no cardioplegia: n = 6; St. Thomas: n = 6; verapamil: n = 6; ($\overline{x}$, ± SEM)

	Control	Cardioplegia Nil	St. Thomas	Verapamil
ATP $\frac{nMol}{mg\ Protein}$	30.6 ±1.5	7.8 ±1.6	15.3 ±1.7	11.8 ±0.9
ADP $\frac{nMol}{mg\ Protein}$	4.7 ±0.5	4.1 ±0.5	4.8 ±0.5	4.8 ±0.5
AMP $\frac{nMol}{mg\ Protein}$	1.6 ±0.5	3.5 ±0.3	2.5 ±0.3	2.3 ±0.3
$\sum$ AN $\frac{nMol}{mg\ Protein}$	35.9 ±1.5	15.4 ±1.9	22.6 ±1.9	18.6 ±1.2
Energy charge	0.89±0.02	0.62±0.04	0.78±0.02	0.75±0.02
ATP/ADP	6.8 ±0.8	2.0 ±0.2	3.4 ±0.4	2.7 ±0.3

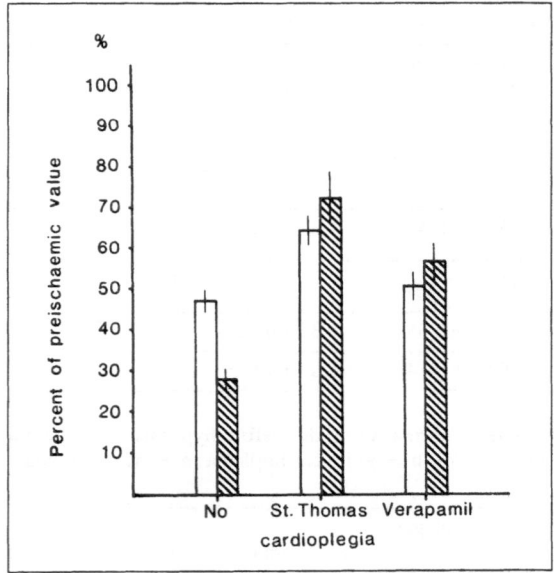

Fig. 2. Pressure-rate-product after hypothermic ischemia 25°C, 120 min and reperfusion (30 min).
White bars: normal ventricle; dark bars: hypertrophied ventricle. No cardioplegia: normal hearts n = 12, hypertrophied hearts n = 8; St. Thomas solution: normal hearts n = 8, hypertrophied hearts n = 10; verapamil: normal hearts n = 11, hypertrophied n = 8; ($\overline{x}$, ± SEM).

Under hypothermic conditions the fall in ATP content and loss of adenine nucleotides was lower in all cases of hypertrophied ventricles than in normal ones, whereas these changes are more pronounced but not significant in verapamil cardioplegia than during the St. Thomas cardioplegic arrest.

The possible cause of this may lie in a different type of compartmentalization of ATP and adenine nucleotides in hypertrophied ventricles. Despite the considerably greater fall in ATP content and greater adenine nucleotide loss "energy charge" was better maintained in normal hearts than in hypertrophied ones after hypothermic ischemia.

On the basis of these experiments it could be stated that only unmodified ischemia strongly damages the hypertrophied ventricle more than the normal one. The statement by Mavroudis (23) that hypertrophied or diseased hearts react to ischemia differently than normal hearts confirms and underlines the necessity for the observed perceptions regarding myocardial protection of the normal hearts to be verified also in diseased hearts.

Whether different results can be obtained by using other models of left ventricular hypertrophy which correspond to "pathological hypertrophy" according to the definition of Wikman-Coffelt, needs further investigation.

Acknowledgment

For technical assistance we thank I. Metzdorf and O.-W. Mensah.

References

1. Alfaro A, Schaible TF, Malhotra A, Yipintsoi T, Scheuer J (1983) Impaired coronary flow and ventricular function in hearts of hypertensive rats. Cardiovasc Res 17: 553–561
2. Arruda JAL, Dytko G, Lubansky H, Mola R, Klebs R, Burt CT (1981) Effect of calcium on intracellular pH. Biochem Biophys Res Commun 102: 891–896
3. Attarian DE, Jones RN, Currie WD, Hill RC, Sink JD, Olsen CO, Chitwood WR Jr, Wechsler AS (1981) Characteristics of chronic left ventricular hypertrophy induced by subcoronary valvular aortic stenosis. I Myocardial blood flow and metabolism. J Thorac Cardiovasc Surg 81: 382–388
4. Attarian DE, Jones RN, Currie WD, Hill RC, Sink JD, Olsen CO, Chitwood WR Jr, Wechsler AS (1981) Characteristics of chronic left ventricular hypertrophy induced by subcoronary valvular aortic stenosis. II. Response to ischemia. J Thorac Cardiovasc Surg 81: 389–395
5. Bing OHL, Matsushita S, Fanburg BL, Levine HJ (1971) Mechanical properties of rat cardiac muscle during experimental hypertrophy. Circ Res 28: 234–245
6. Bürger SB, Strauer BE (1981) Left ventricular hypertrophy in chronic pressure load due to spontaneous essential hypertension. I. Left ventricular function, left ventricular geometry, and wall stress. In: Strauer BE (ed) The Heart in Hypertenson. Springer-Verlag, Berlin Heidelberg New York, pp 13–35
7. Bürger SB, Strauer BE (1981) Left ventricular hypertrophy in chronic pressure overload due to spontaneous hypertension. II. Contractility of the isolated left ventricular myocardium and left ventricular stiffness. In: Strauer BE (ed) The Heart in Hypertension. Springer-Verlag, Berlin Heidelberg New York, pp 37–52
8. Cheung JY, Leaf A, Bonventre JV (1984) Mechanism of protection by verapamil and nifedipine from anoxic injury in isolated cardiac myocytes. Am J Physiol 246: C323–C329
9. Chien KR, Abrams J, Serroni A, Martin JT, Farber JL (1978) Accelerated phospholipid degradation and associated membrane dysfunction in irreversible, ischemic liver cell injury. J Biol Chem 253: 4809–4817
10. Cooley DA, Reul GJ, Wukasch DC (1972) Ischemic contracture of the heart "Stone heart". Am J Cardiol 29: 575–577
11. Coughlin TR, Levitsky S, O'Donoghue M, Williams L, Wright RN, Roper K, Feinberg H (1979) Evaluation of hypothermic cardioplegia in ventricular hypertrophy. Circulation 60 (Suppl I): 164–169
12. Ellis RJ, Pryor W, Ebert PA (1977) Advantages of potassium cardioplegia and perfusion hypothermia in left ventricular hypertrophy. Ann Thorac Surg 24: 299–306
13. Gharagozloo F, Bulkley BH, Hutchins GM, Bixler TJ, Schaff HV, Flaherty JT, Gardner TJ (1979) Potassium-induced cardioplegia during normothermic cardiac arrest. Morphologic study of the

effect of varying concentrations of potassium on myocardial anoxic injury. J Thorac Cardiovasc Surg 77: 602–607

14. Hamrell BB, Alpert NR (1977) The mechanical characteristics of hypertrophied rabbit cardiac muscle in the absence of congestive heart failure. Circ Res 40: 20

15. Hearse DJ, Braimbridge MV, Jynge P (1981) Protection of the ischemic myocardium: cardioplegia. Raven Press, New York

16. Hearse DJ, Yamamoto F, Shattock MJ (1984) Calcium antagonists and hypothermia: the temperature dependency ot the negative inotropic and antiischemic properties of verapamil in the isolated rat heart. Circulation 70 (Suppl I): 54–64

17. Jacob R, Kissling G (1981) Left ventricular dynamics and myocardial function in Goldblatt hypertension of the rat. Biochemical, morphological and electrophysiological correlates. In: Strauer BE (ed) The Heart in Hypertension. Springer-Verlag, Berlin Heidelberg New York, pp 89–106

18. Jolly SR, Menahan LA, Gross GJ (1981) Diltiazem in myocardial recovery from global ischemia and reperfusion. J Mol Cell Cardiol 13: 359–372

19. Jynge P (1980) Protection of the ischemic myocardium. Cold chemical cardioplegia, coronary infusates and the importance of cellular calcium control. Thorac Cardiovasc Surg 28: 310–321

20. Limas CJ, Cohn JN (1977) Defective calcium transport by cardiac sarcoplasmatic reticulum in spontaneously hypertensive rats. Circ Res 40 (Suppl I): 62–69

21. Magee PG, Flaherty JT, Bixler TJ, Glower D, Gardner TJ, Bulkley BH, Gott VL (1979) Comparison of myocardial protection with nifedipine and potassium. Circulation 60 (Suppl I): 151–157

22. Malik AB, Geha AS (1977) Cardiac function, coronary flow and MV02 in hypertrophy in induced by pressure and volume overloading. Cardiovasc Res 11: 310–316

23. Mavroudis C, Ebert PA (1979) Effects of high potassium cardioplegia and hypothermia on myocardial compliance and distribution of water and potassium. II. The hypertrophied canine heart. Surgery 85: 662–670

24. Mayr GW, Bürger S, Strauer BE (1981) Properties of myocardial myosin in left ventricular hypertrophy due to spontaneous essential hypertension. In: Strauer BE (ed) The Heart in Hypertension. Springer-Verlag, Berlin Heidelberg New York, pp 131–141

25. Mundth ED, Goel IP, Morgan RJ, McEnany MT, Austen WG (1975) Effect of potassium cardioplegia and hypothermia on left ventricular function in hypertrophied and nonhypertrophied hearts. Surg Forum 26: 257–258

26. Najafi H, Henson D, Dye WS, Javid H, Hunter JA, Callaghan R, Julian OC (1969) Left ventricular hemorrhagic necrosis. Ann Thorac Surg 7: 550–561

27. Nayler WG, Ferrari R, Williams A (1980) Protective effect of pretreatment with verapamil, nifedipine and propanolol on mitochondrial function in the ischemic and reperfused myocardium. Am J Cardiol 46: 242–248

28. Nayler WG (1981) The role of calcium in the ischemic myocardium. Am J Pathol 102: 262–270

29. Neely JR, Rovetto MJ, Whitmer JT, Morgan HE (1973) Effects of ischemia on function and metabolism of the isolated working rat heart. Am J Physiol 225: 651–658

30. Peyton RB, Jones RN, Attarian D, Sink JD, van Trigt P, Currie WD, Wechsler AS (1982) Depressed high-energy phosphate content in hypertrophied ventricles of animal and man. Ann Surg 196: 278–283

31. Reibel DK, Rovetto MJ (1978) Myocardial ATP synthesis and mechanical function following oxygen deficiency. Am J Physiol 234: H620–H624

32. Rousou JH, Engelman RM, Dobbs WA, Lemeshow S (1981) The optimal potassium concentration in cardioplegic solutions. Ann Thorac Surg 32: 75–79

33. Robb-Nicholson C, Currie WD, Wechsler AS (1976) Effects of Verapamil on myocardial tolerance to ischemic arrest. Comparison to potassium arrest. Circulaton 58 (Suppl I): 119–124

34. Shen AC, Jennings RB (1972) Myocardial calcium and magnesium in acute ischemic injury. Am J Pathol 67: 417–440

35. Shen AC, Jennings RB (1972) Kinetics of calcium accumulation in acute myocardial ischemic injury. Am J Pathol 67: 441–452

36. Sink JD, Pellom GL, Currie WD, Hill RC, Olsen CO, Jones RN, Wechsler AS (1981) Response of hypertrophied myocardium to ischemia. Correlation with biochemical and physiological parameters. J Thorac Cardiovasc Surg 81: 865–872

37. Skou JC (1957) The influence of some cations on an adenosine triphosphatase from peripheral nerves. Biochim Biophys Acta 23: 394–401
38. Swynghedauw B, Schwartz K, Lacombe G, Leger JJ, Thiem NV, Lompre AM (1981) Cardiac myosin in heart overloading. In: Strauer BE (ed) The Heart in Hypertension. Springer-Verlag, Berlin Heidelberg New York, pp 125–130
39. Tomanek RJ, Searls JC, Lachenbruch PA (1982) Quantitative changes in the capillary bed during developing, peak, and stabilized cardiac hypertrophy in the spontaneously hypertensive rat. Cir Res 51: 295–304
40. Vary TC, Angelakos ET, Schaffer SW (1979) Relationship between adenine nucleotide metabolism and irreversible ischemic tissue damage in isolated perfused rat heart. Circ Res 45: 218–225
41. Villalobo A, Lehninger AL (1980) Inhibition of oxidative phosphorylation in ascites tumor mitochondria and cells by intramitochondrial Ca. J Biol Chem 255: 2457–2464
42. Watts JA, Koch CD, La Noue KF (1980) Effects of Ca antagonism on energy metabolism: Ca and heart function after ischemia. Am J Physiol 238: H909–H916
43. Wikman-Coffelt J, Parmley WW, Mason DT (1979) The cardiac hypertrophy process. Analyses of factors determining pathological vs. physiological development. Circ Res 45: 697–707
44. Yamamoto F, Manning AS, Braimbridge MV, Hearse DJ (1983) Cardioplegia and slow calcium-channel blockers. Studies with Verapamil. J Thorac Cardiovasc Surg 86: 252–261
45. Zimmer H, Trendelenburg C, Kammermeier H, Gerlach E (1973) De novo synthesis of myocardial adenine nucleotides in the rat. Circ Res 32: 635–642

Authors' address:

Dr. G. Fenchel, Abt. Thorax-, Herz- u. Gefäßchirurgie, Chirurgische Klinik Tübingen, Calwer Straße 7, D-7400 Tübingen (F.R.G.)

IV. Chronic reactions of the myocardium – Determinants of hypertrophy development and regression

Metabolic aspects of the development of experimental cardiac hypertrophy*

H.-G. Zimmer and H. Peffer

Physiologisches Institut der Universität München, Munich (F. R. G.)

Summary

In three models of cardiac hypertrophy the significance of catecholamines and the adenylate cyclase – cyclic AMP – system was examined. Two approaches were utilized: 1. The time course of cyclic AMP alterations was correlated with the changes in adenine nucleotide and protein biosynthesis. 2. The effect of β-receptor blockade on the obligatory increase in adenine nucleotide and protein synthesis was evaluated. In isoproterenol-elicited cardiac hypertrophy, the elevation of the cyclic AMP content was one of the earliest metabolic alterations preceding the enhancement of the biosynthesis of adenine nucleotides and proteins. β-Receptor blockade with propranolol abolished the increase in adenine nucleotide synthesis. In pressure-induced cardiac hypertrophy due to constriction of the abdominal aorta, catecholamines and the adenylate cyclase – cyclic AMP – system were found not to play a significant role. In triiodothyronine-elicited hypertrophy, the cyclic AMP level was increased very early, but β-receptor blockade did not prevent hypertrophy nor the enhancement of cardiac adenine nucleotide biosynthesis, although the positive chronotropic and inotropic effects of triiodothyronine were abolished. This result can best be interpreted to indicate a direct effect of triiodothyronine on myocardial carbohydrate metabolism including the pentose phosphate pathway.

Key words: adenine nucleotide biosynthesis, aortic constriction, catecholamines, cyclic AMP, pentose phosphate pathway, protein synthesis, triiodothyronine

Introduction

It is well established that the increased synthesis of myocardial ribonucleic acids (RNA) and proteins is one of the key metabolic events underlying the development of cardiac hypertrophy (10, 19, 22, 25). In trying to define the mechanism (or mechanisms) involved in triggering the growth of the heart in various experimental hypertrophy models, it seemed most appropriate to examine those metabolic processes that precede the enhancement of RNA and protein synthesis.

One of these early alterations is the increase in myocardial ornithine decarboxylase activity and the ultimate enhancement of the spermine and spermidine content (3, 4, 18, 23). That spermine may have a trigger function was suggested by experiments in which the addition of spermine to the perfusion medium stimulated RNA synthesis in isolated guinea-pig hearts (4, 21). This concept has recently been examined in a more direct and elegant way by application of α-difluoro-methylornithine which is a potent, selective and irreversible inhibitor of ornithine decarboxylase. It turned out that this inhibitor prevented the increase in ornithine decarboxylase activity both in isoproterenol- and triiodothyronine-induced cardiac hyper-

---

* This study was supported by the Deutsche Forschungsgemeinschaft (Zi 199/4-4)

trophy. However, the increase in heart weight was attenuated only in isoproterenol-induced hypertrophy, whereas cardiac hypertrophy elicited by triiodothyronine was not at all influenced. It thus appears that there are ornithine decarboxylase – dependent and – independent models of cardiac hypertrophy (2).

Another concept is based on the idea that metabolites that originate during increased heart work such as creatine (11, 12) or that the decline of high energy phosphate compounds such as ATP (20) may serve as signals for the stimulation of RNA and protein synthesis. As far as creatine is concerned, it was shown that it does not increase in rat hearts during the development of hyertrophy due to aortic constriction but rather declines quite rapidly (26). Furthermore, the original result that creatine stimulates myosin synthesis in skeletal muscle cell cultures and in embryonic chicken heart cells could not be reproduced (8). Thus, this hypothesis could not be substantiated.

As regards the decline of the ATP content, this is in fact a metabolic feature characteristic for many models of experimental cardiac hypertrophy (33). It is thus not surprising that the decrease of ATP was considered to activate the genetic apparatus of the cardiac cell ultimately resulting in the enhancement of protein synthesis. However, there are several independent lines of evidence to the contrary (17, 28). In a more direct approach, the alleged trigger, the ATP decline, was eliminated. This was achieved in the hypertrophying rat heart due to isoproterenol administration by continuous i. v. infusion of ribose. This pentose stimulates cardiac adenine nucleotide biosynthesis to such an extent that the isoproterenol-induced ATP decline was prevented entirely. Yet, protein synthesis was increased to the same extent. Thus, at least in this hypertrophy model, the diminution of ATP could not be considered to be the trigger for the enhancement of protein synthesis (38).

In this situation the catecholamines deserve serious attention as possible regulators in the processes responsible for the initation of cardiac hypertrophy. In particular, 3′,5′-cyclic AMP (cyclic AMP), the established second messenger of the action of catecholamines (27) is known to be involved in various phosphorylation processes (13, 30). In this contribution, the role of catecholamines and of cyclic AMP will be examined in three models of cardiac hypertrophy in the rat. To do this, two experimental approaches will be applied. In the first, the time course of changes in the content of cardiac cyclic AMP will be compared with the time-dependent alterations of the biosynthesis of adenine nucleotides and of proteins. In previous studies, the enhancement of adenine nucleotide biosynthesis was shown to be an obligatory event in the development of cardiac hypertrophy which always occurred prior to the increase in protein synthesis (33). If cyclic AMP has a role to play, then its content should be elevated before the synthesis of adenine nucleotides and proteins reaches the maximal level. In the second approach, β-receptor blockers were applied in the three cardiac hypertrophy models. It was then examined whether the obligatory stimulation of adenine nucleotide and protein synthesis as well as the development of cardiac hypertrophy was influenced.

Own studies

Methodological procedures

From the many cardiac hypertrophy models three were selected for these studies. Pressure-induced hypertrophy was produced in rats (220–240 g body weight) by constriction of the abdominal aorta to a diameter of 0.65 mm (37). Hypertrophy of both ventricles was elicited by isoproterenol (29) administered as a single s. c. dose of 25 mg/kg. The other chemical hypertrophy model was produced by 3,3′,5-triiodo-L-thyronine which was given every 24 hours s. c. in a dose of 0.2 mg/kg (33).

. The content of cardiac cyclic AMP was determined using the radioimmunoassay of Gilman (9). The biosynthesis of myocardial adenine nucleotides was assessed by relating the total radioactivity of adenine nucleotides due to the incorporation of 1-^{14}C-glycine during their de novo synthesis to the mean specific activity of the glycine precursor pool in the tissue (39). In a similar approach, protein synthesis was expressed by relating the total radioactivity of proteins resulting from the incorporation of 1-^{14}C-glycine to the mean specific activity of glycine (37).

The hemodynamic parameters were measured using the ultraminiature catheter pressure transducer (model PR-249, Millar Instruments, Inc., Houston, Texas) which was inserted via the right carotid artery into the left ventricle of closed-chest rats anesthetized with thiobuta-barbital sodium (Inactin® Byk, 80 mg/kg, i. p.). This method is reliable, rapid, easy to perform and non-destructive (32).

Results

After administration of isoproterenol, the earliest metabolic alteration was the elevation of the cardiac cyclic AMP pool that occurred prior to the enhancement of adenine nucleotide and protein synthesis (Fig. 1). Thus, there was clearly a sequential increase in these three

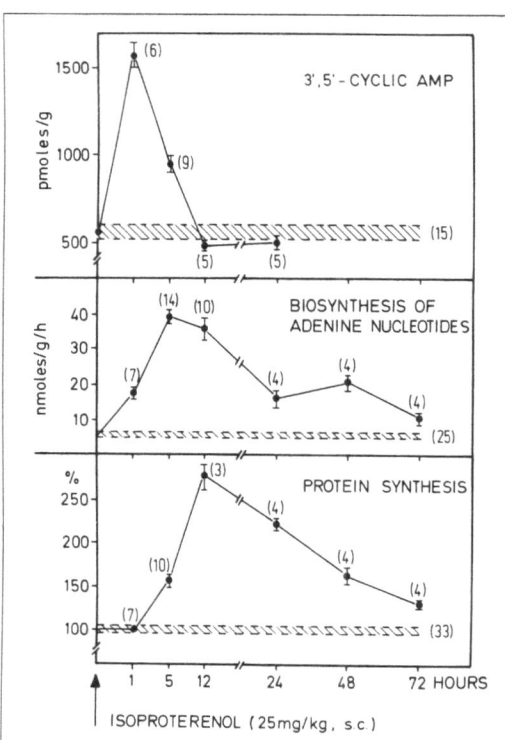

Fig. 1. Changes in the content of myocardial cyclic AMP, in the biosynthesis of adenine nucleotide and in protein synthesis subsequent to a single s. c. injection of isoproterenol. Mean values ± SEM, number of experiments in parentheses.

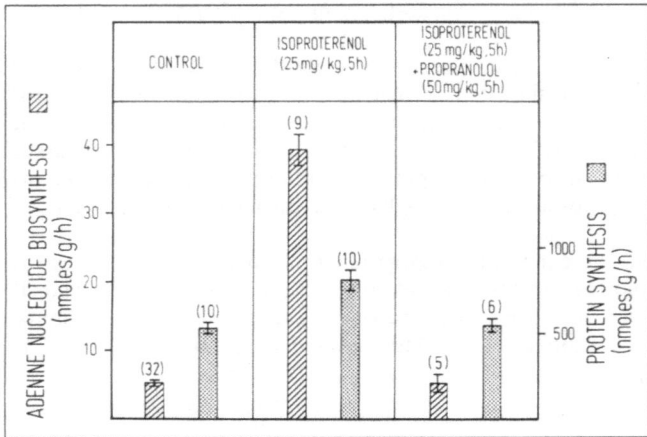

Fig. 2. Increase of the biosynthesis of cardiac adenine nucleotides and of protein synthesis induced by isoproterenol and prevention of the enhancement by propranolol. Measurements were made 5 hours after application of the respective drugs. Mean values ± SEM, number of experiments in parentheses.

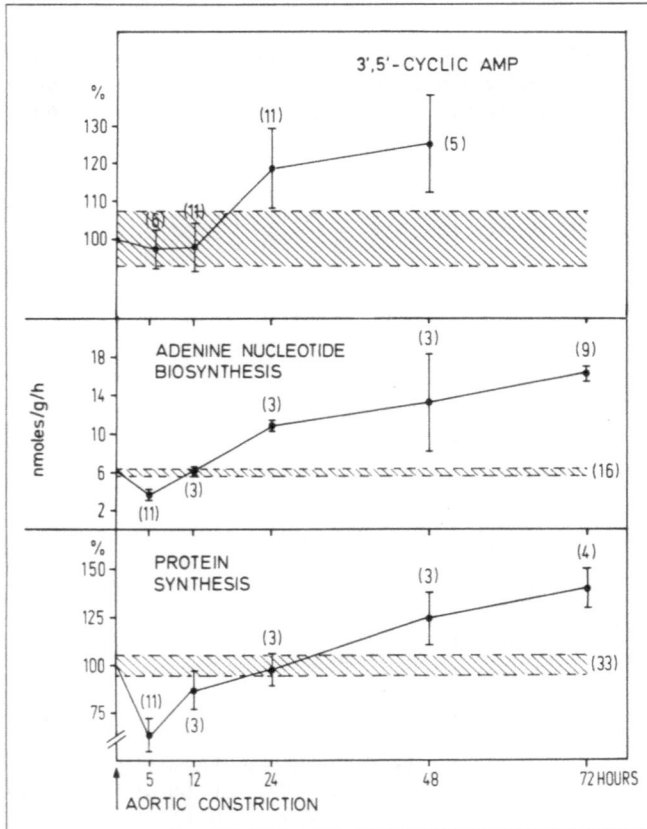

Fig. 3. Alterations in the content of cardiac cyclic AMP, in adenine nucleotide biosynthesis and in protein synthesis during the development of cardiac hypertrophy due to constriction of the abdominal aorta. Mean values ± SEM, number of experiments in parentheses.

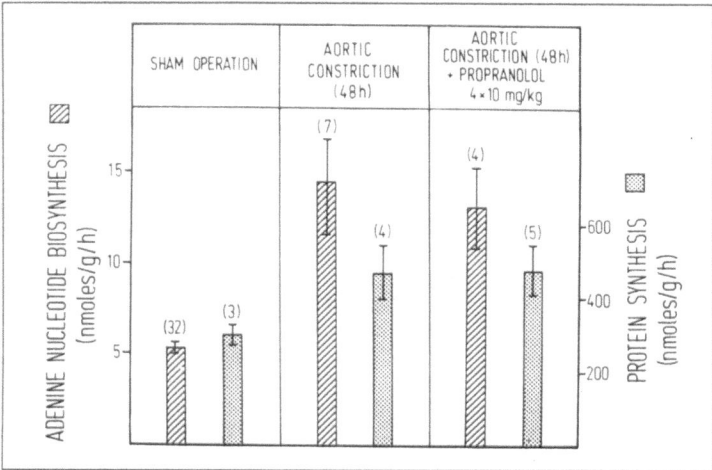

Fig. 4. Changes in myocardial adenine nucleotide and protein synthesis induced by aortic constriction and the effect of propranolol. Measurements were made 48 hours after constriction of the abdominal aorta. Mean values ± SEM, number of experiments in parentheses.

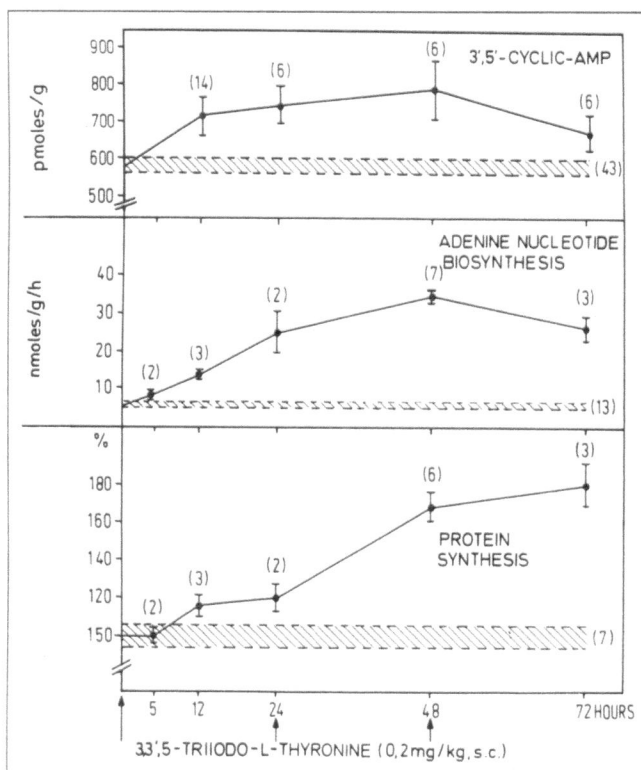

Fig. 5. Time course of changes in the content of cardiac cyclic AMP, in adenine nucleotide biosynthesis and in protein synthesis during the development of hypertrophy elicited by daily s. c. injection of triiodothyronine. Mean values ± SEM, number of experiments in parentheses.

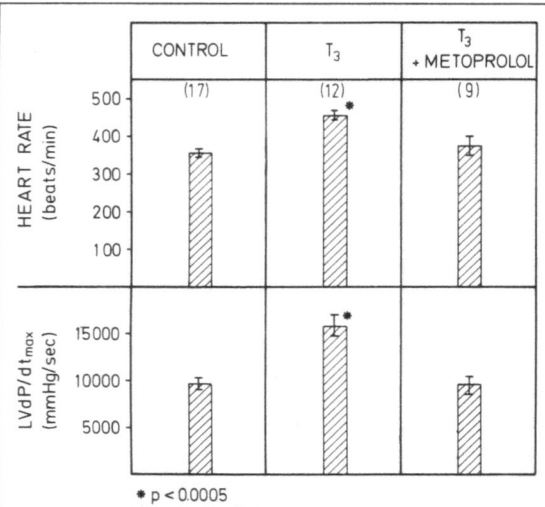

Fig. 6. Changes in heart rate and in LVdP/dt$_{max}$ in rats after 3 days of daily treatment with triiodothyronine given alone or in combination with metoprolol. Metoprolol was administered as continuous i. v. infusion in a dose of 1 mg/kg/h. The hemodynamic parameters were obtained using the Millar ultraminiature catheter pressure transducer (model PR-249) which was implanted in the left ventricle via the right carotid artery. Mean values ± SEM, number of experiments in parentheses.

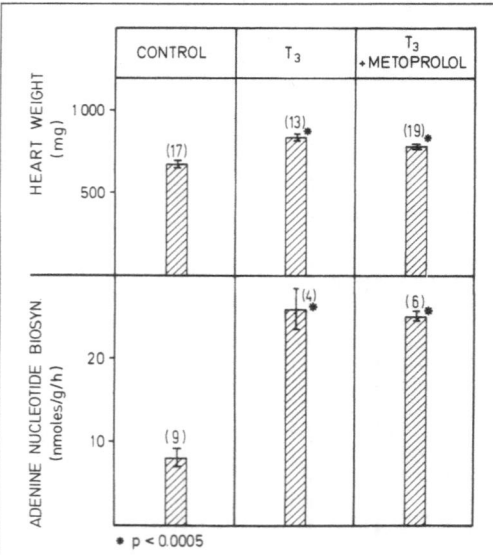

Fig. 7. Effect of triiodothyronine and of triiodothyronine in combination with metoprolol (1 mg/kg/h continuous i. v. infusion) for 3 days on heart weight and on the rates of cardiac adenine nucleotide biosynthesis in rats. Mean values ± SEM, number of experiments in parentheses.

metabolic parameters. From this time course relationship it may be suggested that the enhancement of the cyclic AMP content is the signal triggering the increase of adenine mucleotide and protein synthesis. To test this hypothesis, the increase in the cardiac cyclic AMP level was prevented by β-receptor blockade with propranolol. As a consequence, the biosynthesis of adenine nucleotides and proteins was not enhanced any more (Fig. 2).

The situation was quite different in pressure-induced hypertrophy. In this model, the elevation of the cardiac cyclic AMP pool was only moderate and occurred at the same time as the enhancement of adenine nucleotide biosynthesis which preceded the increase in protein synthesis (Fig. 3). Thus, after constriction of the abdominal aorta, cyclic AMP had obviously no signal function. This was supported by the finding that the enhancement of adenine nucleotide and protein synthesis was not at all influenced by propranolol treatment (Fig. 4).

When triiodothyronine was administered in rats, there was an early elevation of the cyclic AMP pool that occurred before adenine nucleotide and protein synthesis became maximally increased (Fig. 5). Since triiodothyronine induced pronounced hemodynamic alterations, it was first examined whether the β-receptor blocker metoprolol may have an influence. After three days of daily injections of triiodothyronine, heart rate and LV dP/dt$_{max}$ were significantly increased. When metoprolol had been administered as continuous i. v. infusion for three days, these triiodothyronine-evoked hemodynamic changes were entirely prevented (Fig. 6). However, the increase in heart weight induced by triiodothyronine was not affected appreciably by metropolol. Thus, there was a dissociation between the triiodothyronine-elicited increase in the hemodynamic parameters which were normalized by metroprolol and the development of cardiac hypertrophy which was not influenced by metoprolol (Fig. 6, 7). Interestingly, also the enhancement of cardiac adenine nucleotide biosynthesis induced by triiodothyronine was not affected by metropolol (Fig. 7).

Discussion

1. Isoproterenol-induced cardiac hypertrophy

From these studies it appears that the role of catecholamines in the development of cardiac hypertrophy is quite different in the three experimental models examined. The most clear-cut situation was found when cardiac hypertrophy was induced by isoproterenol. In this model, it is the early increase in cyclic AMP which precedes all other metabolic alterations that must be envisaged as obligatory events. Among these, the enhancement of cardiac adenine nucleotide biosynthesis seems to function as the metabolic link between the cyclic AMP signal and the increase in protein synthesis (Fig. 1). This view is substantiated by the finding that the enhancement of adenine nucleotide biosynthesis along with protein synthesis is abolished when the elevation of cyclic AMP is prevented by a β-receptor-blocking agent. The mechanism by which cyclic AMP may exert its trigger function will be discussed from the temporal and causal point of view in regard to two questions. The first is how adenine nucleotide biosynthesis becomes stimulated. There seem to be two distinct phases. During the first few hours, the enhanced glycolysis which occurs as a consequence of the isoproterenol-induced stimulation of glycogenolysis may affect the pentose phosphate pathway either via the oxidative or the non-oxidative branch. In this way, the elevation of the available pool of 5-phosphoribosyl-1-pyrophosphate can be explained which was found throughout the entire period of time following isoproterenol administration (35). Since 5-phosphoribosyl-1-pyrophosphate is an essential precursor substrate for the biosynthesis of adenine nucleotides, it is reasonable to assume that the early increase in this biosynthetic process is brought about via the oxidative or non-oxidative pentose phosphate pathway. However, after 12 hours, the cyclic AMP level and glycogenolysis had returned to control. Thus another mechanism must be envisaged for adenine nucleotide biosynthesis to be maintained at a higher than normal level (Fig. 1). It is exactly at this time that the activity of glucose-6-phosphate dehydrogenase starts to be enhanced reaching a maximum after 48 hours (34, 35). This is the first and rate-limiting enyzme of the oxidative pentose phosphate pathway (6). Since its activity is rather low in the myocardium, the capacity of the oxidative pentose phosphate pathway is limiting for the production of 5-phosphoribosyl-1-pyrophosphate and ultimately for adenine nucleotide biosynthesis. Thus at this stage, when glycogenolysis has come back to normal, glucose-6-phosphate dehydrogenase takes over to keep adenine nucleotide biosynthesis stimulated (Fig. 1). The second question is related to the mechanism by which protein synthesis becomes enhanced. Obviously, the increase in adenine nucleotide biosynthesis plays a substantial role to provide precursors for RNA synthesis which is a prerequisite for protein synthesis. There may, however, also be cyclic AMP-mediated phosphorylation processes that may be involved in the rather rapid stimulation of protein synthesis (13).

2. Pressure-induced cardiac hypertrophy

Compared with the metabolic pattern in the isoproterenol model of cardiac hypertrophy the situation is entirely different in pressure-induced hypertrophy due to aortic constriction. In this type of hypertrophy cyclic AMP does not appear to play a significant role, and the enhancement of adenine nucleotide and protein synthesis does not occur with such rapidity and intensity as in the isoproterenol model (Fig. 3). That catecholamines do not have a role to play in the pressure hypertrophy model is derived from several lines of evidence. First, the increase of cyclic AMP is quite slow and moderate and does not occur prior to the enhancement of adenine nucleotide and protein synthesis. Thus, just taking into consideration the time course studies (Fig. 3), cyclic AMP is very unlikely to be a trigger factor. Furthermore, the increase in adenine nucleotide and protein synthesis does not respond to treatment with the β-receptor blocker propranolol (Fig. 4) so that these metabolic processes appear to become stimulated independently of catecholamines. Finally, the increase in the ratio heart weight/body weight as a measure of cardiac hypertrophy is not influenced by the β-receptor blocker practolol (17). In this context it may be mentioned that depletion of noradrenaline stores with 6-hydroxydopamine did not prevent the development of hypertrophy in hypertensive rats (5). In another hypertrophy model, the spontaneous hypertensive rat (SHR), treatment of pregnant rats with propranolol or timolol and continuation of this treatment in the newborn rats had no effect on the development of cardiac hypertrophy (24).

Since catecholamines do not appear to be involved in pressure-induced hypertrophy, the question arises as to the mechanism responsible for the enhancement of adenine nucleotide and protein synthesis. It is interesting to note that in previous studies glucose-6-phosphate dehydrogenase was found to be stimulated, and this stimulation occurred concomitantly with the increase in adenine nucleotide biosynthesis (36). Since an explanation for this stimulation of the oxidative pentose phosphate pathway in metabolic terms is not easy to find, one may consider mechanical factors to be involved. In fact, it was shown in various experimental models that stretch of muscle fibers is accompanied by an increased transport of amino acids. This was found in isolated papillary muscle (14), in the isolated perfused rat heart (1) and in embryonic skeletal myotubes (31). In the latter preparation, stretch also induced an increase in myosin and total protein synthesis. Thus, there are some examples of metabolic effects evoked by mechanical alterations. Whether these effects are the direct result of mechanical changes or whether they are mediated by some metabolic link, and if so, by what kind of metabolic factors, remains to be elucidated in future studies.

3. Cardiac hypertrophy due to triiodothyronine treatment

There are some particular features that are characteristic for this hypertrophy model. The cyclic AMP level obviously is elevated quite early and remains clearly elevated at least for the first 48 hours. This cyclic AMP increase occurs prior to the maximal enhancement of adenine nucleotide and protein synthesis (Fig. 5). On the other hand, β-receptor blockade with metoprolol does not prevent the development of cardiac hypertrophy and the enhancement of adenine nucleotide biosynthesis (Fig. 7), whereas it absolishes readily the hemodynamic alterations such as the increase in heart rate and in LV dP/dt$_{max}$ (Fig. 6). Thus, there is a dissociation of the development of cardiac hypertrophy from the hemodynamic changes. Cardiac hypertrophy must therefore be triggered by purely metabolic factors. It is interesting to mention that in thyroxine-treated mice 6-hydroxydopamine failed to diminish the degree of cardiac hypertrophy (5).

What distinguishes the cyclic AMP increase in the triiodothyronine model (Fig. 5) from that in the isoproterenol model (Fig. 1), is that it is maintained for some period of time compared with the rapid increase and decline in the isoproterenol model. This prolongation of the elevated cyclic AMP level indicates the maintenance of the stimulation of glycogenolysis. In addition, effects on phosphorylase b kinase and on phosphorylase a were described under the influence of thyroid hormone (7). However, in contrast to the other two experimental models, the activity of glucose-6-phosphate dehydrogenase was not altered when triiodothyronine was administered, although the available pool of 5-phosphoribosyl-1-pyrophosphate turned out to be elevated (36). These findings can best be interpreted to indicate that glycogenolysis and glycolysis are stimulated continuously and that the 5-phosphoribosyl-1-pyrophosphate pool is kept elevated via the non-oxidative pentose phosphate pathway. This would then maintain the enhancement of adenine nucleotide biosynthesis which provides one on of the precursor substrates for RNA synthesis necessary for protein synthesis.

Since adenine nucleotide biosynthesis remains elevated when metoprolol is administered as continuous i. v. infusion, it can be concluded that this postulated sequence of metabolic events may take place even in the presence of β-receptor blockade. In fact, it was demonstrated by other authors in earlier studies that the adenylate cyclase – cyclic AMP – system is stimulated by thyroid hormone when the β-receptors are blocked (15). On the other hand, it is known that thyroid hormone has an intracellular receptor at the nucleus and can thereby trigger metabolic processes related to RNA and protein synthesis (16).

Conclusions

Obviously, there are different mechanisms operative in the three models of experimental cardiac hypertrophy examined in this study. The isoproterenol-induced hypertrophy is clearly dependent on the cyclic AMP increase, since the elevation of cyclic AMP is the first metabolic alteration preceding adenine nucleotide and protein synthesis stimulation and since these metabolic alterations characteristic for cardiac hypertrophy can be prevented by β-receptor blockade. On the other hand, pressure-induced hypertrophy, as judged by the same criteria, appears to be independent of catecholamines and the adenylate cyclase – cyclic AMP – system. Cardiac hypertrophy elicited by daily injections of triiodothyronine is accompanied by an early cyclic AMP increase, however, it cannot be prevented by β-receptor blockade which abolishes the positive chronotropic and inotropic effects of triiodothyronine. This finding is compatible with the stimulation of carbohydrate metabolism including the pentose phosphate pathway which contributes to the maintenance of the enhancement of adenine nucleotide biosynthesis and ultimately of protein synthesis.

Acknowledgements

The expert technical assistance of Ms G. Steinkopff and Ms M. Sagstetter is gratefully acknowledged. Dr. H. Peffer was a fellow of the Deutsche Forschungsgemeinschaft during this study (Zi 199/4-4).

136

References

1. Ahren K, Hjalmarson A, Isaksson O (1972) In vitro work load and rat heart metabolism. II. Effect on amino acid transport. Acta Physiol Scand 86: 257–270
2. Bartolome J, Huguenard J, Slotkin TA (1980) Role of ornithine decarboxylase in cardiac growth and hypertrophy. Science 210: 793–794
3. Caldarera CM, Casti A, Rossoni C, Visioli O (1971) Polyamines and noradrenaline following myocardial hypertrophy. J Mol Cell Cardiol 3: 121–126
4. Caldarera CM, Orlandini G, Casti A, Moruzzi G (1974) Polyamine and nucleic acid metabolism in myocardial hypertrophy of the overloaded heart. J Mol Cell Cardiol 6: 95–104
5. Cohen J (1974) Role of endocrine factors in the pathogenesis of cardiac hypertrophy. Circ Res 34, 35: II 49–II 57
6. Eggleston LV, Krebs HA (1974) Regulation of the pentose phosphate cycle. Biochem J 138: 425–435
7. Frazer A, Hess ME, Shanfeld J (1969) The effects of thyroxine on rat heart adenosine 3',5'-monophosphate, phosphorylase b kinase and phosphorylase a activity. J Pharmacol Exp Ther 170: 10–16
8. Fry DM, Morales MF (1980) A reexamination of the effects of creatine on muscle protein synthesis in tissue culture. J Cell Biol 84: 294–297
9. Gilman AG (1970) A protein binding assay for adenosine 3',5'-cyclic monophosphate. Proc Natl Acad Sci 78: 305–312
10. Gudbjarnason S, Telerman M, Bing RJ (1964) Protein metabolism in cardiac hypertrophy and heart failure. Am J Physiol 206: 294–298
11. Ingwall JS (1976) Creatine and the control of muscle-specific protein synthesis in cardiac and skeletal muscle. Circ Res 38: I 115–I 122
12. Ingwall JS, Weiner CD, Morales MF, Davis E, Stockdale FE (1974) Specificity of creatine in the control of muscle protein synthesis. J Cell Biol 63: 145–151
13. Langan TA (1968) Histone phosphorylation: Stimulation by adenosine 3',5'-monophosphate. Science 162: 579–580
14. Lesch M, Gorlin R, Sonnenblick EH (1970) Myocardial amino acid transport in the isolated rabbit right ventricular papillary muscle. Circ Res 27: 445–460
15. Levey GS, Epstein SE (1969) Myocardial adenyl cyclase: activation by thyroid hormones and evidence for two adenyl cyclase systems. J Clin Invest 48: 1663–1669
16. Limas CJ, Chan-Stier C (1978) Myocardial chromatin activation in experimental hyperthyroidism in rats. Role of nuclear non-histone proteins. Circ Res 42: 311–316
17. Malik AB, Geha AS (1975) Role of adrenergic mechanisms in the development of cardiac hypertrophy. Proc Soc Exp Biol Med 150: 796–800
18. Matsushita S, Sogani RK, Raben MS (1972) Ornithine decarboxylase in cardiac hypertrophy in the rat. Circ Res 31: 699–709
19. Meerson FZ (1962) Compensatory hyperfunction of the heart and cardiac insufficiency. Circ Res 10: 250–258
20. Meerson FZ, Pomoinitsky VD (1972) The role of high-energy phosphate compounds in the development of cardiac hypertrophy. J Mol Cell Cardiol 4: 571–597
21. Moruzzi G, Caldarera CM, Casti A (1974) The biological effect of polyamines on heart RNA and histone metabolism. Mol Cell Biochem 3: 153–161
22. Nair KG, Cutilleta AF, Zak R, Koide T, Rabinowitz M (1968) Biochemical correlates of cardiac hypertrophy. I. Experimental model; changes in heart weight, RNA content, and nuclear RNA polymerase activity. Circ Res 23: 451–462
23. Pegg AE, Hibasami H (1980) Polyamine metabolism during cardiac hypertrophy. Am J Physiol 239: E 372–E 378
24. Pfeffer MA, Pfeffer JM, Weiss AK, Frohlich ED (1977) Development of SHR hypertension and cardiac hypertrophy during prolonged beta blockade. Am J Physiol 232: H 639–H 644
25. Rabinowitz M, Zak R (1972) Biochemical and cellular changes in cardiac hypertrophy. Ann Rev Med 23: 245–262
26. Reilly PJ. Cooksey JD (1979) Cardiac energy stores and creatine in experimental cardiac hypertrophy, Proc Soc Exp Biol Med 161: 193–198

Authors' address:

H.-G. Zimmer, Physiologisches Institut der Universität München, Pettenkoferstraße 12, D-8000 München 2 (F.R.G.)

Intracellular turnover and cardiac hypertrophy

U. Pfeifer and J. Dämmrich

Pathologisches Institut der Unviersität Würzburg, Würzburg (F.R.G.)

Summary

Ultrastructural evidence is presented that intracellular autophagic degradation of cytoplasmic constituents is reduced during perssure induced hypertropy of left ventricular myocardium after supravalvular aortic constriction in rats. This anti-catabolic reaction has to be considered as an important mechanism for shifting the balance between synthesis and degradation to the positive side. Short term studies after administration of isoproterenol suggest a close functional relationship between work load on the one hand and the anti-catabolic reaction on the other.

Key words: cellular autophagy, protein turnover, hypertrophy, aortic constriction, isoproterenol, electron microscopy, morphometry

Introduction

The term cardiac hypertrophy is commonly used in a static sense, i. e. to characterize the state of increased mass of myocardium. From this aspect, questions as to how structural and functional properties of heart muscle are altered in the hypertrophic state may be well to the fore. Hypertrophy can also be taken, however, to designate the process of increase in size of cardiomyocytes and increase in number of the subcellular structures. In this case the general question of growth and its regulation has to be considered.

The constituents of cytoplasm do not exist as stable structures – although more or less they are often considered to do so – but are continuously synthesized and assembled on the one hand, and degraded on the other (40). In view of this permanent turnover growth is not necessarily only the result of increased synthesis, but has to be considered as the consequence of shifting the balance between synthesis and degradation to the positive side. This may be achieved by a stimulation of the synthetic machinery to build up additional structures, as is commonly presumed. The same effect would also result, however, from the inhibition of degradation of cytoplasmic components, i. e. by increasing their life time (35).

Most assessments of intracellular turnover are based on biochemical measurements concerning protein turnover (26). The results of those observations are controversial as to whether or not inhibition of degradation, i. e. the anti-catabolic mechanism, plays a role in the process of myocardial hypertrophy. In a number of investigations no decrease in the rate of protein degradation (8, 9, 15, 19, 42), or even an increase (25) was observed. On the other hand a decrease in the rate of degradation, especially of mitochondrial proteins has been described by others (1, 21, 34, 39, 49).

Intracellular turnover does not take place exclusively at the molecular level of organization, but also has its structural correlation. It is generally accepted now that the main site of intracellular degradation is the lysosomal compartment (13). Cytoplasmic components to be degraded are translocated to this compartment by the process of cellular autophagy (6, 7, 31). Small portions of cytoplasm are segregated in this process by a membraneous border apt to fuse with the membrane of a lysosome. By this way the lysosomal hydrolytic enzymes obtain contact with the cytoplasmic portion which is eventually degraded to its low molecular constituents (16). As long as the structural integrity of the segregated cytoplasmic portions is preserved, they can be identified in the electron microscope as the so-called autophagic vacuoles (AVs) which have been shown to occur regularly in untreated myocardium of the rat (38). Since the morphological half-life of AVs as assessed from time sequential electron microscopic studies in the whole animal and in vitro, has turned out to be rather constant (22, 30, 32, 44), the fractional volume of AVs can be taken under certain presumptions as a relative measure of the rate of intracellular degradation by autophagy.

The following report is based on two series of experiments. In the first, the AV volume fraction was determined during the process of pressure induced hypertrophy resulting from supravalvular aortic constriction (4, 5). Secondly, short term experiments with low dose isoproterenol (10, 48) were aimed to the question if the inhibition of autophagic degradation could be considered as an early reaction to work load, which appears to represent the most relevant stimulus for myocardial hypertrophy.

Experiments

Male Sprague-Dawley rats weighing between 170 and 250 g were used for the experiments. Since the AV volume fraction is subject to circadian variations (38), all animals were killed between 10 a. m. and 1 p. m. The hearts were fixed by perfusion via the abdominal aorta (11) with 2.5% glutaraldehyde in 0.05 M cacodylate buffer pH 7.2, with the addition of 4% dextran for oncotic protection (3). Tissue cubes from the subepicardial myocardium of the left anterior wall were postfixed with 2% OSO_4, and were embedded in epon via propylene oxide after dehydration in graded series of ethanol. In the isoproterenol experiments tissue cubes from the right ventricular myocardium were prepared in addition.

Supravalvular aortic constriction was performed as described in detail elsewhere (4). The cross sectional area of the aorta ascendens was reduced in these experiments to 18% of the control values. No differences in the postoperative course of body weight were seen between operated (n = 33) and sham operated (n = 25) animals. Perfusion fixation was performed 3, 7, 14, 21, and 35 days after the operations.

DL-isoproterenol-HCL (Serva, Heidelberg, F.R.G.) dissolved in Ringer solution (3 mg/ml) was administered to anesthesized rats (n = 15) 1.5 mg/kg body weight intravenously and, at the same time, 1.5 mg/kg body weight subcutaneously. Ringer solution without additions was injected into control animals (n = 15). The animals were killed by perfusion fixation 10, 20 and 30 min after the injections.

The *morphometric evaluation* was performed by examining large test areas for AVs directly at the fluorescent screen of the electron microscope (34). Only vacuoles with contents that could be clearly identified as being derived from the cytoplasm were included in the evaluation. AV profiles containing mitochondria (AV mito) and those containing other components, such as endoplasmatic reticulum, t-tubules, glycogen and cytosolic ground substance (AV ergs) were registered separately. By relating the AV surface area to the total surface area of sectioned cytoplasm, the fractional volume of AVs was calculated according to basic stereological principles (47). The numerical density of AVs was calculated according to the Weibel and Gomez formula (47).

Results and discussion

The AVs observed in these experiments (Fig. 1) fulfilled the structural criteria described elsewhere (5, 32, 38) and did not show qualitative differences between experimental and control animals. In both experiments, pressure induced hypertrophy, as well as short term stimulation by isoproterenol, a significant reduction of the AV volume fractions was observed.

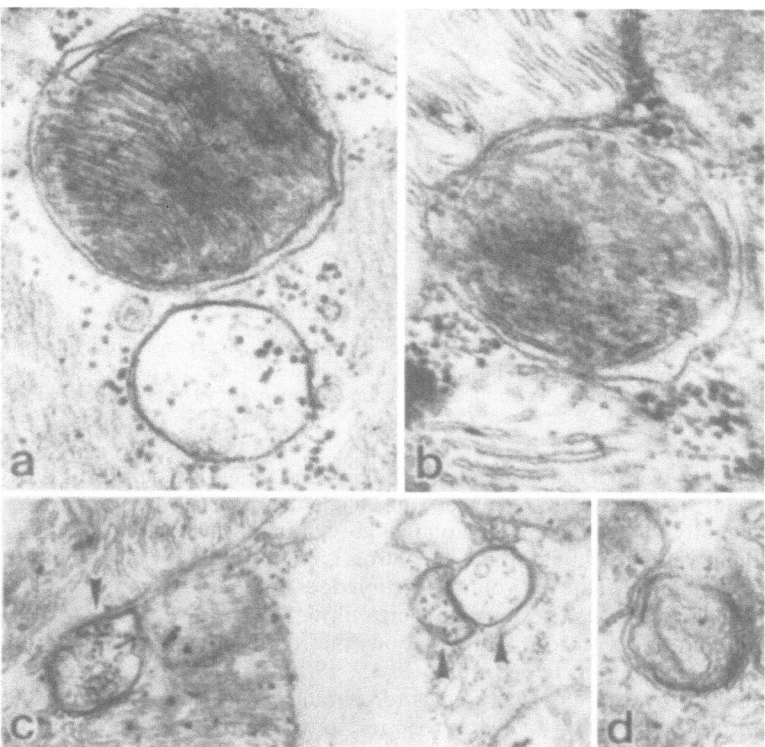

Fig. 1a–c. Typical examples of autophagic vacuoles (AVs) in cardiomyocytes are shown. a: Two AVs can be seen, the upper containing a mitochondrion (AV$_{mito}$) which is slightly condensed but still has intact cristae membranes, the lower containing cytosolic ground substance together with a few vesicles and glycogen granules (AV$_{ergs}$). b: Showing an AV$_{mito}$ at a later stage where part of the cristae membranes are already disintegrated. c: Three AV$_{ergs}$ with well preserved contents are shown. d: A profile of the t-tubular system is enclosed in this AV$_{ergs}$. a 49,000 ×, b 58,000 ×, c 36,000 ×, d 47,000 ×.

Supravalvular aortic constriction

The mass of left ventricular myocardium and the mean cardiomyocyte volume increased up to 70 % over controls within 21 days after supravalvular aortic constriction. No significant further increase was observed between 21 and 35 days. The growth rate, expressed as the difference between the rates of increase in cardiomyocyte volume in experimental and in control animals reached a maximum of about 5 percent per day 7 days after the aortic constriction (Fig. 2) but slowed down to zero between 22 and 35 days.

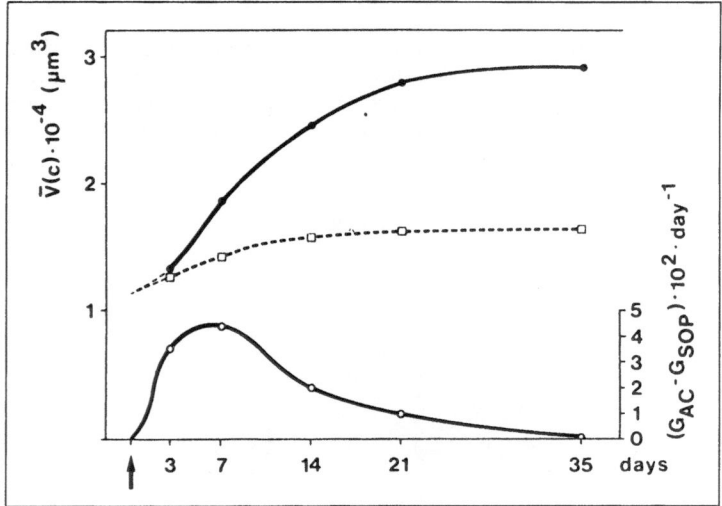

Fig. 2. From the increase of the average single cardiomyocyte volume $\bar{V}_{(c)}$ after aortic constriction (——•——) and after sham operation (---□---) (values from [4]), the differential growth rate ($G_{AC} - G_{SOP}$) was calculated (——○——) which has its maximum at about 7 days after the operations (from [5], with kind permission of Springer-Verlag).

An exactly inverse course was obtained for volume fraction and numerical density of AVs relative to controls (Fig. 3). These data show that autophagic degradation of cytoplasmic components is significantly reduced during adaptive growth of cardiomyocytes. In this way, already the normal synthetic activity which in controls is counteracted by degradation, contributes to growth. As expected, the AV volume fraction does not return to control values before growth has ceased in the state of sustained hypertrophy.

The data are not in contradiction to the observations that the synthetic machinery of cardiomyocytes is stimulated during hypertrophy (8, 15, 19, 42, 43). The simultaneous inhibition of degradative processes, however, seems to guarantee a maximum of effect at lowest expenditure of metabolic energy, which is required for both synthesis and degradation.

The use of the anticatabolic mechanism for growth is not a special feature of cardiac muscle. AV volume fractions have been found to be significantly reduced in hepatocytes of rats re-fed after starvation (36), in growing liver after partial hepatectomy (33), in hypertrophying kidney after unilateral nephrectomy (18, 37), as well as in hyperplasia of adrenal cortex stimulated by ACTH (27). The extent of inhibition of autophagy seems to be correlated with the growth rate. In fast growing organs, such as liver and adrenal cortex, the maximal reduction of AV volume fraction amounts to 90–100%, whereas in slower growing systems, e. g. kidney and myocardium, the inhibition is only 40–50%.

Short term effects of isoproterenol

The results of the isoproterenol experiments indicate that the anticatabolic response to increased work load is a rather fast reaction. 10 min after the injection of isoproterenol the AV volume fraction is already reduced to about 45% of control values, both in left and right ventricular myocardium (Table 1). This result is well in agreement with biochemical studies

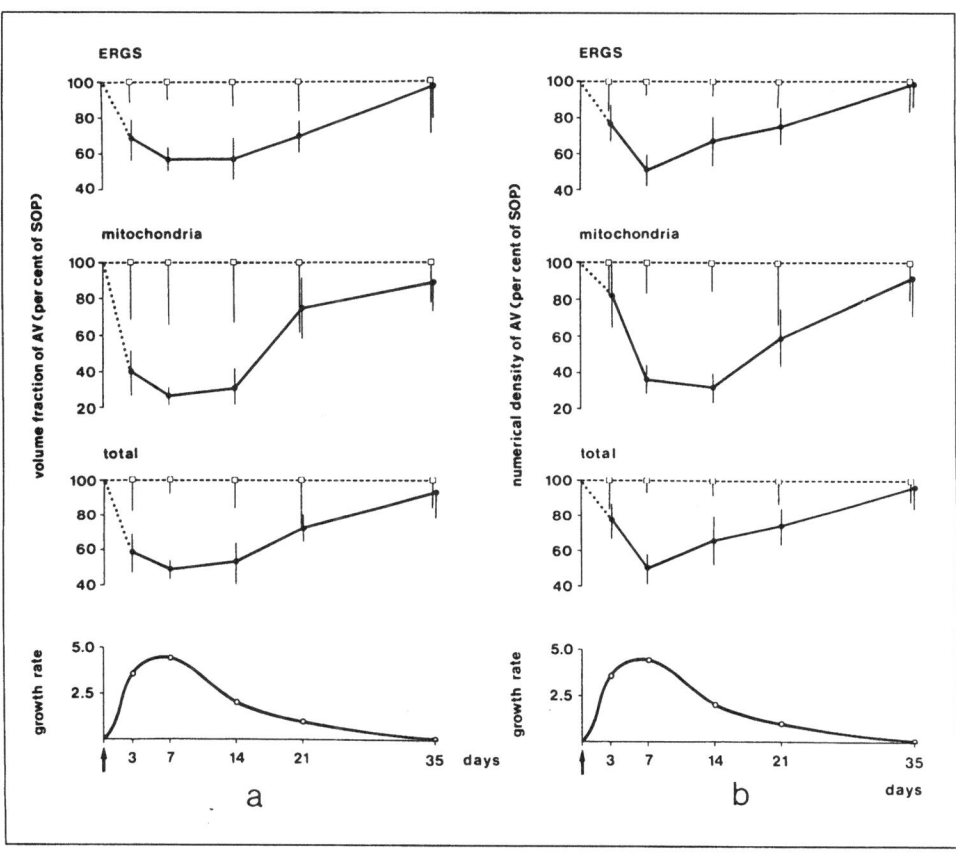

Fig. 3. AV volume fractions (a) and numerical densities (b) in cardiomyocytes after aortic constriction (——●——) expressed as percent of sham-operated controls (----□----). Maximal reduction is seen 7 days after aortic constriction, the degree of reduction being higher for AV_{mito} than for AV_{ergs}. The curves are inverse to the differential growth rate (bottom) as exemplified in Fig. 2 (from [5] with the kind permission of Springer-Verlag).

Table 1. Volume fraction of total autophagic vacuoles in cardiomyocytes of rats injected with Ringer solution or with DL-isoproterenol (1.5 mg/kg i. v. + 1.5 mg/kg s. c.)
The values given are mean values from 5–7 animals ± standard error of the mean. %changes were calculated as (isoproterenol − Ringer) × 100/Ringer.

	Time after Injection	Ringer	Isoproterenol	%change	t-test
Left ventricle	10 min	1.71 ± 0.17	0.80 ± 0.15	−56%	p < 0.01
	20 min	1.46 ± 0.40	1.02 ± 0.19	−30%	n. s.
	30 min	1.52 ± 0.29	1.16 ± 0.18	−24%	n. s.
Right ventricle	10 min	0.82 ± 0.15	0.34 ± 0.08	−55%	p < 0.02
	20 min	1.59 ± 0.43	0.44 ± 0.16	−72%	p < 0.05
	30 min	2.56 ± 0.93	1.63 ± 0.15	−76%	p < 0.05

showing that in addition to its well known stimulating effect on cardiac protein synthesis isoproterenol also inhibits protein degradation (23, 29). 20 and 30 min after the administration of isoproterenol, the AV volume fraction relative to controls seems to take a different course in the left and in the right ventricular myocardium. It amounts to 70 and 75% of control values in the left ventricular myocardium, but to only 30 and 25% in the right ventricular myocardium, respectively. From the absolute values shown in Table 1 it becomes clear that these differences are probably to be explained by a rather high variability between the control groups.

Since it is well known that long term administration of isoproterenol induces myocardial hypertrophy (2, 45) the immediate anticatabolic reaction appears to represent an important functional link between work load on the one hand and adaptative hypertrophy on the other.

Additional comment

It should be mentioned that the morphometric evaluations presented do not allow estimates on the rates of degradation of the main cytoplasmic components, the myofibrils. These have never been observed as contents of autophagic vacuoles, either in cardiomyocytes (38) or in skeletal muscle (41). A number of biochemical investigations suggest that myofibrils first undergo disassembly by neutral or alkaline proteases (14, 17, 20, 26) followed by final degradation of the myofibrillar proteines within the lysosomal compartment (12, 28). It remains an open question and may be a topic for further disputation , whether or not the anticatabolic mechanism is also of relevance in the increase in myofibrillar mass during hypertrophy.

References

1. Albin R, Dowell RT, Zak R, Rabinowitz M (1973) Synthesis and degradation of mitochondrial components in hypertrophied rat hearts. Biochem J 136: 629–637
2. Alderman EL, Harrison DC (1971) Myocardial hypertrophy resulting from low dosage isoproterenol administration in rats. Proc Soc Exp Biol Med 136: 268–270
3. Bohmann SO, Maunsbach AB (1970) Effects on tissue fine structure of variations in colloid osmotic pressure of glutaraldehyde fixatives. U Ultrastruct Res 30: 195–208
4. Dämmrich J, Pfeifer U (1983a) Cardiac hypertrophy in rats after supravalvular aortic constriction. I. Size and number of cardiomyocytes, endothelial and interstitial cells. Virchows Arch (Cell Pathol) 43: 265–286
5. Dämmrich J, Pfeifer U (1983b) Cardiac hypertrophy in rats after supravalvular aortic contriction. II. Inhibition of cellular autophagy in hypertrophying cardiomyocytes. Virchows Arch (Cell Pathol) 43: 287–307
6. De Duve C, Wattiaux R (1966) Functions of lysosomes. Ann Rev Physiol 28: 435–492
7. Ericsson JLE (1969) Mechanismus of cellular autophagy. In: lysosomic in Biology and Pathology (eds J. T. Dingle and H. B. Fell), Vol II, 345–394. North Holland, Amsterdam
8. Everett AW, Taylor RR, Sparrow MP (1977) Protein synthesis during right ventricular hypertrophy after pulmonary-artery stenosis in the dog. Biochem J 166: 315–321
9. Everett AW, Sparrow MP, Taylor RR (1979) Early changes in myocardial protein synthesis in vivo in response to right ventricular pressure overload in the dog. J Mol Cell Cardiol 11: 1253–1263
10. Föhr J (1984) Akute Hemmung der zellulären Autophagie im Herzmuskel nach Isoproterenol. Inauguraldissertation, Universität Würzburg
11. Forssmann WG, Siegrist G, Orci L, Girardier L, Pictet R, Rouiller C (1967) Fixation par perfusion pour la microscopie électronique. Eassai de généralisation. J. Microsc 6: 279–304
12. Gerhard KW, Schneider DL (1979) Evidence for degradation of myofibrillar proteins in lysosomes. Myofibrillar proteins derivatized by intramuscular injection of N-ethylmaleimide are sequestered in lysosomes. J Biol Chem 254: 11798–11805

13. Glaumann H, Ballard FJ (eds) (1986) Lysosomes: Their role in protein degradation. Academic Press, London (in press)
14. Griffin WST, Wildenthal K (1978) Myofibrillar alkaline protease activity in rat heart and its response to some interventions that alter cardiac size. J Mol Cell Cardiol 10: 669–676
15. Gudbjarnason S, Telerman M, Bing RJ (1964) Protein metabolism in cardiac hypertrophy and heart failure. Am J Physiol 206: 294–298
16. Henell R, Glaumann H (1984) Effect of leupeptin on the autophagic vacuolar system in rat hepatocytes. Correlation between ultrastructure and degradation of membrane and cytosolic proteins. Lab Invest 51: 46–56
17. Jenkins AB, Whittaker M, Schofield PJ (1979) The starvation induced increase in muscle protein degradation is non-lysosomal in origin. Biochem. Biophys Res Comm 86: 1014–1019
18. Jurilj N, Pfeifer U (1985) Hemmung der cellulären Autophagie im Nierentubulus als frühe Reaktion nach unilateraler Nephrektomie. Ver Dtsch Ges Pathol 69 (in press)
19. Kao RL, Rannels DE, Whitman V, Morgan HE (1978) Factors accounting for growth and atrophy of the heart. Re Adv Stud Cardiac Struct Metab 12: 105–113
20. Kay J, Siemankowski RF, Greweling JA, Siemankowski LM, Goll DE (1981) Proteolysis of myofibrillar proteins at neutral pH. Acta Biol Med Germ 40: 1323–1331
21. Kelly FJ, Goldspink DF (1983) The differing response of four muscle types to dexamethasone treatment in the rat. Biochem J 208: 147–151
22. Kovács J (1983) Regression of autophagic vacuoles in seminal vesicle cells following cycloheximide treatment. Exp Cell Res 144: 231
23. Lockwood TD (1985) Minute to minute neuroendocrine control of a major nonlysosomal pathway of myocardial protein degradation by β-receptor occupancy. Progr Clin Biol Res 180: 619–622
24. Martin AF, Reddy MK, Zak R, Dowell RT, Rabinowitz M (1974) Protein metabolism in hypertrophied heart muscle. Circ Res 35: 32–40
25. Millward DJ (1980) Protein turnover in skeletal and cardiac muscle during normal growth and hypertrophy. In: Wildenthal K (ed) Degradative processes in heart and skeletal muscle. Elsevier/North-Holland Biomedical Press, Amsterdam, pp 161–199
26. Morgan HE, Chua B, Beinlich CJ (1980) Regulation of protein degradation in heart. In: Wildenthal K (ed) Research monographs in cell and tissue physiology 3/4. Degradative processes in heart and skeletal muscle. Elsevier/North-Holland Biomedical Press, Amsterdam, pp 87–113
27. Müller J (1985) Autophagie beim ACTH-skuntierten Wachstum der Nebennierenrinde. Inaugerwal dissertation, Würzburg
28. Murakami U, Uchida K (1979) Degradation of rat cardiac myofibrils and myofibrillar proteins by a myosin-cleaving protease. J Biochem 86: 553–562
29. O'Hara DS, Curfman GD (1978) Suppression of protein degradation by beta-adrenergic stimulation on isolated cardiac muscle. J Cell Biol 79: 193a
30. Papadopoulos T, Pfeifer U (1986) Regression of rat liver autophagic vacuoles by locally applied cycloheximide. Lab Invest 54 (in press)
31. Pfeifer U (1976) Lysosomen and Autophagie. Verh Dtsch Ges Pathol 60: 28–64
32. Pfeifer U (1978) Inhibition by insulin of the formation of autophagic vacuoles in rat liver. J Cell Biol 78: 152–167
33. Pfeifer U (1979) Inhibited autophagic degradation of cytoplasm during compensatory growth of liver cells after partial hepatectomy. Virchows Arch (Cell Path) 30: 313–333
34. Pfeifer U (1980) The evaluation of large test fields for morphometric studies in electron microscopy. Pathol Res Pract 166: 188–202
35. Pfeifer U (1982) Kinetic and subcellular aspects of hypertrophy and atrophy. Int Rev Exp Pathol 23: 1–45
36. Pfeifer U, Bertling J (1977) A morphometric study of the inhibition of autophagic degradation during restorative growth of liver cells in rats re-fed after starvation. Virchows Arch (Cell Pathol) 24: 109–120
37. Pfeifer, U, Jurilj N (1979) Hemmung des intrazellulären Organellenabbaus als Prinzip der Wachstumsregulation in Leber und Niere. Verh Dtsch Ges Pathol 63: 505
38. Pfeifer U, Strauss P (1981) Autophagic vacuoles in heart muscle and liver. A comparative morphometric study including circadian variations in meal fed rats. J Mol Cell Cardiol 13: 37–49

39. Rabinowitz M (1973) Protein synthesis and turnover in normal and hypertrophied heart. Am J Cardiol 31: 202–210
40. Schoenheimer R (1942) The dynamic state of body constituents. Harvard University Press, London Cambridge
41. Schiaffiano S, Hanzilkova V (1972) Studies on the effect of denervation in developing muscle. II. The lysosomal system. J Ultrastruct Res 39: 1–14
42. Schreiber SS, Oratz M, Evans C, Reff F, Klein J, Rothschild MA (1973) Cardiac protein degradation in acute overload in vitro: Re-utilization of amino acids. Am J Physiol 224: 338–345
43. Schreiber SS, Evans CD, Oratz M, Rothschild MA (1981) Protein synthesis and degradation in cardiac stress. Circ Res 48: 601–611
44. Schworer CM, Shiffer KA, Mortimore GE (1981) Quantitative relationship between autophagy and proteolysis during graded amino acid deprivation in perfused rat liver. J Biol Chem 256: 7652–7658
45. Stanton HC, Brenner G, Mayfield ED (1969) Studies on isoproterenol-induced cardiomegaly in rats. Am Heart J 77: 72–80
46. Topping TM, Travis DF (1974) An electron cytochemical study of mechanism of lysosomal activity in the rat left ventricular mural myocardium. J Ultrastruct Res 46: 1–22
47. Weibel ER (1969) Sterological principles for morphometry in electron microscopy. Int Rev Cytol 26: 235–302
48. Wilhelm W (1986) Inauguraldissertation, Universität Würzburg, in Vorbereitung
49. Zak R (1976) Protein metabolism in the work-overloaded myocardium. Adv Cardiol 18: 46–56

Authors' address:
U. Pfeifer, Pathologisches Institut der Universität Würzburg, Luitpoldkrankenhaus, D-8700 Würzburg (F.R.G.)

Correlation between total catecholamine content and redistribution of myosin isoenzymes in pressure loaded ventricular myocardium of the spontaneously hypertensive rat*

H. Rupp and R. Jacob

Physiologisches Institut II, Universität Tübingen, Tübingen (F.R.G.)

Summary

In the spontaneously hypertensive rat (SHR) with established hypertension left ventricular mass closely correlated with the proportion of ventricular myosin (VM)-3. A 60% VM-3 content was reached corresponding, under the present housing conditions, to an average age of 40 weeks without any significant change in total noradrenaline content. However, all 72-week-old SHR showed marked reduction in total noradrenaline content which corresponded to noradrenaline depletion. At this stage, the proportion of VM-3 varied greatly; some of the SHR exhibited a higher proportion of VM-3 than would be expected from their ventricular weight. The excessive redistribution in the direction of VM-3 might, therefore, be considered as a reaction secondary to noradrenaline depletion. Total dopamine content was also reduced in 72-week-old SHR. In younger SHR, a positive correlation was found for dopamine content and left ventricular weight. It is concluded that a redistribution of the myosin isoenzymes up to 60% VM-3 in SHR is not associated with deterioration of ventricular performance to the extent that an excessive neurohumoral drive ensues. However, in the late stage of haemodynamic overload, a functional state is reached which is prone to noradrenaline depletion. A causative factor involved in this process could be the extreme redistribution of the myosin isoenzyme population, besides other factors such as fibrosis and dilatation. Which functional determinants or structural elements are finally decisive for the transition into a myocardium with depleted noradrenaline stores requires further investigation.

Key words: hypertrophy, noradrenaline, myosin, spontaneous hypertension, catecholamine

Introduction

Ventricular myocardium of the spontaneously hypertensive rat (SHR) reacts to prolonged increased pressure load with hypertrophy of the myocytes in order to normalize wall stress. This increase in mass is associated with redistribution of the ventricular myosin isoenzymes towards ventricular myosin (VM)-3 (21, 26), the enzyme of low ATPase activity (20, 23, 25), low shortening velocity (5, 34) and increased economy of tension development of isolated fibres (2, 3) and whole heart (13, 16, 17). Although such reactions are considered advantageous for counteracting the imposed load, impaired performance is often encountered in the advanced stage of pressure load (10–14, 22). Despite much inquiry into the matter in the past, it is still controversial why the state of compensation cannot be maintained in the pressure

* This study was supported by the Deutsche Forschungsgemeinschaft (Ja 172/12-1)

loaded heart. To trace the characteristic reactions involved in the deterioration of heart performance, we measured the total catecholamine content of pressure loaded left ventricles of SHR. Whenever heart performance drops below a certain level that is determined by an intrinsic regulatory system of the circulation (1), neurohumoral drive is increased on a longer term basis finally leading to cardiac noradrenaline depletion (30). In the present approach, we determined the time course of changes in blood pressure, ventricular weight, myosin isoenzyme population and catecholamine content in SHR and normotensive Wistar rats. It is shown that a VM-3 proportion of up to 60 % can be reached in SHR without any detectable loss in total noradrenaline content. The hearts of older SHR are, however, prone to noradrenaline depletion. Noteworthy is that a reduction in total noradrenaline content was observed before the limit of possible redistribution towards VM-3 was reached.

Experimental procedure

Male SHR/Kissleg (Okamoto-Aoki strain) and Wistar/WU rats from Ivanovas, Kissleg, F.R.G. were housed under standard conditions (21–23°C, 12 h light : 12 h dark cycle), fed "Ssniff" pellet diet containing 0.45 % sodium (Plange, Soest, F.R.G.) and received tap water ad libitum. Blood pressure was determined in the conscious rat using a piezo-resistive pressure transducer. Rats were sacrificed by decapitation.

Catecholamines were determined using a Waters M 6000 A high performance liquid chromatograph (Waters Ass., Milford, U.S.A.) and a Metrohm 64 electrochemical detector (Metrohm, Herisau, Switzerland) operating at + 0.7 V versus Ag/AgCl reference electrode. Separation of catecholamines was carried out on a Nucleosil 5 C_{18} column (Macherey-Nagel, Düren, F.R.G.), the eluent contained 60 mM citric acid/acetate buffer (pH 4.0) 1 mM di-n-butylamine, 0.1 mM disodium EDTA, 0.9 mM 1-octanesulfonic acid in 95 : 5 (v/v) water-methanol. Sample preparation using the alumina extraction procedure was performed as given by Refshauge et al. (24). Alternatively, the supernatant of the homogenate was injected after centrifugation at 160,000 × g for 20 min (Airfuge of Beckman, Palo Alto, U.S.A.).

Myosin isoenzyme populations were determined by non-dissociating gel electrophoresis in the presence of sodium pyrophosphate as described previously (26, 28). In case of considerable overlap of the components, the densitometric profile was simulated based on Gaussian components (27). Multiple statistical comparisons were performed using the rank test of Kruskal and Wallis (32). Statistical significance was assumed at P < 0.05.

Results

Blood pressure, left ventricular weight, myosin isoenzyme population and total noradrenaline content of SHR and Wistar rats of different age are given in Table 1. Ventricular weight and the proportion of VM-3 continued to increase up to approximately 40 weeks of age in SHR. 72-week-old SHR did not exhibit under our conditions a further increase in ventricular weight, although blood pressure continued to increase significantly. The myosin isoenzyme population in the latter group varied markedly. Total noradrenaline content was not lower in SHR than in age-matched Wistar rats up to the age of 40 weeks, but it was markedly reduced in 72-week-old SHR.

To analyze the cause of the marked variation in the proportion of VM-3 in 72-week-old SHR, left ventricular weight was plotted versus VM-3 content expressed as a percentage (Fig. 1). Some of the rats among the 72-week-old SHR exhibited a proportion of VM-3 that corresponded to their ventricular weight, but there were also rats with a nearly homogeneous

Table 1. Age-dependent changes in blood pressure, left ventricular weight (LVW), myosin isoenzyme population and total noradrenaline content of SHR and Wistar rats; n, number of animals.

	n	Blood pressure (mm Hg)	LVW (mg)	VM-3 (%)	VM-2 (%)	VM-1 (%)	Noradrenaline (ng/left ventricle)
SHR, 21 wk	18	161 ± 6[a]+++	1059 ± 49[a]+++	41.1 ± 9.0[a]+++	30.0 ± 1.6[a]+++	28.9 ± 6.5[a]+++	681.6 ± 115.0[a]++
Wistar, 21 wk	25	107 ± 6	699 ± 54	17.4 ± 5.8	26.8 ± 3.3	55.8 ± 8.6	572.8 ± 94.7
SHR, 34 wk	9	198 ± 8[a][b]+++	1228 ± 153[a][b]+	52.5 ± 5.0[a][b]+++	27.8 ± 1.7[a] ns	19.7 ± 3.3[a][b]+++	733.0 ± 121.9[a] ns
Wistar, 34 wk	13	109 ± 14[b] ns	823 ± 62[b]+++	23.2 ± 5.8[b]+	27.8 ± 2.5[b] ns	49.0 ± 8.2[b]+	653.8 ± 122.0[b] ns
SHR, 40 wk	7	193 ± 13[a]+++	1351 ± 193[a]+++	58.9 ± 6.5[a]+++	25.1 ± 2.5[a]+++	16.0 ± 4.1[a]+++	530.7 ± 100.8[a] ns
Wistar, 40 wk	7	108 ± 9[c] ns	830 ± 48[c] ns	30.9 ± 3.6[c]+	31.9 ± 0.9[c]+++	37.2 ± 4.1[c]++	501.2 ± 68.0[c]++
SHR, 72 wk	4	225 ± 13[a]+++	1306 ± 160[a]+++	76.0 ± 18.2[a]+++	17.8 ± 12.6[a] ns	6.2 ± 6.1[a]+++	148.0 ± 85.4[a]+++
Wistar, 60 wk	5	109 ± 12[d] ns	904 ± 40[d]+	34.1 ± 6.4[d] ns	33.5 ± 2.1[d] ns	32.4 ± 7.1[d] ns	563.8 ± 112.2[d] ns

Statistical comparisons were made between (a) age-matched SHR and Wistar rats as well as between 72-week-old SHR and 60-week-old Wistar rats. Furthermore, between the following groups of different age consisting of either SHR or Wistar rats: (b) 34-week-old versus 21-week-old; (c) 40-week-old versus 34-week-old or 60-week-old versus 40-week-old; (d) 72-week-old versus 40-week-old. + P < 0.05, + + P < 0.01, + + + P < 0.001, ns P > 0.05.

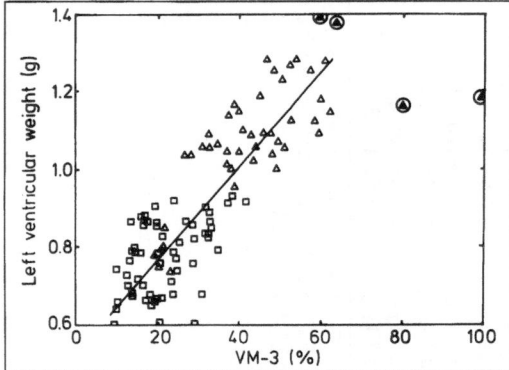

Fig. 1. Weight of left ventricles (including septum) is plotted versus the proportion of VM-3 for individual ($\triangle$) SHR and ($\square$) Wistar rats. 72-week-old SHR are represented by filled-in triangles surrounded by a circle. A linear regression ($y = 0.01 \times + 0.52$, $r = 0.84$, $P < 0.01$) was calculated using the data points of all SHR and Wistar rats with the exception of 72-week-old SHR.

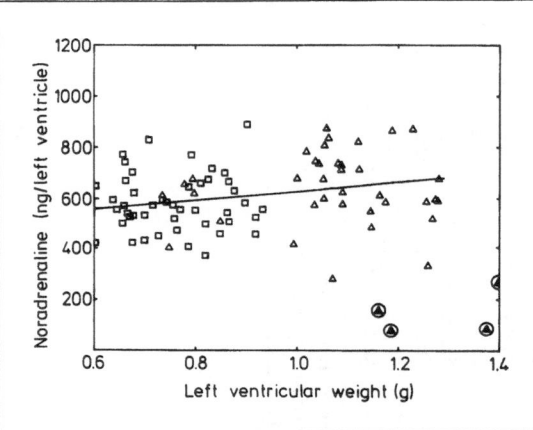

Fig. 2. Total noradrenaline content of left ventricles is given versus left ventricular weight for individual ($\triangle$) SHR and ($\square$) Wistar rats. A linear regression ($y = 0.18 \times + 453.3$, $r = 0.28$, $P < 0.05$) was calculated using the data points of all rats with the exception of 72-week-old SHR (filled-in triangles surrounded by a circle).

VM-3 population. Thus, whereas younger rats exhibited a close correlation between ventricular weight and the proportion of VM-3, additional reactions responsible for the nearly homogeneous VM-3 have to be assumed in some of the 72-week-old SHR.

Regarding the interrelationship between total noradrenaline content and left ventricular weight, it follows that noradrenaline depletion occurred in all of the 72-week-old SHR, although some of the rats exhibited a ventricular weight comparable with that of younger rats (Fig. 2). Thus, the process of noradrenaline depletion does not seem to be linked to a critical ventricular mass. In order to follow the interrelationship between noradrenaline depletion and redistribution of the myosin isoenzymes, total noradrenaline content is given as a function of the proportion of VM-3 in Fig. 3. Noradrenaline depletion occurred also in those 72-week-old SHR where the proportion of VM-3 still corresponded to a given ventricular mass. The process of transmitter depletion is, therefore, an event which occurs prior to the excessive redistribution of myosin isoenzymes in the direction of VM-3.

In contrast to noradrenaline, dopamine content was positively correlated with ventricular

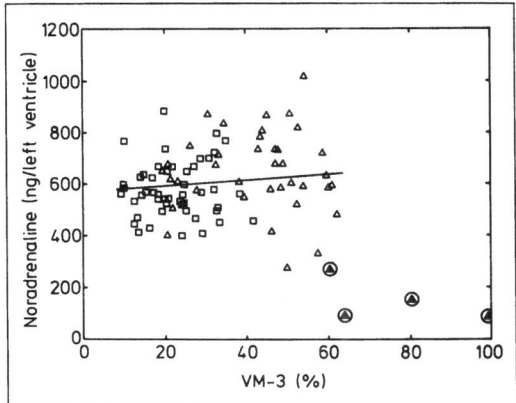

Fig. 3. The interrelationship between total noradrenaline content and the proportion of VM-3 for individual (△) SHR and (□) Wistar rats. A linear regression (y = 1.06 × + 572.7, r = 0.12, n. s.) was calculated using the data points of all rats with the exception of 72-week-old SHR (filled-in triangles surrounded by a circle).

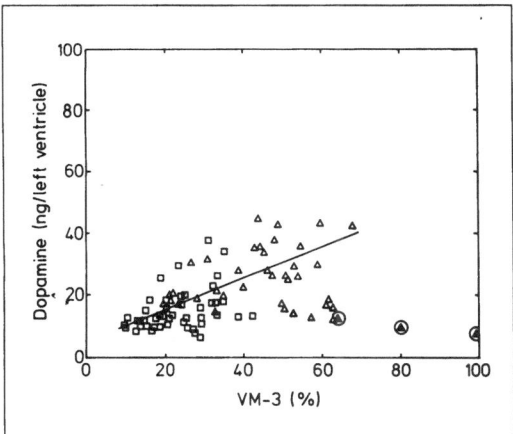

Fig. 4. The interrelationship between total dopamine content and the proportion of VM-3 for individual (△) SHR and (□) Wistar rats. A linear regression (y = 0.48 × + 5.08, r = 0.68, P < 0.01) was calculated using the data points of all rats with the exception of 72-week-old SHR (filled-in triangles surrounded by a circle).

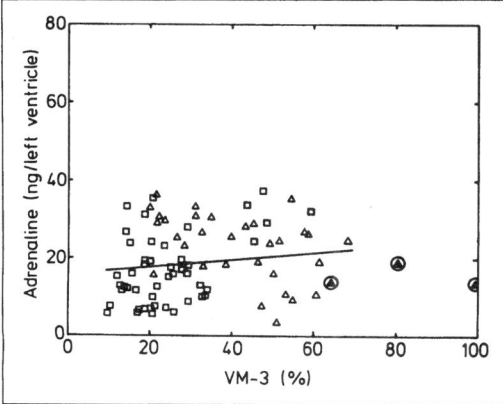

Fig. 5. The interrelationship between total adrenaline content and the proportion of VM-3 for individual (△) SHR and (□) Wistar rats. A linear regression (y = 0.09 × + 16.02, r = 0.17, n. s.) was calculated using the data points of all rats with the exception of 72-week-old SHR (filled-in triangles surrounded by a circle).

mass (Fig. 4). Since young SHR exhibited a dopamine content comparable to that of older Wistar rats with similar ventricular weight, it is most likely that the higher dopamine content observed in older SHR is characteristic for the increased ventricular mass and cannot be attributed to strain differences independent of ventricular mass. 72-week-old SHR exhibited both a reduced dopamine and noradrenaline content. The total content of adrenaline did not depend in any significant way on the proportion of VM-3 in Wistar rats or SHR (Fig. 5).

Discussion

The ventricle reacts to an increased pressure load with hypertrophy of the myofibres and redistribution of the myosin isoenzyme population towards VM-3. Because a close correlation between left ventricular weight and the proportion of VM-3 common to both Wistar rats and SHR was observed (31), an increased proportion of VM-3 is unlikely to have, a priori, a detrimental influence on myocardial performance. Rather it seems likely that pressure overload only extends the range of ventricular mass and the proportion of VM-3 encountered in normotensive rats. Furthermore, redistribution of the myosin isoenzyme population should not be regarded as an isolated event in the pressure-loaded myocardium, but as the best studied representative example, to date, of a general transformational reaction towards a slow-type muscle. Thus, Ca^{2+}-uptake of sarcoplasmic reticulum is affected in parallel with the myosin isoenzyme population in the pressure loaded ventricle with apparently compensated hypertrophy (29).

The present data demonstrate that a proportion of VM-3 up to 60% in SHR is not associated with an altered total noradrenaline content of left ventricles. This proportion of VM-3 is even higher than that observed in old Wistar rats kept under the same conditions as SHR. This increase in VM-3 which is typical for the overloaded ventricle does not lead to a functional state of myocardium which is associated with a prolonged, markedly increased sympathetic drive. In the 40-week-old SHR, the myocardium still performs adequately enough for the circulatory system involving cardiac and arterial baroreceptors (1) not to elicit prolonged elevated neurohumoral drive. Accordingly, heart performance was reported not to be impaired until 52 weeks of age (22). In the subsequent months, additional processes involving fibrosis and dilatation most probably occur leading to a prolonged higher peripheral sympathetic activity giving rise to cardiac noradrenaline depletion. During this period, the response of ventricular mass to the overload is apparently variable. Although under the present conditions ventricular weight did not change, other studies have reported a decrease (6) or an increase (22) in ventricular weight. Since noradrenaline was considered to be involved in the process of hypertrophy (18, 35), it is an intriguing possibility that the absence of hypertrophy, despite increased blood pressure, might be related to noradrenaline depletion or marked loss in adrenergic receptors.

In 72-week-old SHR noradrenaline depletion occurred, but was not necessarily accompanied by further redistribution of myosin isoenzymes towards VM-3. The nearly homogeneous VM-3 population observed in some of the 72-week-old SHR is considered to be a reaction secondary to processes associated with noradrenaline depletion. Noteworthy is that noradrenaline depletion was not accompanied by an increased proportion of dopamine as might be inferred from hamsters with cardiomyopathy. In the late stage of this model, the rate-limiting step of catecholamine biosynthesis was shifted from tyrosine hydroxylase to hydroxylation of dopamine, resulting in accumulation of dopamine (36–38). However, with the exception of 72-week-old SHR, increasing ventricular mass of SHR was associated with a higher content of dopamine. Whether this increase in dopamine content should be viewed as indicative of an increase in sympathetic drive of the heart at a stage when total noradrenaline content is still unchanged requires further validation. Particularly, since part of cardiac dopamine was reported not to be associated with noradrenergic nerves (4) and to be released independently of sympathetic noradrenergic activity (9). Given that the higher dopamine content in SHR of approximately 21 weeks and older is indeed indicative of an increased sympathetic activity, then obviously the conditions leading to a higher peripheral sympathetic activity would already be fulfilled much earlier, as might be inferred also from a diminished contractile reserve on 20–24 weeks SHR (33). Nevertheless, the still unchanged noradrenaline stores suggest that, at this stage, the potential of the sympathetic nervous system to compensate for lower myocardial performance by increasing cardiac noradrenaline release is not reduced.

Irrespective of the time-course of cardiac noradrenaline depletion in SHR, abnormalities in noradrenaline metabolism of younger SHR have been demonstrated. In 4-week-old SHR peripheral sympathetic activity was found to be increased (7, 39) and even cardiac hypertrophy was observed (39). In established hypertension, sympathoadrenal activity was also enhanced (7, 8, 15). Despite a possible increase in noradrenaline turnover in the heart of SHR the outcome is not a reduction in cardiac noradrenaline content. Only in the late stage of pressure load does noradrenaline depletion occur. We do not consider this process as being typical of spontaneous hypertension alone, but as diagnostic of a myocardium with long-standing overload in the transition to impaired performance.

In conclusion, we are able to demonstrate that a marked redistribution of the myosin isoenzymes in pressure loaded heart is not necessarily associated with a reduction in total noradrenaline content. The redistribution in favour of VM-3 cannot, therefore, be considered a priori as a process with detrimental consequences. This is in accordance with data on mechanics and haemodynamics of pressure loaded heart (10–14). However, in the late stage of haemodynamic overload a functional state is reached which gives rise to a prolonged excessive neurohumoral drive eventually resulting in noradrenaline depletion and loss of adrenergic receptors in heart (19, 30). Besides other factors, such as fibrosis and dilatation, the extreme redistribution towards VM-3 could be regarded as a causative factor contributing to this process. The elucidation of the reactions which induce the transition of a heart that is not subjected to a prolonged enhanced sympathetic drive to one that is subjected to such a drive presents a great challenge. At present, neither the origin of the trigger reactions of this transition nor the functional demands or structural parameters favourable for such a transition are known. In the final analysis, changes that occur at the organ level, particularly those involving ventricular geometry should be taken into account. The reactions which lead to noradrenaline depletion are probably associated with dilatation which greatly restricts pumping function (11). Progress towards the understanding of the crucial process of decompensation of pressure loaded heart requires an integrative approach which involves parallel characterization of the changes that occur at the molecular level and the performance of the heart as a whole (10–14). In view of the high incidence of heart failure, it is hoped that this problem can be resolved in the near future.

Acknowledgement

The expert assistance of L. Schwarz is greatly appreciated.

References

1. Abboud FM, Thames MD (1983) Interaction of cardiovascular reflexes in circulatory control. In: Shepherd JT, Abboud FM (eds) Handbook of Physiology, Section 2: The cardiovascular system, Vol III. American Physiological Society, Bethesda, pp 675–753
2. Alpert NR, Mulieri LA, Litten RZ, Holubarsch C (1984) A myothermal analysis of the myosin crossbridge cycling rate during isometric tetanus in normal and hypothyroid rat hearts. Eur Heart J 5 (Suppl F): 3–11
3. Alpert NR, Mulieri LA (1986) Intrinsic determinants of myocardial energetics in normal and hypertrophied hearts. In: Rupp H (ed) Regulation of heart function – Basic concepts and clinical applications. Thieme Inc, New York, pp 292–304
4. Drake AJ, Templeton WW, Stanford SC (1982) Evidence for a role of dopamine in cardiac function. Neurochem Internat 4: 435–439
5. Ebrecht G, Rupp H, Jacob R (1982) Alterations of mechanical parameters in chemically skinned preparations of rat myocardium as a function of isoenzyme pattern of myosin. Basic Res Cardiol 77: 220–234
6. Farmer BB, Harris RA, Jolly WW, Vail WJ (1974) Studies on the cardiomegaly of the spontaneously hypertensive rat. Circ Res 35: 102–110
7. Grobecker H, Saavedra JM, Weise VK (1982) Biosynthetic enzyme activities and catecholamines in adrenal glands of genetic and experimental hypertensive rats. Circ Res 50: 742–746
8. Howe PRC, Provis JC, West MJ, Chalmers JP (1979) Changes in cardiac norepinephrine in spontaneously hypertensive and stroke-prone rats. J Cardiovasc Pharmacol 1: 115–122
9. Ilebekk A, Andersen FR, Kjeldsen SE, Eide I (1983) Dopamine release from the porcine myocardium. Acta Physiol Scand 119: 197–201
10. Jacob R (1985) Chronische Reaktionen des Herzmuskels: Probleme der Interpretation am Beispiel der Myofibrillenfunktion. In: Mall G, Otto HF (eds) Herzhypertrophie. Springer-Verlag, Berlin New York, pp 1–23
11. Jacob R (1986) Cardiac responses to hypertension. Reactions of the heart to experimental chronic pressure overload – Adaptation or damage? In: Tarazi RC, Zanchetti A (eds) Handbook of Hypertension, Vol VII. Elsevier/North Holland Biomedical Press (in press)
12. Jacob R, Kissling G, Ebrecht G, Holubarsch C, Medugorac I, Rupp H (1983) Adaptive and pathological alterations in experimental cardiac hypertrophy. In: Chazov E, Saks V, Rona G (eds) Advances in Moycardiology, Vol 4. Plenum Publishing Corporation, New York, pp 55–77
13. Jacob R, Kissling G, Ebrecht G, Jörg E, Rupp H, Takeda N (1984) Cardiac alterations at the myofibrillar level: Is a redistribution of the myosin isoenzyme pattern decisive for cardiac failure in haemodynamic overload? Eur Heart J 5 (Suppl F): 13–26
14. Jacob R, Ebrecht G, Kissling G, Rupp H, Takeda N (1986) Functional consequences of cardiac myosin isoenzyme redistribution. In: Rupp H (ed) Regulation of heart function – Basic concepts and clinical applications. Thieme Inc, New York, pp 305–326
15. Judy WV, Watanabe AM, Murphy WR, Aprison BS, Yu P-L (1979) Sympathetic nerve activity and blood pressure in normotensive backcross rats genetically related to the spontaneously hypertensive rat. Hypertension 1: 598–604
16. Kissling G, Rupp H, Malloy L, Jacob R (1982) Alterations in cardiac oxygen consumption under chronic pressure overload. Significance of the isoenzyme pattern of myosin. Basic Res Cardiol 77: 255–269
17. Kissling G, Malloy L, Rupp H (1983) Energetics of the rat heart in chronic pressure overload. In: Jacob R, Gülch RW, Kissling G (eds) Cardiac adaptation to hemodynamic overload, training and stress. Steinkopff Verlag, Darmstadt, pp 167–173
18. Laks MM, Morady F (1976) Norepinephrine – The myocardial hypertrophy hormone? Am Heart J 91: 674–675
19. Limas CJ, Limas C (1984) Beta-adrenergic hormone-receptor interactions in the hypertrophied and failing myocardium. Eur Heart J 5 (Suppl F): 329–337
20. Lompré A-M, Schwartz K, d'Albis A, Lacombe G, van Thiem N, Swynghedauw B (1979) Myosin isoenzyme redistribution in chronic heart overload. Nature (London) 282: 105–107
21. Mercadier J-J, Lompré A-M, Wisnewsky C, Samuel J-L, Bercovici J, Swynghedauw B, Schwartz K

(1981) Myosin isoenzymic changes in several models of rat cardiac hypertrophy. Circ Res 49: 525–532

22. Pfeffer JM, Pfeffer MA, Fishbein MC, Frohlich ED (1979) Cardiac function and morphology with aging in the spontaneously hypertensive rat. Am J Physiol 237: H461–H468
23. Pope B, Hoh JFY, Weeds A (1980) The ATPase activities of rat cardiac myosin isoenzymes. FEBS Lett 118: 205–208
24. Refshauge C, Kissinger PT, Dreiling R, Blank L, Freeman R, Adams RN (1974) New high performance liquid chromatographic analysis of brain catecholamines. Life Sci 14: 311–322
25. Rupp H (1983) The determinants of the calcium-dependent activation of myofibrils from rat heart as judged by myofibrillar adenosine triphosphatase and superprecipitation of natural actomyosin. Mol Physiol 3: 249–263
26. Rupp H, Jacob R (1982) Response of blood pressure and cardiac myosin polymorphism to swimming training in the spontaneously hypertensive rat. Can J Physiol Pharmacol 60: 1098–1103
27. Rupp H, Kissling G, Jacob R (1983) Hormonal and hemodynamic determinants of polymorphic myosin. In: Alpert NR (ed) Perspectives in cardiovascular research, Vol 7, Myocardial hypertrophy and failure. Raven Press, New York, pp 373–383
28. Rupp H, Felbier H-R, Bukhari AR, Jacob R (1984) Modulation of myosin isoenzyme populations and activities of monoamine oxidase and phenylethanolamine-N-methyltransferase in pressure loaded and normal rat heart by swimming exercise and stress arising from electrostimulation in pairs. Can J Physiol Pharmacol 62: 1209–1218
29. Rupp H, Jacob R (1985) Ventricular myocardium as a fast- or slow-type muscle as inferred from rate of Ca-uptake of sarcoplasmic reticulum. J Mol Cell Cardiol 17 (Suppl 3): 18
30. Rupp H, Jacob R (1986) The autonomic nervous system of the heart: Adaptation, deadaptation, and impaired nervous control of heart performance. In: Rupp H (ed) Regulation of heart function – Basic concepts and clinical applications. Thieme Inc, New York, pp 53–70
31. Rupp H, Jacob R (1986) Myocardial transitions between fast- and slow-type muscle as monitored by the population of myosin isoenzymes. In: Rupp H (ed) Regulation of heart function – Basic concepts and clinical applications. Thieme Inc, New York, pp 271–291
32. Sachs L (1984) Applied Statistics. Springer-Verlag, Berlin New York
33. Saragoca MA, Tarazi RC (1980) Cardiac contractile reserve in spontaneously hypertensive rats. Clin Sci 59: 365s–368s
34. Schwartz K, Lecarpentier Y, Martin JL, Lompré AM, Mercadier JJ, Swynghedauw B (1981) Myosin isoenzymic distribution correlates with speed of myocardial contraction. J Mol Cell Cardiol 13: 1071–1075
35. Sen S, Tarazi RC (1983) Regression of myocardial hypertrophy and influence of adrenergic system. Am J Physiol 244: H97–H101
36. Sole MJ, Kamble AB, Hussain MN (1977) A possible change in the rate-limiting step for cardiac norepinephrine synthesis in the cardiomyopathic Syrian hamster. Circ Res 41: 814–817
37. Sole MJ (1982) Alterations in sympathetic and parasympathetic neurotransmitter activity. In: Braunwald E, Mock MB, Watson J (eds) Congestive heart failure. Grune & Stratton Inc, New York, p 1
38. Strobeck JE, Factor SM, Bhan A, Sole M, Liew CC, Fein F, Sonnenblick EH (1979) Hereditary and acquired cardiomyopathies in experimental animals: Mechanical, biochemical, and structural features. Ann NY Acad Sci 317: 59–88
39. Yamori Y, Mori C, Nishio T, Ooshima A, Horie R, Ohtaka M, Soeda T, Saito M, Abe K, Nara Y, Nakao Y, Kihara M (1979) Cardiac hypertrophy in early hypertension. Am J Cardiol 44: 964–969

Authors' address:

Heinz Rupp, Physiologisches Institut II, Universität Tübingen, Gmelinstraße 5, D-7400 Tübingen (F.R.G.)

Significance of physical exercise in hypertension. Influence of water temperature and beta-blockade on blood pressure, degree of cardiac hypertrophy and cardiac function in swimming training of spontaneously hypertensive rats*

M. Vogt, B. Ott, H. Rupp, and R. Jacob

Physiologisches Institut II, Universität Tübingen, Tübingen (F.R.G.)

Summary

In previous studies swimming training (ST) of spontaneously hypertensive rats (SHR) at 36° water temperature (WT) led to a decrease in blood pressure (BP). A similar effect of ST has not been described in human hypertension. Our purpose was to investigate the influence of WT on this training effect, the influence of ST on LV hypertrophy and the involvement of adrenergic stimuli in the latter. Male SHR (20 weeks old) were divided randomly into 4 groups. 1) SHR sedentary 2) SHR ST 36° 3) SHR ST 26° 4) SHR ST 36° + atenolol (50 mg/kg/die). ST was performed 2 × 90 min/day for 31 days and then reduced to 2 × 60 min/day. After 7 weeks of ST BP was lower in all ST groups compared with SHR sed entary (p < 0.001). BP was higher in ST 26° than in ST 36° (p < 0.05). No additional effect of atenolol on BP was observed. The increase in the degree of LV hypertrophy during ST (ST 36°: +15%; ST 26°: +26%) could be prevented by atenolol (ST 36° + atenolol: −1.5%). ST 36° led to improved ventricular and myocardial performance with decreased LV wall stress ("luxury hypertrophy"), while in ST 26° ventricular dilatation occurred with increased stystolic wall stress and elevated LVEDP. It was uncertain whether this should be interpreted as a state of LV pre-insufficiency in ST 26° in spite of no indications of impaired myocardial contractile capability. Peripheral vascular resistance (PVR) was significantly reduced by ST. The reduction was more evident in ST 26°, but was partially compensated for by an increased cardiac output. The weights of adrenal glands increased (p < 0.001), most markedly for ST 26°. The level of thyroid hormones (T_3 and fT_3) was increased in ST 26°. In summary, ST proved to be effective in lowering BP of SHR. WT had great influence with respect to cardiovascular adaptation and mechanisms involved in ST of SHR. Cardioadrenergic drive was of great significance for the process of hypertrophy during ST in SHR.

Key words: atenolol, cardiac adaptation, cardiac hypertrophy, hypertension, peripheral vascular resistance, physical exercise, SHR

Introduction

During the last 15 years growing attention has been paid to the influence of physical exercise on blood pressure modulation in essential hypertension in man. Two main topics can be emphasized. Firstly physical exercise as a preventive measure (2, 21, 27) and secondly as a conceivable therapeutical principle in the management of essential hypertension (13, 19,

* The study was supported by the Deutsche Forschungsgemeinschaft (Ja 172/12-1)

29). In 1970 Hanson and Nedde (13) achieved some indications of a favourable effect of physical training on blood pressure in essential hypertension. Although a series of investigations followed (15, 19, 21, 29), most of them failed to prove the pressure-reducing effect of training per se on account of the lack of randomization or controls or of additional interventions (19). Although the SHR (Aoki-Okamoto strain) is disputed as a model of human essential hypertension (23), it is a model of primary hypertension which closely resembles the course of essential hypertension in man (12, 37). Therefore we used SHR to evaluate the effect of exercise training on primary hypertension under controlled conditions.

In our previous studies swimming training at 36° led to a considerable decrease in blood pressure of SHR (30, 31). Since a similar effect of swimming training has not been described in man, the purpose of the present study was to investigate the influence of water temperature on this training effect. In addition, the consequence of reduced blood pressure elicited by training on the degree of left ventricular hypertrophy and the involvement of adrenergic stimuli in the latter were studied.

Methods

The experiments were carried out on 40 male SHR of the Aoki-Okamoto strain. At the beginning of the training the animals were 20 weeks old. The rats received standard dry meal and tap water ad libitum. The SHR were randomly divided into 4 groups. One group remained sedentary, was restrictively fed to avoid differences in body weight as compared to trained SHR and served as control (SHR sed.). One group swam at a water temperature of 26°C (ST 26°), two groups at 36°C, one of which received additionally the β-receptor blocking agent atenolol (at.) (50 mg/kg b. w. and day, applied to the drinking water) (ST 36° and ST 36° + at.). The daily duration of ST was gradually increased up to 2 × 90 min, and reduced to 2 × 60 min after 31 days. Total duration of training was about 100 h. The number of swimmers per given surface area was 24/m².

Systolic blood pressure (BP) was measured at regular intervals by plethysmographic tail cuff method in conscious rats as described elsewhere (30).

At the end of the training period hemodynamic measurements were carried out. After anesthetization with urethane (1.2 g/kg b. w.), intubation and setting of venous infusion the chest was opened by a parasternal incision. An electromagnetic flow probe was placed around the ascending aorta, the left ventricle was pierced with a steel cannula No. 1 and the right arteria carotis communis was cannulated with a silicon tube. LVP, LVEDP, LV dP/dt, flow signal and phasic or mean systemic pressure were registered on a Hellige multichannel recorder. Isovolumetric beats were performed by clamping the ascending aorta. End-diastolic pressure-volume relationships were measured at the end of each experiment according to the method of Ullrich et al. (40). Finally LV weight, the weight of adrenal glands and tibia length were determined.

Assuming a thick-walled spherical shell LV wall stress was calculated for midwall region according to Gülch in (14) and to (24). Peripheral vascular resistance (PVR) was computed by means of mean arterial pressure and cardiac output.

Statistical analysis was performed by using Student's t-test for normally distributed values and H-test (Kruskal and Wallis) or analysis of variance for multiple comparisons. The degree of LV hypertrophy was evaluated by means of linear regression analysis.

Results

A. Systolic blood pressure

While the systolic BP of SHR sed. rose continuously during observation, the BP of all ST-groups dropped under swimming training, even if to different degrees. After 7 weeks of

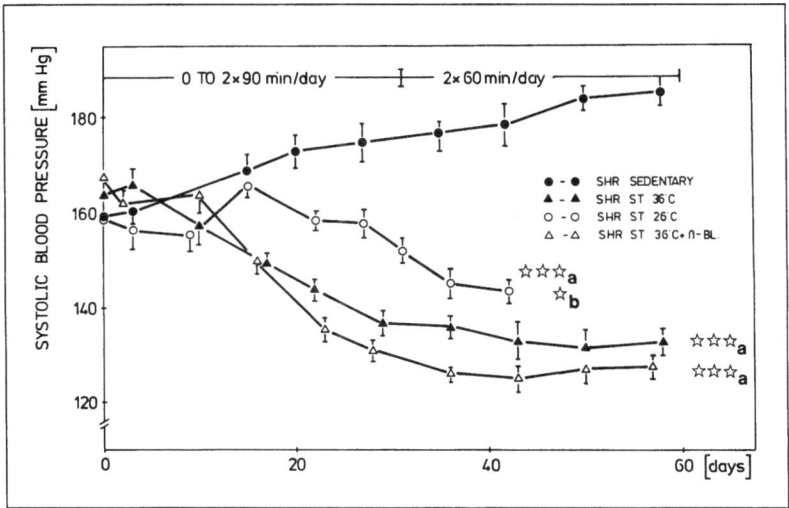

Fig. 1. Influence of chronic swimming training at different water temperatures (26° and 36°) and of additional beta-blockade (atenolol 50 mg/kg b. w. × die) on systolic blood pressure in SHR. Values are means ± SEM

☆☆☆a — p <0.001 (as related to SHR sedentary)
☆b — p <0.05 (as related to SHR ST 36°)

training BP reached a new steady state and was significantly lower for all ST-groups compared to SHR sed. (p <0.001) (Fig. 1). The onset of reduction in BP was clearly delayed for ST 26°, there being even an initial increase in BP. After 7 weeks BP of ST 26° was significantly above that of ST 36° (p <0.05). The additional application of atenolol had no further significant effect on reduction of BP during ST 36°.

B. Body weight and tibia length

Initially the trained rats lost some weight, but grew heavier again at a later stage of training. As a result of restrictive feed the body weight of the sedentary SHR increased only slowly, so that there was no significant difference between the groups. Only the body weight of ST 36° + at. was significantly lower than that of SHR sed. (p <0.05).

The growth of the tibia was retarded for all the trained groups (SHR sed.: 39.2 ± 0.2 mm, ST 36°: 38.4 ± 0.4 mm, ST 26°: 38.3 ± 0.4 mm, ST 36° + at.: 38.1 ± 0.4 mm; p <0.01).

C. Degree of cardiac hypertrophy

ST 36° and ST 26°, but not ST 36° + at. resulted in an increase in LV weight (SHR sed.: 1128 ± 79 mg; ST 36°: 1250 ± 128 mg, n. s.; ST 26°: 1357 ± 168 mg, p <0.01; ST 36° + at.: 1050 ± 48 mg, n. s.; compared with SHR sed. respectively). To evaluate the degree of hypertrophy regression analysis of LV weight to body weight and tibia length, respectively, was performed (Fig. 2). Degree of hypertrophy was significantly greater after ST 26° (+26%) as compared with ST 36° (+15%, p. <0.05). Application of atenolol was effective in preventing further increase of cardiac hypertrophy during ST, failed, however, to induce regression of hypertrophy (−1.5%, n. s.).

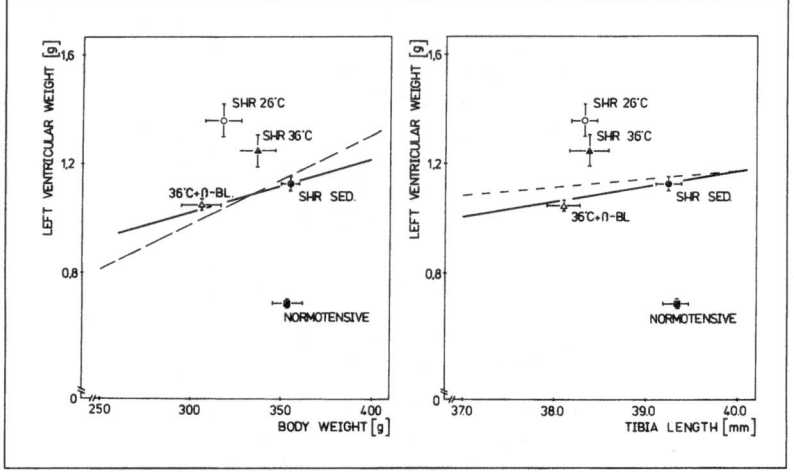

Fig. 2. Effect of swimming training and beta-blockade on cardiac hypertrophy of SHR. The degree of cardiac hypertrophy was evaluated by means of regression analysis of left ventricular weight of SHR sedentary to body weight and tibia length, respectively. The difference in the degree of hypertrophy between ST 36° and ST 26° was significant (p < 0.05).

D. Cardiac dynamics

Essential parameters of cardiac function are depicted in Table 1 A and B. In the ST SHR a flattening of the LV end-diastolic pressure-volume relationship with increasing diastolic

Table 1. Influence of swimming training at different water temperatures on essential hemodynamic parameters in SHR.

A. Auxotonic conditions at regular diastolic filling

	SHR sed.		SHR ST 36°		SHR ST 26°	
LVEDP (mm Hg)	3.2 ±	1.0	3.4 ±	0.3	5.3 ±	1.2 a☆☆
σ_{diast} (10^{-4} N/mm^2)	2.5 ±	0.3	2.4 ±	0.2	5.2 ±	1.2 a☆☆ b☆☆
V_{ED} (ml)	0.30±	0.02	0.33±	0.01a☆	0.57±	0.15a☆☆ b☆☆
LVP (mm HG)	175.8 ±	10.9	145.3 ±	8.5a☆☆☆	152.1 ±	9.6a☆☆
σ_{syst} (10^{-4} N/mm^2)	107.9 ±	9.7	93.5 ±	12.1a☆	144.9 ±	22.4a☆☆ b☆☆
dP/dt max. pos. (mm Hg/s)	10372.9 ±1097.2		10909.2 ±861.4		10335.0 ±838.0	
dσ/dt max. pos. (10^{-3} N/mm^2/s)	776.5 ±	102.4	790.4 ±	94.9	1027.5 ±107.6a☆☆	
V_S (ml)	0.12±	0.02	0.14±	0.02	0.23±	0.07a☆☆ b☆
EF (%)	39.8 ±	4.9	43.0 ±	6.0	41.1 ±	3.2
Cardiac output (ml/min)	30.9 ±	4.8	31.9 ±	5.9	52.5 ±	11.9a☆☆ b☆☆
Heart rate (min^{-1})	246.0 ±	35.0	225.0 ±	47.0	220.0 ±	37.0
V_{CF} (circ/s)	2.05±	0.35	2.19±	0.40	1.76±	0.26b☆
Systolic SR (%)	52.2 ±	3.3	61.1 ±	3.2a☆☆	56.8 ±	3.1

Table 1. B. Isovolumetric conditions at optimal diastolic filling

	SHR sed.	SHR ST 36°	SHR ST 26°
LVP (mm Hg)	327.0 ± 19.3	351.7 ± 7.4a☆☆b☆☆	328.8 ± 11.7b☆☆
σ_{syst} (10^{-4} N/mm²)	286.6 ± 31.8	308.3 ± 31.3	353.2 ± 25.8a☆☆☆b☆
dP/dt max. pos. (mm Hg/s)	11077.0 ± 1584.0	11925.0 ± 187.0	9937.5 ± 1251.4b☆☆
dσ/dt max. pos. (10^{-3} N/mm²/s)	978.7 ± 202.6	1044.5 ± 93.4	1066.7 ± 138.4

LVEDP	= left ventricular end-diastolic pressure; LVP = left ventricular pressure;
σ_{diast}	= diastolic wall stress; σ_{syst} = systolic wall stress;
dP/dt max. pos.	= maximum rate of pressure rise; dσ/dt max. pos. = maximum rate of wall stress rise;
V_{ED}	= end-diastolic volume; V_S = stroke volume; EF = ejection fraction;
V_{CF}	= circumferential shortening velocity; systolic SR = systolic stress reserve.

Statistical comparisons: Values are mean ± SD ☆p < 0.05, ☆☆p < 0.01, ☆☆☆p < 0.001
Comparisons between swimming trained and sedentary SHR are indicated by a, comparisons between
SHR ST 36° and SHR ST 26° are indicated by b.

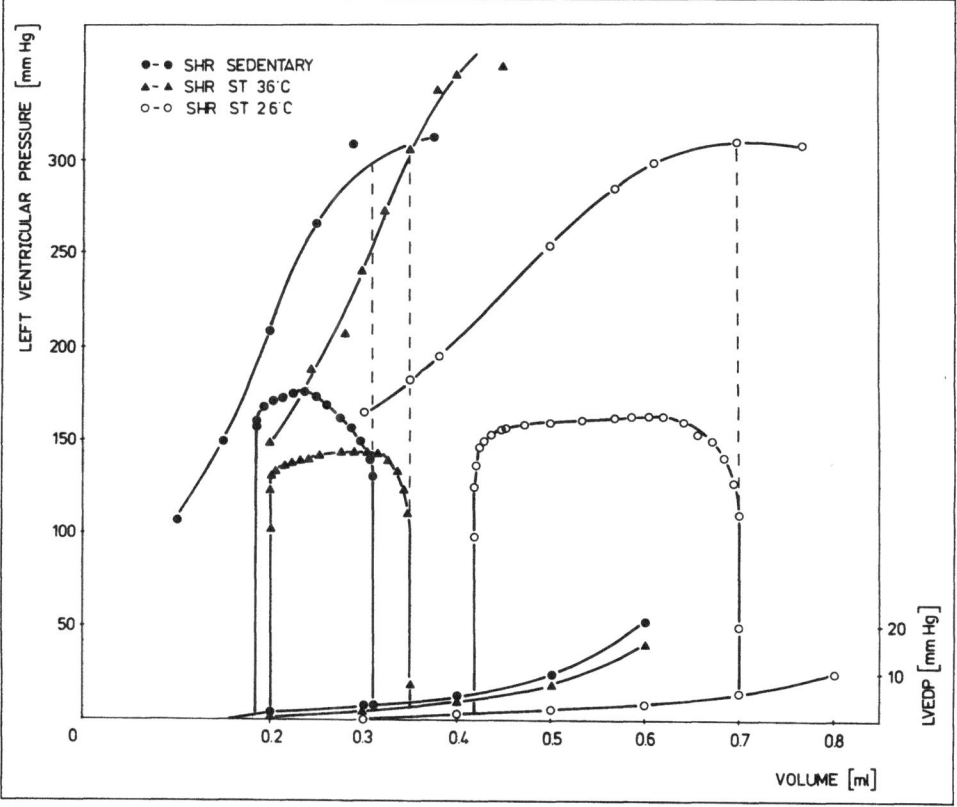

Fig. 3. Pressure-volume diagram. Isovolumetric maxima and pressure-volume loops of ejecting beats at the "working point" are presented for sedentary SHR and swimming trained SHR at 36° and 26° water temperature (SHR ST 36° and SHR ST 26°, resp.).

ventricular capacity was apparent (Fig. 3). The transformation towards volume type of hypertrophy was significantly more pronounced after ST 26° than after ST 36°. Consequently the working point was shifted to greater end-diastolic volumes, whereat an increase in LV filling pressure occurred in ST 26°.

According to the altered ventricular geometry the isovolumetric pressure-volume relationship shifted to the right for the ST collectives. In the range of high filling pressures isovolumetric pressure development as well as peak isovolumetric pressure were increased in ST 36° (p < 0.01), but not in ST 26° as compared with the sedentary group (Figs. 3 and 5 A). At optimal ventricular filling maximum rate of pressure rise (dP/dt max. pos.) was slightly increased for ST 36° and decreased for ST 26°, presumably due to geometric conditions (Fig. 5C). Peak isovolumetric wall stress and its maximum rate of rise, calculated for the midwall region were increased for both ST 36° and ST 26° (Figs. 4 and 5 B and D; Table 1 B).

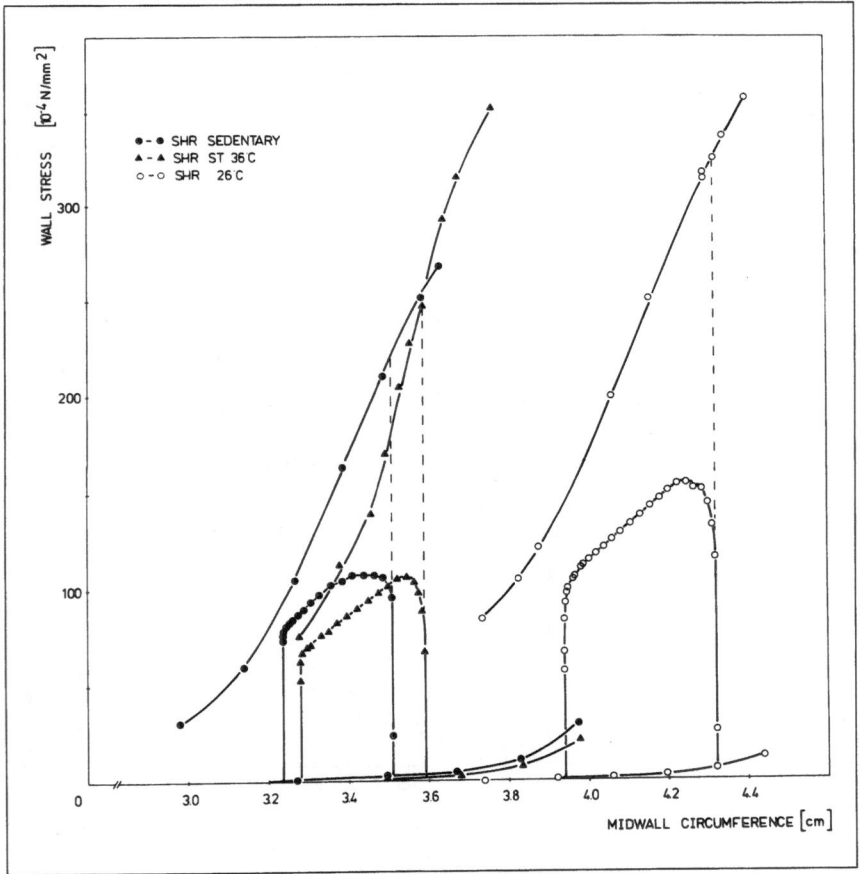

Fig. 4. Length-tension diagram, calculated on the basis of a thick-walled spherical shell corresponding to the data in Fig. 3. Note the increased systolic wall stress in SHR ST 26°.

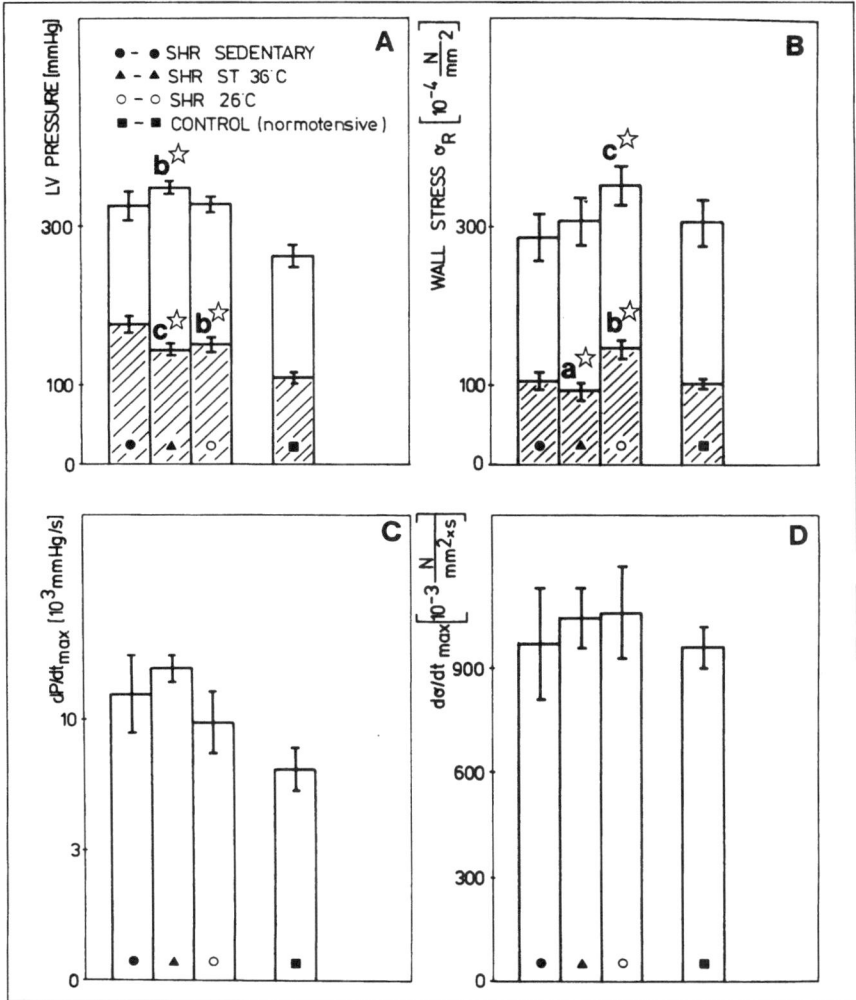

Fig. 5.
A and B: Auxotonic (hatched columns) and maximum isovolumetric pressure and wall stress as influenced by swimming training at different water temperatures (26° and 36°). For comparison age-matched normotensive nontrained controls are depicted.

C and D: Maximal values of left ventricular rate of pressure and wall stress rise.

Statistical comparisons: values are means ± SD. a☆ − p <0.05, b ☆ − p <0.01, c ☆ − p <0.001 (as compared to SHR sedentary).

Under auxotonic conditions at regular diastolic ventricular filling LV pressure was reduced significantly for ST 36° and ST 26° as compared to SHR sed. (p <0.001, p <0.01, respectively) Fig. 3; Table 1 A). This reduction was more marked after ST 36° than after ST 26°. Maximum rate of LV pressure rise was only slightly increased for ST 36°. Ejection fraction remained unaltered. However, as a result of greater diastolic ventricular capacity, stroke volume was increased and thus despite reduced heart rate, cardiac output was enhanced in ST SHR. The changes were more pronounced and only significant for ST 26° (Table 1 A).

Under regular auxotonic working conditions peak systolic LV wall stress of SHR sed. lay in the range of normotensive controls, indicating a fully compensated stage. As a result of the increase in LV muscle mass, only slight eccentricity and reduced LV pressure, peak systolic wall stress was decreased in ST 36° ($p < 0.05$; however not to be seen in Fig. 4). On the other hand, due to greater dilatation and inadequate increase in myocardial mass, it was markedly increased in ST 26° ($p < 0.01$) (Figs. 4 and 5 B; Table 1 A).

LV systolic stress reserve (%) was evaluated by: (isovolumetric systolic wall stress – auxotonic peak systolic wall stress) × 100/isovolumetric systolic wall stress. Auxotonic and isovolumetric beats were performed at the same end-diastolic wall stress. ST 36°, as a result of "luxury hypertrophy", led to a significant increase in LV systolic stress reserve ($p < 0.01$), while after ST 26° stress reserve showed a tendency to be already reduced compared to ST 36°.

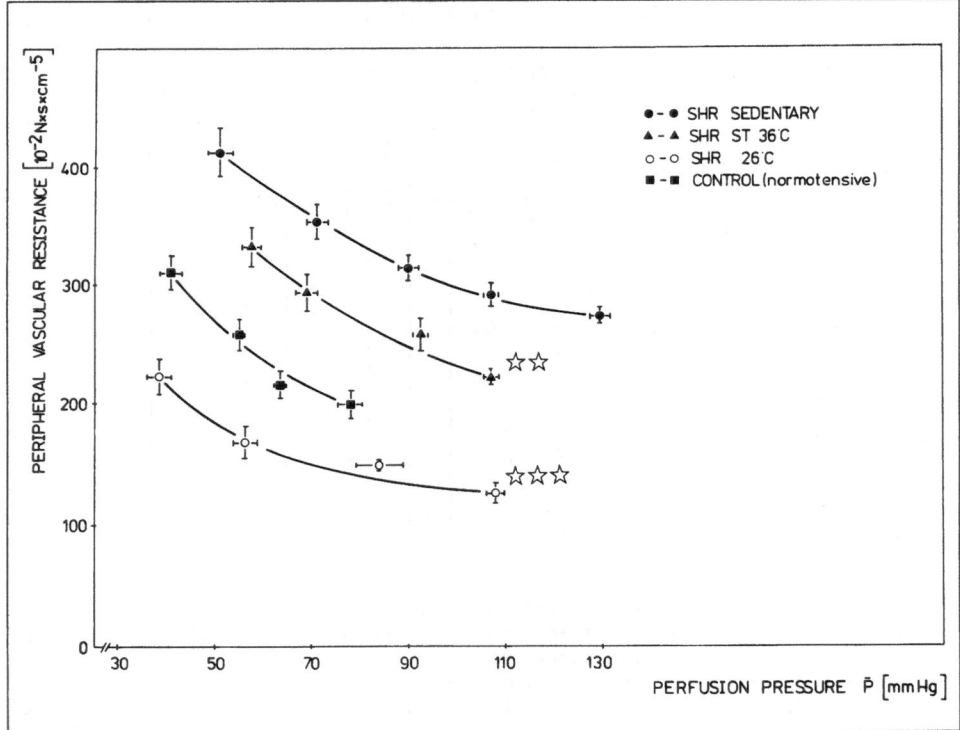

Fig. 6. Peripheral vascular resistance as influenced by swimming training.
Calculated PVR was fitted as a function of perfusion pressure $\bar{P}$. Different perfusion pressures were obtained by variation in volume loading.

Statistical comparisons: values are means ± SEM; ☆☆-$p < 0.01$, ☆☆☆-$p < 0.001$ (in comparison to SHR sedentary).

E. Peripheral vascular resistance (PVR)

PVR was plotted as a function of perfusion pressure $\bar{P}$ (Fig. 6). ST 36° reduced PVR significantly ($p < 0.01$), but failed to normalize it to the same value in normotensive rats. On the other hand, following ST 26°, the reduction in PVR was more pronounced. PVR values were even lower than those of normotensive controls ($p < 0.01$) over the whole range of perfusion pressure.

F. Alterations in endocrine state

In all ST groups the adrenal glands were massively increased compared to SHR sedentary (SHR sed.: 39.8 ± 6.0 mg; SHR ST 36°: 59.7 ± 5.6 mg; SHR ST 26°: 79.6 ± 8.6 mg; SHR ST 36° + at.: 67.3 ± 3.1 mg; $p < 0.001$; weights of left and right adrenal glands). This increase was most marked in ST 26°.

For the SHR ST 26° the plasma levels of thyroid hormones were determined and compared with the values of sedentary SHR of the same age from a previous study. While T_4 and fT_4 remained nearly unaltered, the values of T_3 (SHR sed.: 66.1 ± 3.1 ng/dl; SHR ST 26°: 82.8 ± 1.1 ng/dl; $p < 0.05$) and fT_3 (SHR sed.: 265.2 ± 8.8 pg/dl; SHR ST 26°: 428.1 ± 1.0 pg/dl; $p < 0.001$) were significantly elevated.

Discussion

While there is agreement that training is ineffective in modulating BP in secondary hypertension (9, 13), the influence of training on resting BP in primary hypertension is frequently described as a controversial topic (3, 19, 33, 41). Some of the contradictions in trained SHR may be due to differences in type, duration and intensity of training, in sex of the rats and to the fact that ST in itself is a complex stress (4). In an attempt to unravel some of the discrepancies regarding the effect of ST on BP in SHR and in hypertensive man, we included an additional thermal factor in our study by using different water temperatures. While ST 36°, as previously seen (30, 31), again led to a rapid decrease in systolic BP within the first few days, the time-course of BP during ST 26° was biphasic with an initial increase, followed by a delayed and less reduction in BP. The initial increase in BP was probably due to prolonged adrenergic stimulation induced by cold stress and overriding the diminution of sympathetic tone, usually observed during adaptation to physical exercise (3). Considering the water temperature at which humans usually swim, this could be an explanation for the ineffectiveness of ST to lower BP in hypertensive man. With increasing daily duration of ST, i. e. in the later stages of ST 26°, extensive alterations in the endocrine system, indicated by increased levels of circulating T_3 and fT_3 and marked increase in the weight of adrenal glands, were involved in the rat. Differences in the ability to maintain constant body temperature as well as in the response of the thyroid gland (5, 8) prohibit the transfer of these alterations in the late stage of ST 26° to man.

Mechanisms underlying the training-induced lowering of BP

The diminution of body weight can result in reduction of BP in essential hypertension (15) and thus could be cited as a cause of training-induced reduction of BP in SHR. In our present study, however, by restrictive feeding of the sedentary group, we ensured that no significant difference in body weight existed between the groups. This indicates that training per se is effective on BP, independent of the effect of reduced body weight.

Since resting cardiac output of the ST 36° SHR did not decrease, the reduction in systolic BP was a result of reduced PVR. Calculated PVR of ST 26° was most markedly reduced to values even below those of normotensive controls, but was partially compensated for by an enhanced cardiac output. Thus hypertension due to increased PVR, prevailing in that stage of SHR has turned into hypertension due to increased cardiac output, following long-term ST at 26°. Presumably, increased plasma levels of thyroid hormones are involved in the scope of adaptation to cold.

The mechanisms underlying the training-induced reduction of resting BP of SHR still appear enigmatic. Training-induced increase in vagal tone and diminution of sympathetic activity at rest (3, 33), changes in response of baro- or chemoreceptors (16, 38, 39), decrease in precapillary resistance (6), modification in the tone of vascular smooth muscles (6), possibly as a result of altered density or sensitivity of adrenergic receptors, increase in total vascular cross-sectional area (26) and involvement of the atrial natriuretic factor (10) must all be considered.

Cardiac adaptation: changes in degree of hypertrophy

The mode and the degree of cardiac hypertrophy during physical exercise are also controversial issues (32, 41). Increased LV weight as observed in trained normotensive, but not in trained SHR or trained rats with aortic stenosis, at times led to the conclusion that a ventricle, once adapted to pressure-overload, became less capable of reacting to volume-loading (7, 22). Our results, however, clearly indicate that the pressure-loaded left ventricle of SHR still has the potential to cope with the additional stimulus of volume-loading by increasing its myocardial mass and by transition into an eccentric type of hypertrophy. On the other hand, it was astonishing that during ST 36° in spite of drastic reduction of systolic BP, no regression of LV hypertrophy was observed, although eccentricity of the ventricles was only modestly pronounced. However, the degree of LV hypertrophy in SHR does not strictly correlate with systolic BP (34) as it does in rats with renovascular hypertension (35). The prevention of increase in LV weight during ST at 36° by additional application of atenolol, as shown by our present investigation, suggests that cardioadrenergic drive plays an important role in the hypertrophy process in SHR. These conclusions are supported by findings in literature which reveal that reduction of BP by pharmacological interventions without control of sympathetic activity fail to reduce the degree of hypertrophy in SHR (25, 36). Thus intermittently increased sympathetic activity has to be considered as a decisive factor for the increase in cardiac hypertrophy during ST of SHR.

In ST 26° two additional factors which influence the degree of hypertrophy have to be discussed. Beneath higher sympathetic activity – the one induced by exposition to cold is superimposed to the one induced by physical exercise – a permissive effect of thyroid hormones may be responsible for greater increase in cardiac hypertrophy in ST 26° as compared with ST 36° (11). Additionally, after a short time of swimming at low water temperatures, a decrease in body temperature of the rat was accompanied by a direct depressing effect of cooling on pacemaker activity that could not be overridden by exercise (1). Thus no adequate chronotropic reaction during exercise was possible and the required increase in cardiac output has to be achieved by enhanced stroke volume. The resultant emphasized significance of the Frank-Starling mechanism in this event could be responsible for the dilatation of the ventricles in ST 26°.

Cardiac performance

The increase in LV working capacity and in essential hemodynamic parameters as well as the enhanced LV systolic wall stress reserve all speak for improved ventricular and myocardial performance after ST at 36°. Thus our results confirm former studies (18, 20, 28, 32). In spite of a moderate change in ventricular shape towards eccentric hypertrophy, complying with the necessity of being able to expel a temporarily increased stroke volume, peak systolic wall stress in ejecting beats was reduced. Thus reduction in BP and increase in LV mass led to a state of "luxury hypertrophy" in ST 36°.

Also after ST 26° LV working capacity was enhanced primarily due to altered geometric conditions. Augmentation of LV inner diameter with, however, inadequate increase in myocardial mass occurred along with an increase in systolic wall stress. This type of unfavourable configuration with enhanced mechanical loading of the myocardium corresponds, strictly speaking, to the term "ventricular dilatation" (17). Since end-diastolic ventricular pressure was also moderately elevated, further investigation is necessary to clarify whether, under these conditions, LV pre-insufficiency had set in despite no indications of impaired myocardial contractility.

In summary, ST proved to be effective in lowering resting BP of SHR. Water temperature was of great influence with respect to cardiovascular adaptation and mechanisms involved in SHR. The early phase of ST 26° could provide some clue to the cause of the discrepancy in findings regarding the effects of ST in hypertensive man and SHR.

Cardioadrenergic drive was of great significance for the process of cardiac hypertrophy. Physical exercise could reveal new aspects in the treatment of essential hypertension. However, further investigation is needed to probe the effectiveness of physical training in reducing BP at rest and during exercise. Furthermore, the consequence of training on the process of cardiac hypertrophy in essential hypertensive man must be clarified.

References

1. Baker MA, Horvath SM (1964) Influence of water temperature on heart rate and rectal temperature of swimming rats. Am J Physiol 207: 1073–1076
2. Berglund G, Wilhelmsen L (1975) Factors related to blood pressure in a general population sample of Swedish men. Acta Med Scand 198: 291–298
3. Conway J (1984) Hemodynamic aspects of essential hypertension in humans. Physiol Rev 64: 617–660
4. Dawson CA, Horvath SM (1970) Swimming in small laboratory animals. Med Sci Sports 2: 51–78
5. Ducommun P, Sakiz E, Guillemin R (1966) Dissociation of the acute secretions of thyrotropin and adrenocorticotropin. Am J Physiol 210: 1257–1259
6. Edwards MT, Diana FN (1978) Effect of exercise on pre- and postcapillary resistance in the spontaneously hypertensive rat. Am J Physiol 234: H439–H446
7. Evenwel R, Struyker-Boudier H (1979) Effect of physical training on the development of hypertension in the spontaneously hypertensive rats. Pflügers Arch 381: 19–24
8. Fisher AD, Odell WD (1971) Effect of cold on TSH secretion in man. J Clin Endocr 33: 859–862
9. Fregly MJ (1984) Effect of an exercise regimen on development of hypertension in rats. J Appl Physiol 56: 381–387
10. Genest J (1984) Atrial natriuretic factor: Biochemistry and Physiopathology. Ther Woche 34: 6387–6388
11. Greenberg AH, Najjar S, Blizzard RM (1974) Effects of thyroid hormone on growth, differentiation and development. In: Greer MA, Solomon DH (eds) Handbook of Physiology. American Physiological Society, Washington, Vol III, pp 377–389
12. Grollman A (1972) The spontaneous hypertensive rat: an experimental analogue of essential hypertension in human being. In: Okamoto K (ed) Spontaneous hypertension. Springer-Verlag, New York, pp 238–242

168

13. Hanson JS, Nedde WH (1970) Preliminary observations on physical training for hypertensive males. Circ Res 26 (Suppl I): 49–53
14. Hepp A, Hansis M, Gülch R, Jacob R (1974) Left ventricular isovolumetric pressure-volume relations, "diastolic tone" and contractility in the rat heart after physical training. Basic Res Cardiol 69: 516–532
15. Horton ES (1981) The role of exercise in the treatment of hypertension in obesity. Int J Obes 5 (Suppl 1): 165–171
16. Huang TF, Peng FI (1976) Role of the chemoreceptor in diving bradycardia in rat. Jpn J Physiol 26: 395–401
17. Jacob R, Kissling G, Ebrecht G, Holubarsch C, Medugorac I, Rupp H (1983) Adaptive and pathological alterations in experimental cardiac hypertrophy. In: Chazov E, Saks V, Rona G (eds) Advances in myocardiology. Plenum Publishing Corporation, New York, Vol 4, pp 55–77
18. Jacob R, Kissling G, Ebrecht G, Holubarsch C, Rupp H (1984) Das Sportherz im Tierversuch: Einfluß eines chronischen Schwimmtrainings auf Herzdynamik, Myokardfunktion und kontraktile Proteine bei der Ratte. In: Jeschke D (ed) Stellenwert der Sportmedizin in Medizin und Sportwissenschaft. Springer-Verlag, Berlin Heidelberg New York, pp 34–47
19. Jeschke D, Bauer KE, Heitkamp HCh (1985) Die Bedeutung körperlichen Trainings in der Hochdruckbehandlung aus epidemiologischer und klinischer Sicht. Fortschr Med 103: 35–42
20. Kissling G, Wendt-Gallitelli MF (1977) Dynamics of the hypertrophied left ventricle in the rat. Effects of physical training and chronic pressure-load. Basic Res Cardiol 72: 178–183
21. Leon AS, Blackburn H (1982) Physical activity and hypertension. In: Sleight P, Freis E (eds) Hypertension. Butterworths, London, pp 14–36
22. Ljungquist A, Unge G, Carlsson S (1976) The myocardial capillary vasculature in exercising animals with increased cardiac pressure load. Acta Path Microbiol Scand, Sect A, 84: 244–246
23. McGiff JC, Quilley CP (1981) The rat with spontaneous genetic hypertension is not a suitable model of human essential hypertension. Circ Res 48: 455–463
24. Mirsky I, Parmley WW (1973) Assessment of passive elastic stiffness for isolated heart muscle and the intact heart. Circ Res 33: 233–243
25. Östman-Smith I (1981) Cardiac sympathetic nerves as the final common pathway in the induction of adaptive cardiac hypertrophy. Clin Sci 61: 265–272
26. Oppliger RA, Hodgins T, Tipton CM, Vailas AC, Marcus KD (1980) The influence of training on wall – lumen ratios of WKY and SHR populations. (Abstr) Med Sci Sports Exerc 12: 130
27. Paffenbarger RS, Wing AL, Hyde RT, Jung DL (1983) Physical activity and incidence of hypertension in college Alumni. Am J Epidemiol 117: 245–357
28. Pfeffer MA, Ferrell BA, Pfeffer JM, Weiss AK, Fishbein MC, Frohlich ED (1978) Ventricular morphology and pumping ability of exercised spontaneously hypertensive rats. Am J Physiol 235: H193–H199
29. Rost R, Hollmann W, Liesen H (1976) Körperliches Training mit Hochdruckpatienten, Ziele und Probleme. Herz/Kreislauf 8: 680–686
30. Rupp H, Jacob R (1982) Response of blood pressure and cardiac myosin polymorphism to swimming training in the spontaneously hypertensive rat. Can J Physiol Pharmacol 60: 1098–1103
31. Rupp H, Fellbier HR, Bukhari AR, Jacob R (1984) Modulation of myosin isoenzyme populations and activities of monoamine oxidase and phenylethanolamine-N-methyltransferase in pressure loaded and normal rat heart by swimming exercise and stress arising from electrostimulation in pairs. Can J Physiol Pharmacol 62: 1209–1218
32. Scheuer J, Penpargkul S, Bhan AK (1974) Experimental observations on the effects of physical training upon intrinsic cardiac physiology and biochemistry. Am J Cardiol 33: 744–751
33. Scheuer J, Tipton CM (1977) Cardiovascular adaptations to physical training. Ann Rev Physiol 39: 221–251
34. Sen S, Tarazi RC, Khairallah PA, Bumpus FM (1974) Cardiac hypertrophy in SHR. Circ Res 35: 775–781
35. Sen S, Tarazi RC, Bumpus FM (1981) Reversal of cardiac hypertrophy in renal hypertensive rats: medical vs. surgical therapy. Am J Physiol 240: H408–H412
36. Sen S, Tarazi RC (1983) Regression of myocardial hypertrophy and influence of adrenergic system. Am J Physiol 244: H97–H101

37. Smirk FH (1970) The neurogenically maintained component in hypertension. Circ Res 36 and 37 (Suppl II): 55–63
38. Tipton CM, Matthes RD, Marcus KD, Rowlett KA, Leininger JR (1983) Influences of exercise intensity, age, and medication on resting systolic blood pressure of SHR populations. J Appl Physiol: Respir Env Ex Physiol 55: 1 5–1310
39. Trzebski A, Malgorzata T, Zoltowski M, Przybylski J (1982) Increased sensitivity of the arterial chemoreceptor drive in young men with mild hypertension. Cardiovasc Res 16: 163–172
40. Ullrich JK, Riecker G, Kramer K (1954) Das Druck-Volumendiagramm des Warmblüterherzen. Isometrische Gleichgewichtskurven. Pflügers Arch 259: 481–498
41. Weiss L (1978) Adaptive cardiovascular changes to physical training in spontaneously hypertensive and normotensive rats. Cardiovasc Res 12: 329–333

Authors' address:

Dr. Martin Vogt, Physiologisches Institut II, Universität Tübingen, Gmelinstraße 5, D-7400 Tübingen (F.R.G.)

Basis and clinical significance of regression of hypertensive hypertrophy

W. Motz, J. Zähringer*, and B. E. Strauer

Zentrum für Innere Medizin der Philipps-Universität Marburg and *Medizinische Klinik I der Universität München (F.R.G.)

Summary

The basis of every therapy in hypertensive heart disease is blood pressure normalization. However, blood pressure should be lowered through antihypertensive drugs, which can a) regress LV hypertrophy, b) increase myocardial perfusion and c) improve LV function depending on the stage of hypertensive heart disease. Such a step-care of hypertensive heart disease must not be understood as a therapeutic scheme, but should be considered as an attempt to cover the clinical therapy of common hypertensive cardiac complications.

Key words: LV hypertrophy, antihypertensive therapy, myocardial protein synthesis

Introduction

Left ventricular (LV) hypertrophy presents the structural adaptation of the heart in response to a chronic arterial pressure burden. This mechanism enables the heart to maintain systemic perfusion in spite of excessive increased systolic pressures. However, concentric LV hypertrophy is not a permanent mechanism of compensation, because the hypertrophied heart cannot sustain the increased pressure load indefinitely and cardiac function will become impaired in the time course of cardiac hypertrophy (21, 22). Consequently, a medical therapy which prevents the development of LV hypertrophy or regresses an already established LV hypertrophy equals a causative treatment of hypertensive heart failure

Beznak (2) demonstrated that experimentally induced cardiac hypertrophy in response to an LV pressure overload due to renal hypertension, chronic thyroxine administration, aortic coarctation as well as nutrional anaemia was completely reversible after removal of the inciting stimulus. Since the aetiology of primary arterial hypertension in man as well as in spontaneously hypertensive rats (SHR) is unknown by definition, blood pressure has to be lowered more or less unspecifically by medical treatment. Recently, most clinically used antihypertensive drugs have been studied in SHR in respect of their ability to regress myocardial hypertrophy (13). The most interesting finding was that blood pressure normalization did not always lead to control of cardiac hypertrophy. Sen found after blood pressure normalization by hydralazine treatment no concomitant reversal of LV hypertrophy (18). After blood pressure lowering by minoxidil LV muscle mass was even found to be increased (19). Only a methyldopa treatment lead to regression of LV hypertrophy along with blood pressure reduction (20). These unexpected results raised questions on the hypothesis that progression and regression of LV hypertrophy are the mere consequences of physical forces acting on the myocytes.

Due to an increase in wall thickness, LV wall tension per cross-sectional area, i. e. LV systolic wall stress, can be preserved, even in the presence of an excessive LV systolic pressure load. Regarding LV ejection fraction and myocardial oxygen consumption per weight unit, such a hypertrophied ventricle does not differ from a non-hypertrophied one (21, 22).

When LV systolic pressure is lowered by medical therapy, corresponding to the processes of hypertrophy development, a complete structural remodeling of the ventricle is expected. Since experimental studies revealed that regression of LV hypertrophy is not always associated with blood pressure control, it has been suggested that extra-cardiac humoral factors may play an important part in developing and reversing LV hypertrophy. Since alpha-methyldopa therapy, which was found to induce regression of LV hypertrophy, leads to diminished myocardial catecholamine concentrations, it was argued that catecholamines and the sympathetic nervous system play the deciding role in LV hypertrophy apart from LV systolic pressure. This hypothesis was supported by experiments in dogs, which indicated that subhypertensive doses of norepinephrine could actually induce myocardial hypertrophy (10).

Experimental studies

After treatment of SHRs with metoprolol in combination with hydralazine a significantly lower LV muscle mass was found than after monotherapy with hydralazine. After this 40 week treatment with hydralazine, LV hypertrophy was found to be significantly lower than in untreated SHR (14) (Fig. 1). This finding is in line with data of Pfeffer et al., who could prevent a further increase in LV muscle mass from 12 to 18 months of age by hydralazine treatment (17). The failure of Sen et al. (18) to show this effect in spite of blood pressure normalization may be due to the short duration of treatment (6 weeks) in their study. They argued that reflex-raised catecholamines through hydralazine may offset the mechanical effect of systolic unloading on cardiac hypertrophy. The finding that after an additional therapy with metoprolol at almost identical blood pressure levels, LV muscle mass was quantitatively lower than after hydralazine alone, supports the hypothesis that, at least in SHR, adrenergic influences on the myocardium may play a part in the development of cardiac hypertrophy besides systolic blood pressure. Moreover, the influence of antihypertensive drugs on heart rate may also modulate their efficacy in respect of LV hypertrophy. A higher heart rate means a higher frequency of peak systolic pressure events and may also contribute to the fact that LV hypertrophy was less expressed after additional metoprolol treatment (heart rate: 380 beats/min) than after hydralazine alone (heart rate: 414/min). A 20 week long antihypertensive therapy with the calcium channel blocker nifedipine was found to regress LV muscle mass in SHRs even when therapy was started in the fully established phase of LV hypertrophy.

Along with blood pressure normalization due to nifedipine treatment LV muscle mass was reduced (Fig. 2). It is conceivable that regression of LV hypertrophy extends only to contractile proteins of the myocardium, whereas non-contractile proteins such as collagen may persist. In this event, a therapeutically induced reversal of muscle mass would cause an increment in myocardial collagen concentration and therefore deteriorate diastolic distensibility due to an increase in stiffness (9). Since after the nifedipine treatment myocardial collagen concentration remained unaltered, total LV collagen mass decreased along with muscle mass reduction (12). Consequently, regression of LV hypertrophy through nifedipine treatment also affects LV collagen mass contrary to a methyldopa therapy which leaves LV collagen unchanged in spite of myocardial mass reduction. To determine whether reversal of LV collagen is commonly associated with reversal of LV hypertrophy or whether drug specific effects play a role in controlling myocardial collagen mass, further studies are

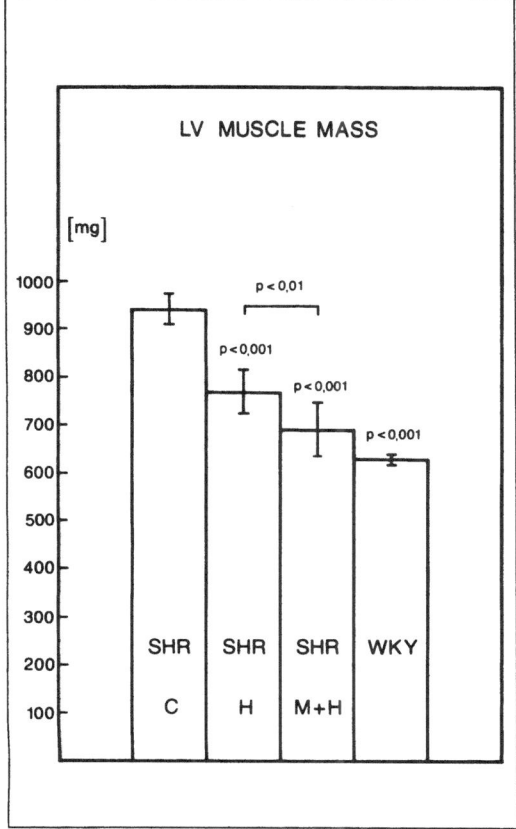

Fig. 1. Mean data (± standard deviation) for LV muscle mass of untreated SHR (C), SHR treated with hydralazine (H), SHR treated with metoprolol and hydralazine (M + H), and normotensive Wistar-Kyoto control rats (WKY).

necessary. Myocardial protein synthesis is primarily regulated by the myocardial messenger RNS concentration, whereas degradation processes play only a minor part. Since messenger RNA concentration was significantly lower in nifedipine treated hearts than in untreated controls, a medical treatment with nifedipine extends also to cardiac gene-expression for cardiac protein synsthesis (Fig. 3) (3).

Clinical studies

Comparable to experimental investigations clinical studies also revealed a wide scatter in respect of the ability of antihypertensive agents in inducing reversal of LV hypertrophy. Whereas blood pressure control through phtalazine derivates such as hydralazine and trimazosine was not associated with reversal of LV hypertrophy (4, 5), antihypertensive treatment with sympatholytic substances such as alpha-methyldopa, resperine and clonidine caused a marked decrease in LV muscle mass (1, 7, 23, 26). A therapy with the calcium channel blocker nifedipine also induced reversal of myocardial hypertrophy along with blood pressure reduction (24). So did angiotensin converting enzyme inhibitors such as captopril and enalapril (8, 11, 15, 16), whereas diuretics have no hypertrophy reversing

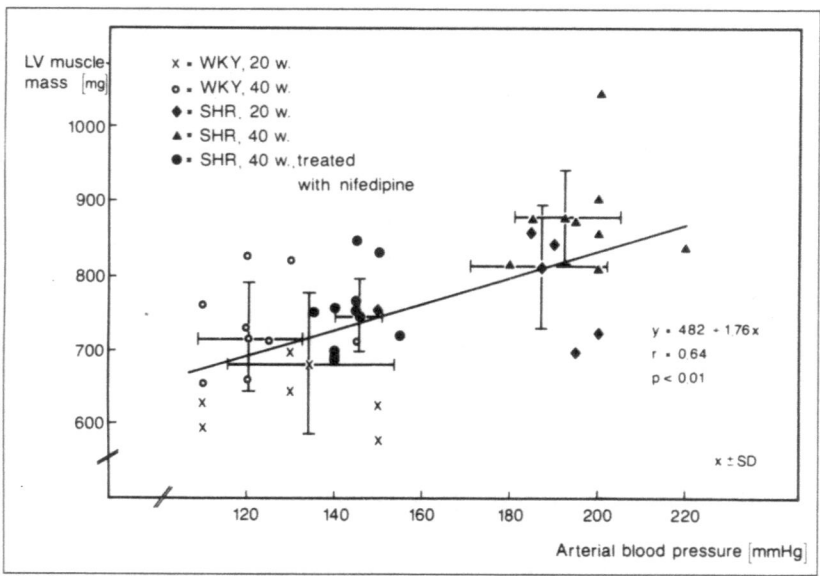

Fig. 2. A direct correlation between systolic arterial blood pressure and left ventricular (LV) muscle after treatment with nifedipine exists. LV muscle mass decreased along with a reduction in blood pressure.

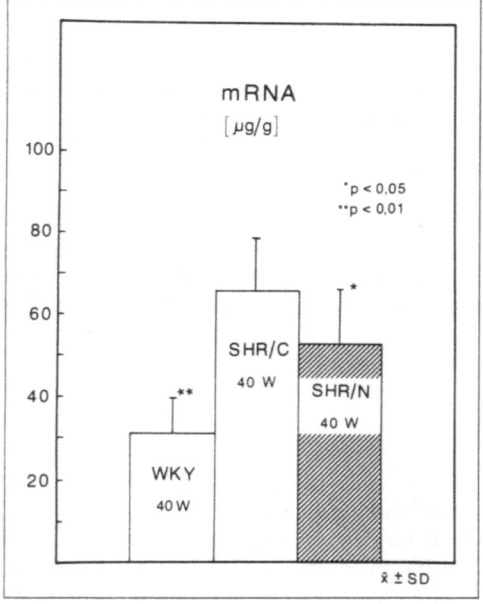

Fig. 3. Mean data ($\pm$ standard deviation) for mRNA ($\mu g/g$) of normotensive Wistar-Kyoto control rats (WKY), untreated spontaneously hypertensive rats (SHR/C) and SHR treated with nifedipine (SHR/N).

potency or they reverse LV hypertrophy to a small extent only (4, 6). A beta-receptor blocker is also effective in diminution of LV mass, although regression of hypertrophy occurred only after a very prolonged treatment (> 8 months) (25).

That cathecholamines may also play a part in reversal of hypertrophy in man is underlined by studies with clonidine and prazosin (23). In relation to the amount of blood pressure decrease a clonidine treatment, which reduced peripheral norepinephrine levels, reduced LV muscle mass to a greater proportion than a prazosin therapy, which left peripheral catecholamines unchanged. When considering the individual response of norepinephrine to clonidine therapy and dividing the clonidine collective into responders and non-responders, responders did reveal a larger drop in LV mass than non-responders (Fig. 4) (23).

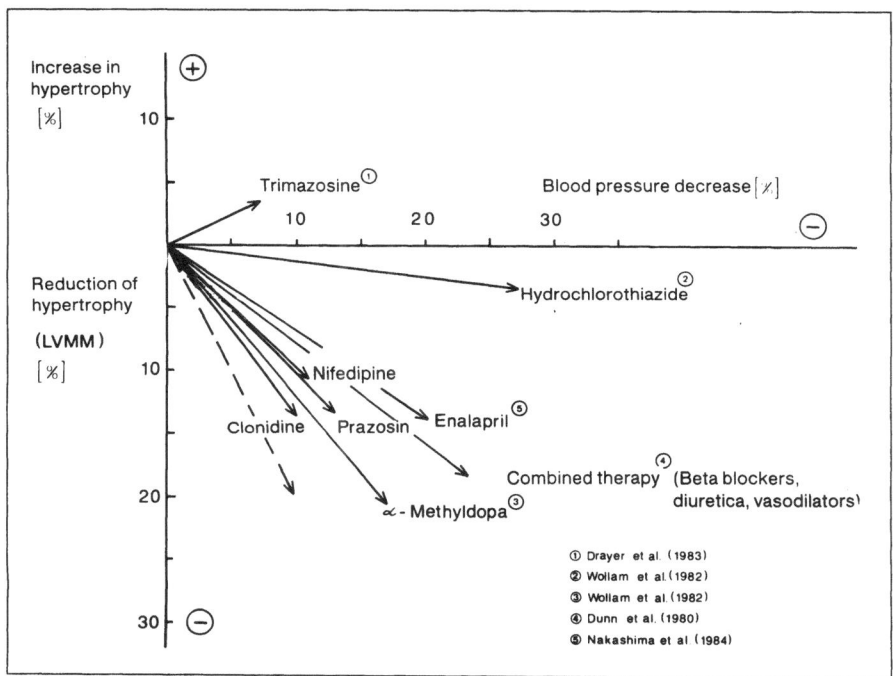

Fig. 4. Relationship between the amount of blood pressure decrease and the extent of reversal of hypertrophy after various antihypertensive agents. The dotted line represents patients who under clonidine therapy revealed a significant decrease of plasma-norepinephrine concentration. Notice the most pronounced regression of hypertrophy under this therapy in comparison to the other treatments.

In summary, drug specific effects of the different antihypertensive agents seem to modulate the structural cardiac changes following systolic relief due to systemic blood pressure lowering.

For example an antihypertensive therapy with the ganglion-blocking agent guanethidine, which usually causes fluid retention, increases end-diastolic volume. Accordingly, a new stimulus for LV hypertrophy – eccentric LV hypertrophy –, is generated, which is the typical structural response of the heart to a volume load (17). Consequently, an antihypertensive treatment with hydralazine and minoxidil (18, 19), which leads to hypercirculation, diminishes the favourable mechanical effects of blood pressure control on LV hypertrophy or compensates for those effects completely.

176

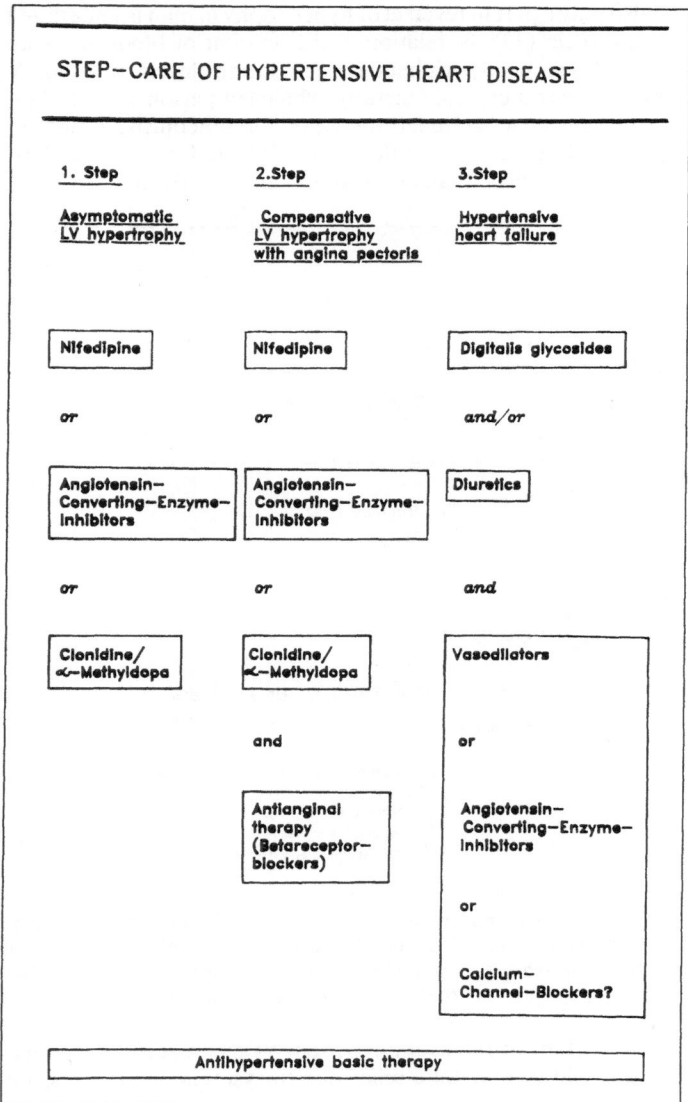

Fig. 5. Step-care of hypertensive heart disease according to the specific stage of disease.

Therapeutic consequences

The analysis of the experimental and clinical data point to the possibility of a specific therapy of hypertensive heart disease, which is naturally distinctly different from treatment of mere arterial hypertension. Whereas established antihypertensive step care aims at normalization of hypertensive blood pressure, the therapy of hypertensive heart disease aims at completely reversing hypertensive cardiac organ manifestations such as LV hypertrophy and coronary microangiopathy. In analogy to the different stages of hypertensive heart disease (haemodynamically compensated LV hypertrophy with or without angina pectoris, hypertensive heart failure) a step care specifically designed for hypertensive heart disease should be performed. In the case of haemodynamically compensated LV hypertrophy with or without angina pectoris, regression of both myocardial hypertrophy and coronary micro-angiopathy should be the main therapeutical goal (step 1).

In the event of additional hypertensive coronary insufficiency a decreased myocardial energy consumption and an enhanced coronary perfusion is aimed at (step 2). When hypertensive heart disease has progressed to the stage of heart failure, improvement of LV function through inotropic stimulation and systolic unloading should be at the center of therapeutic considerations (step 3). Consequently, such a differentiated step care of hypertensive heart disease differs from an antihypertensive treatment using primarily diuretics and beta-receptor blockers (Fig. 5). Since diuretic and beta-receptor blockers, which are first line drugs in arterial hypertension, have no pronounced effects on reducing LV hypertrophy, they have only minor importance in the therapy of hypertensive heart disease. On the other hand calcium channel blockers, sympatholytic drugs and angiotensin converting enzyme inhibitors, which are drugs of second and third choice in arterial hypertension appear to be first line agents in the step care of hypertensive heart disease.

References

1. Alcocer L, Aspe J (1979) The effect of antihypertensive treatment with alpha-methyldopa on left ventricular mass. In: Robertson JIS, Caldwell ADS (eds) Left ventricular hypertrophy in hypertension. Royal Society of Medicine International Congress and Symposium Series No. 9 Academic Press (London), and Grune & Stratton, pp 94–97
2. Beznak M, Korecky B, Thomas G (1969) Regression of cardiac hypertrophies of various origin. Can J Physiol Pharmacol 47: 579–586
3. Danninger B, Stangl E, Aschauer W, Motz W, Strauer BE, Zähringer J (1985) Herzmuskelhypertrophie – Regression und Veränderungen der myokardialen Genexpression unter Nifedipin-Gabe. Z Kardiol 74 (Suppl 3): 62
4. Devereux RB, Savage DD, Sachs J, Laragh JH (1980) Effect of blood pressure control on left ventricular hypertrophy and function in hypertension. Circulation 62 (Suppl II): II-36
5. Drayer JIM, Gardin JM, Weber MA, Aronow WS (1982) Changes in cardiac anatomy and function during therapy with alpha-methyldopa: an echocardiographic study. Curr Ther Res 32: 856–865
6. Drayer JIM, Weber MA, Gardin JM, Lipson JL (1983) Effect of long-term antihypertensive therapy on cardiac anatomy in patients with essential hypertension. Am J Med 75 (Suppl 3A): 116
7. Fouad FM, Nakashima Y, Tarazi RC, Salcedo EE (1982) Reversal of left ventricular hypertrophy in hypertensive patients treated with alpha-methyldopa: lack of association with blood pressure control. Am J Cardiol 49: 795
8. Fouad FM, Tarazi RC, Bravo EL (1983) Hemodynamic and cardiac effects of enalapril. J. Hypertension 1 (Suppl 1): 135
9. Hess OM, Riter M, Schneider J, Grimm J, Turina M, Krayenbühl HP (1983) Diastolic myocardial stiffness and myocardial structure in aortic valve disease before and after value replacement. J Am Coll Cardiol 1 (2): 640
10. Laks MN, Morady F (1976) Norepinephrine – the myocardial hypertrophy hormone? Am Heart J 91: 674–675

11. Lederle RM, Klaus D, Tegenthoff M (1984) Die Rückbildung der Linksherzhypertrophie unter Captopril bei Patienten mit therapieresistenter Hypertonie. Herz/Kreislauf 2: 73
12. Motz W, Ploeger M, Strauer BE (1983) The effect of nifedipine on cardiac function in acute pulmonary embolism. Circulation 68 (Suppl III): 36
13. Motz W, Strauer BE (1984) Regression of structural cardiovascular changes by antihypertensive therapy. Hypertension 6 (Suppl III): 133–139
14. Motz W, Strauer BE (1985) Prevention of left ventricular hypertrophy by antihypertensive therapy in spontaneously hypertensive rats: effects on systolic wall stress and systolic function. Basic Res Cardiol (in press)
15. Mujais SK, Tarazi RC, Rouad FM, Bravo EL (1983) Reversal of left ventricular hypertrophy with captopril. Clin Cardiol 6: 595
16. Nakashima MAJ, Fouad FM, Tarazi RC (1984) Regression of left ventricular hypertrophy from systemic hypertension by enalapril. Am J Cardiol 53: 1044
17. Pfeffer JM, Pfeffer MA, Fletcher P, Fishbein M, Brawald E (1982) Favorable effects of therapy on cardiac performance in spontaneously hypertensive rats. Am J Physiol 242: H 776
18. Sen S, Tarazi RC, Khairallah PA, Bumpus FM (1974) Cardiac hypertrophy in spontaneously hypertensive rats. Circ Res 35: 775
19. Sen S, Tarazi RC, Bumpus FM (1977) Cardiac hypertrophy and antihypertensive therapy. Cardiovasc Res 11: 427
20. Spech M, Ferrario CM, Tarazi RC (1980) Cardiac pumping ability following reversal of hypertrophy and hypertension in spontaneously hypertensive rats. Hypertension 2: 75
21. Strauer BE (1979) Myocardial oxygen consumption in chronic heart disease: Role of wall stress, hypertrophy and coronary reserve. Am J Cardiol 44: 730
22. Strauer BE (1983) Das Hochdruckherz, 2nd ed. Springer-Verlag, Berlin
23. Strauer BE (1985) Neue Ergebnisse in der Therapie der hypertensiven Herzkrankheit. Therapiewoche (in press)
24. Strauer BE, Mahmoud MA, Bayer F, Bohn I, Motz U (1984) Reversal of left ventricular hypertrophy and improvement of cardiac function in man by nifedipine. Eur Heart 5 (Suppl I): 53
25. Trimarco B, Wikstrand J (1984) Regression of cardiovascular structural changes by antihypertensive treatment. Hypertension 6 (Suppl III): III–150
26. Wollam GL et al. (1982) Diuretic potency of combined hydrochlorothiazide and furosemide therapy in patients with azotemia. Am J Med 72 (6): 929

Authors' address:

Dr. W. Motz, Lehrstuhl für innere Medizin, Schwerpunkt Kardiologie, Philipps-Universität Marburg, Klinikum Lahnberge, Baldinger Straße, D-3550 Marburg/Lahn (F.R.G.)

V. Morphology and pathophysiology of the failing heart

Histochemically determinable changes in cardiac insufficiency and their functional significance*

C. P. Adler

Institute of Pathology, Ludwig-Aschoff-Haus, University of Freiburg (F.R.G.)

Summary

Chronic cardiac insufficiency can be produced by a variety of causes which may be partly determined by means of macroscopic, histological and electron microscopic investigations. By using quantitative histochemical methods, changes of substances in the myocardium can be observed indicating myocardial insufficiency and giving an explanation of its cause. Hypertrophied hearts without insufficiency show cardiac muscle fibres having increased in width, volume and dry weight up to a maximum value which will not be exceeded even in further progressing cardiac hypertrophy. The biochemically determined amount of collagen increases significantly with the growing weight of the myocardium. Both the myocardial amount of DNA and the amount of myoglobin, correlated with the width of the fibres, have also increased. The heart muscle nuclei showed a polyploidization which is also correlated with the weight of the myocardium. In insufficient hearts suffering from myocardial hypertrophy, the increase of the total DNA content is significantly decreased as compared to non-insufficient hearts. The mean ploidy level is increased in case of lower weights of the myocardium and decreased in higher weights in comparison to non-insufficient hearts of the same weight. In insufficient hearts a more significantly increased amount of the connective tissue cells is observed than in the case of cardiac hypertrophy alone. In contrast to this, the increase of the heart muscle cells is significantly reduced. A lack of contractile proteins, decreased DNA synthesis, increased fibrozation and, in particular, the reduced number of cardiac muscle cells must be considered as essential factors for cardiac insufficiency.

Key words: heart hypertrophy, heart insufficiency, DNA cytophotometry, cell number, fibres dry weight, hydroxyprolin estimation, morphometry

Introduction

Cardiac insufficiency is characterized by a condition in which the heart fails to supply the organism with abundant blood both at rest and during physical strain although sufficient blood is available and blood pressure is satisfactory. This condition is usually produced in the myocardium itself because a reduced pumping rate is due to a decreased contractility of the heart muscle in myocardial insufficiency. Cardiac insufficiency may be produced by many causes, and in some cases the underlying condition may be determined at patho-anatomic level (for instance: cardiac malformation, stenosis of the aortic valve, myocarditis, myocardial infarction). In many other cases, however, the functional status is only roughly reflected by the morphological changes seen in the myocardium.

The results obtained from various patho-anatomic investigations depend on the respective

* This study was supported by grants from the Deutsche Forschungsgemeinschaft.

cardiac disease (21). Metabolic disturbances mainly show changes at the submicroscopic level, while macroscopic and microscopic findings only allow a tentative diagnosis to be established. Microscopic studies play a decisive role in myocarditis. Changes influencing the shape and size of the heart can easily be analysed macroscopically and will also reveal characteristic changes at the submicroscopical level. Hearts showing chronic insuffiency are usually considerably enlarged macroscopically. Histologically a loosened myocardium showing myocytolyses, disseminated myocardial necroses, an interstitial edema associated with cellular infiltrates or a finely maculated interstitial fibrosis is observed. Due to this, a loss of coordination capacity of the heart muscle cells is seen followed by a reduced effectiveness of myocytic contraction. The extent of these microscopic changes is correlated with the degree of cardiac insufficiency.

In myocardial insufficiency pathological changes are determined ultrastructurally in the cellular membranes, in the basic sarcoplasm and its cellular organelles, in the nucleus as well as in the interstitium. Frequently a dehiscence of the intercalated disks is observed producing mainly a disturbed ventricular stimulus conduction as well as a loss of coordination within the individual heart muscle cells (14, 19, 20). In addition, a more or less pronounced swelling of the mitochondria and the endosarcoplasmic reticulum, showing dilated transversal tubuli, is recognized.

By means of quantitative histochemical measurements we have been investigating insufficient hearts over a long period of time and our compiled data were helpful in clarifying some problems of cardiac insufficiency.

Methodological procedures

Human hearts of all ages (autopsy material) with hypertrophy and cardiac insufficiency were analysed histochemically using different methods: The width of muscle cell fibres was estimated by *morphometric measurements* and from the measurement data the volume of heart muscle fibres could be calculated. The *dry weight* of heart muscle fibres measuring 10 μ was determined by means of X-ray historadiographs (30). The *amount of collagen*, as a measure of fibrous tissue, was estimated by determination of hydroxyprolin (31). Quantitative measurements of *DNA* were also performed by biochemical methods (diphenylamine reaction [11, 12, 13]) and by Feulgen-cytophotometry (1, 23). On the basis of quantitative ultraviolet-cytophotometric examinations we determined the *amount of myoglobin* in the heart muscle cells (8). The absolute number of connective tissue and heart muscle cells was calculated by the method developed by Adler (1, 2) based upon biochemical and cytophotometric DNA measurements.

Our own studies

A. Cardiac hypertrophy without insufficiency

Width and volume of fibres: In hypertrophic hearts, myocardial fibres differing greatly in width can be observed histologically (2). The width of fibres may increase from normally 15 μ up to 23.6 μ (Fig. 1 a). In the right ventricle the width of fibres is reduced by 12% in comparison with the left ventricle. In cardiac hypertrophy of the left ventricle the difference is 28%. Our morphometric measurements also showed that the maximum width of fibres in the right ventricle is found to be 18.6 μ, and 23.6 μ in the left ventricle. Even in higher degrees of cardiac hypertrophy the width of fibres will not exceed these values (7). In hypertrophic hearts the volume of the heart muscle fibres increases up to a maximum of 37% (Fig. 1 b). This increase is more pronounced in the left than in the right ventricle. The maximum value of 2550 μ^3 presents a marginal volume which will not be exceeded even in the case of more excessive cardiac hypertrophy.

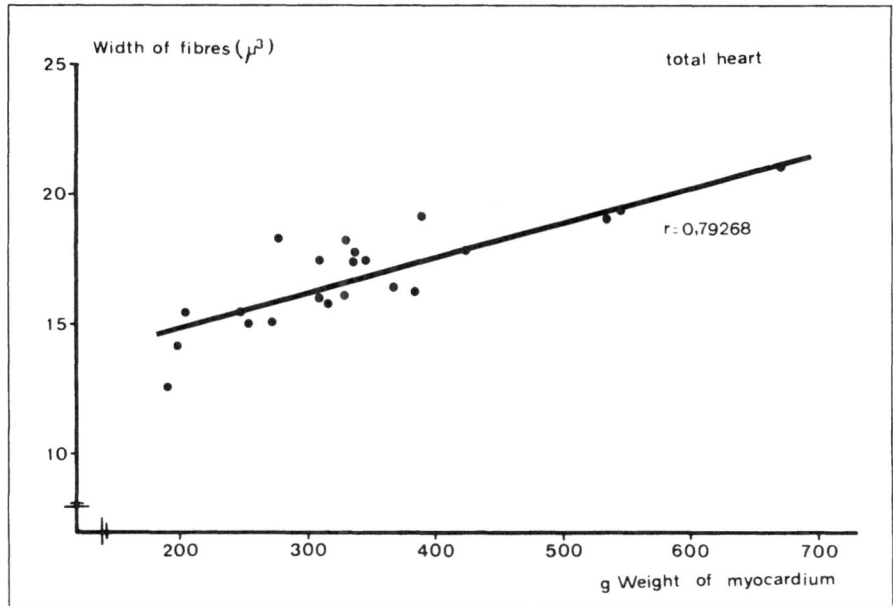

Fig. 1a.

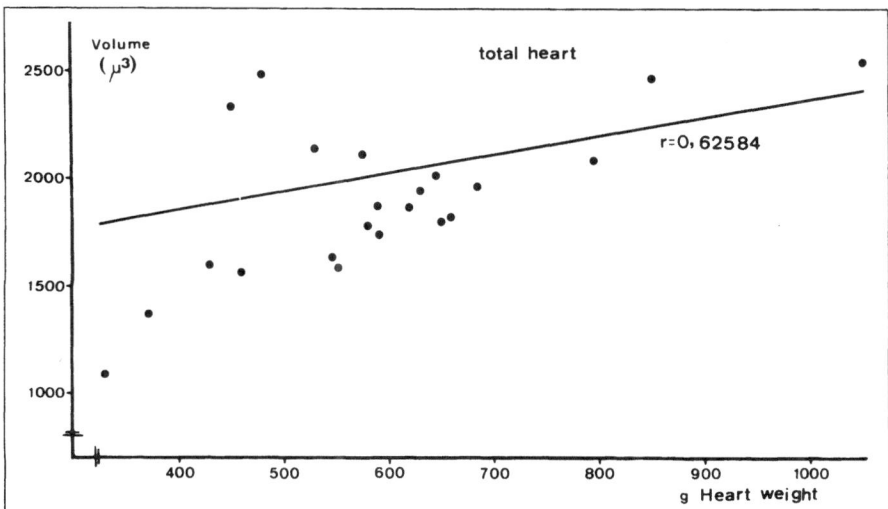

Fig. 1b

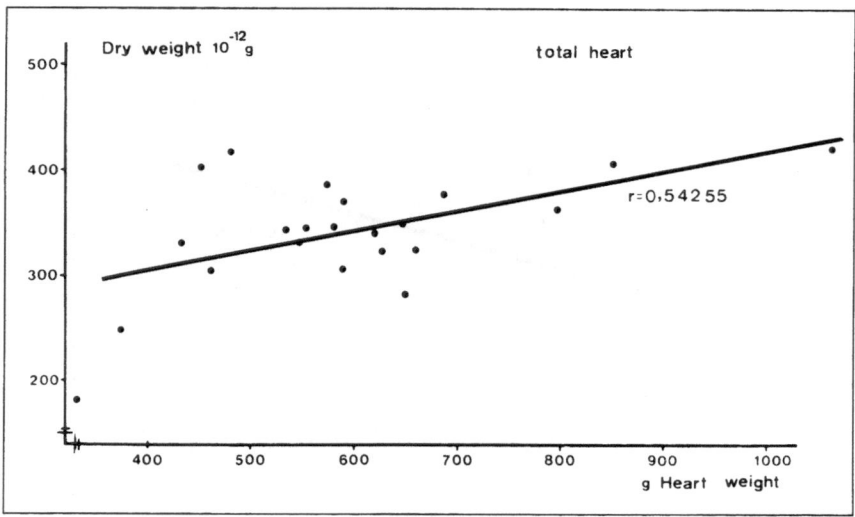

Fig. 1c

Fig. 1a, 1b, 1c. a) Increase of the fibre width of the heart muscle cells in cardiac hypertrophy from 15 μm to a maximum value of 23.6 μm.

b) Increase of the volume of the heart muscle fibres – referring to a length of fibre sections of 10 μm – in cardiac hypertrophy, up to a maximum volume of 2550 μm³.

c) Increase of the dry weight of the fibres – reffering to a length of fibre sections of 10 μm – in cardiac hypertrophy, from 250 $\times$ 10⁻¹² g to a maximum value of 450 $\times$ 10⁻¹² g.

Dry weight of fibres: The dry weight of sections of heart muscle fibres from normal hearts measuring 10 μ is about 250 $\times$ 10⁻¹² g (Fig. 1 c). We were able to demonstrate a significant increase of the dry weight of fibres obtained from hypertrophic hearts weighing up to 500 g. In a heart weighing 480 g, we found the dry weight of the fibres to be 418 $\times$ 10⁻¹²g. With progressing cardiac hypertrophy no further increase of the dry weight of the fibres was observed. In a heart weighing 850 g and in a heart weighing 1060 g, we found a somewhat lower dry weight of 407 $\times$ 10⁻¹² g than in hearts weighing 500 g. These findings suggest that in hearts weighing up to 500 g the increased mass of the hypertrophied heart may be explained by a considerable increased weight and size of the individual heart muscle cells (7, 25, 29). In more excessive degrees of hypertrophy an additional multiplication of the heart muscle cells must, however, be assumed.

Morphology of heart muscle cells: The structural transformation of the myocardium in cardiac hypertrophy due to hyperfunction has a morphologic equivalent in the structures of the heart muscle nuclei (9). This shows an increasing euchromatinization indicating a stimulated cellular function (24). Excessively hypertrophied hearts characteristically show so-called "inguinal nuclei" with longitudinally oriented, deep grooves which were described by Aschoff as early as 1905. "Inguinal nuclei" are produced by an impression of the clotted myofibrils (17). Newly formed myofilaments, an occurrence of membranes of the ergastoplasm as well as an increase of ribosomes and glycogenic granules in the basal sarcoplasm can be observed (20, 22, 32). Frequently an intermediary sarcolemma is found to be lying between two intercalated disks which must not be mistaken for a dehiscence of the intercalated disks (20). Finally, a mitochondriosis can be observed composed of a great number of small polymorphic mitochondria which are probably of little functional value because they do not possess any vital mitochondrial granules (16).

Connective tissue: In progressing cardiac hypertrophy the content of connective tissue of the myocardium is seen to increase. By means of the determination method for hydroxyprolin (31), we defined biochemically the content of collagen in normal and hypertrophied hearts. Our findings revealed that the total myocardial amount of collagen increases significantly in correlation with the growing weight of the pure myocardium. In a normal heart weighing 360 g, we found 1325 mg collagen, whereas in a heart weighing 900 g, 6162 mg collagen was found.

DNA: A prerequisite for myocardial growth is a synthesis of DNA. Quantitative biochemical determinations of the DNA in hearts of children revealed that the total amount of DNA increases with the growing heart weight. From the time of birth until adult age, the amount of DNA increases from 20 mg to 100 mg (6). In hypertrophic hearts weighing up to 900 g the amount of DNA is increased as much as threefold in comparison with normal hearts. The amount of DNA obtained from the heart muscle nuclei alone, which was determined by means of cytophotometric measurements, reveals that in cardiac hypertrophy the progressing weight of the myocardium is accompanied by a drastic and highly significant increase of DNA from 3×10^{-9} g in normal hearts up to 9.7×10^{-9} g in excessively hypertrophied hearts (7).

Myoglobin: By means of quantitative ultraviolet cytophotometric investigations we additionally found an augmentation of the amount of myoglobin (4, 8). In hearts weighing less than 500 g the amount of myoglobin equals 6 arbitrary units (AU), whereas in hearts weighing more than 500 g 10–14 AU were observed. Thus an amount of myoglobin showing a difference of about 100 % in normal human hearts as compared to hypertrophied hearts can be noted above the critical heart weight of 500 g. With progressing weight of the heart no further increase of the amount of myoglobin in the muscle fibres is seen (5, 18). If the measurement values are based on the respective width of the fibres it becomes evident that the amount of myoglobin is correlated with the width of the fibres. Fibres of hypertropied hearts contain significantly more myoglobin as compared to those of normotrophic hearts.

Polyploidization: All our quantitative histochemical investigations have revealed that the growth of the individual heart muscle fibres in hyperfunctional cardiac hypertrophy does not exceed a critical limit. If a functional overload in the myocardium were to continue this would lead to insufficiency unless a further multiplication of the heart muscle cells provided a final reserve for compensation. An increased synthesis of DNA is necessary for numeric hyperplasia of the myocardial cells (28). A comparison of the percentage distribution of the ploidy levels in normal and hypertrophied hearts shows the interdependence of the DNA content of the heart muscle nuclei in correlation with the heart weight. Whereas in normal hearts tetraploid cells dominate with a value of 50–55 % in the presence of 20 % diploid and octoploid nuclei, an increased polyploidization occurs with progressing hypertrophy. In a heart weighing 850 g, no diploid heart muscle cells remain to be seen. Besides 29 % tetraploid cells, only higher ploidy levels are found to be present.

Cell number: After having defined the basic underlying conditions leading to an increase of the myocardial cells, we elaborated a method which allows the determination of the total cell number in the heart (1, 27): after determining the weight of the heart during autopsy, the pure weight of the myocardium is estimated. Representative muscle samples are removed for biochemical determination of DNA was well as for cytophotometric measurements and for the preparation of histological sections. By applying the biochemical method for determining DNA the total amount of DNA in the respective heart is obtained. By means of cytophotometric measurements the ploidy levels of the heart muscle nuclei and their percentage distribution are estimated. By counting the nuclei in the histological sections, the quantitative relationship between heart muscle nuclei and connective tissue nuclei is obtain-

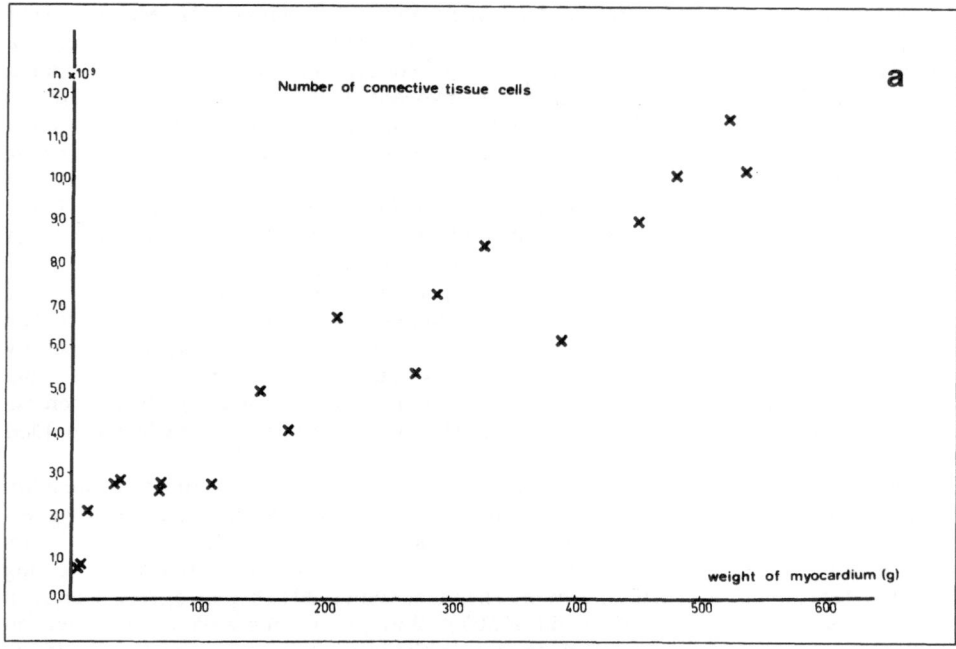

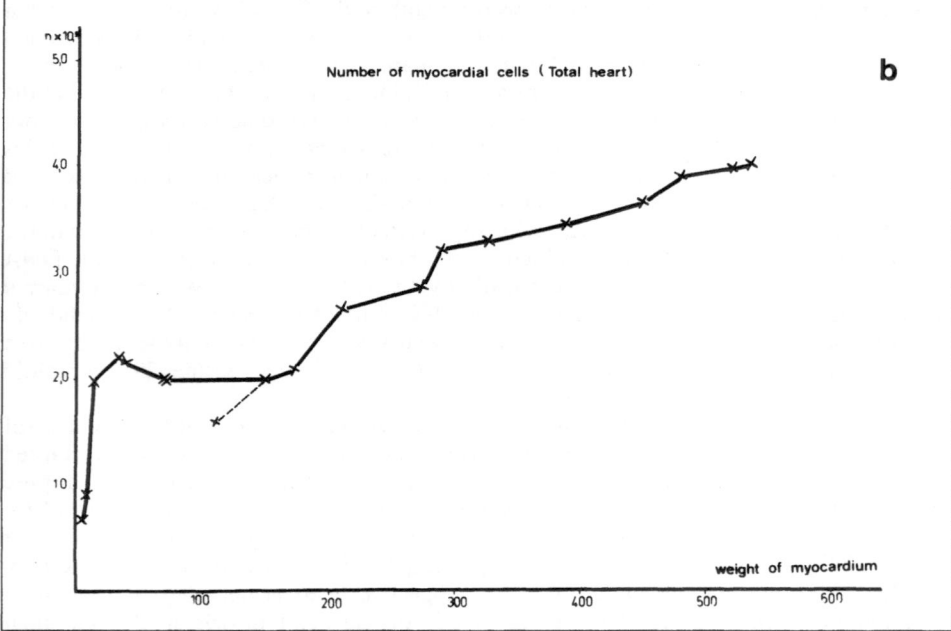

Fig. 2. Connective tissue cells (a) and heart muscle cells (b) increase in number during physiological heart growth and in cardiac hypertrophy.

ed. By using these three parameters and by making a calculation based on the weight of the myocardium, the absolute number of heart muscle nuclei and connective tissue nuclei in the heart will be established.

When applying this method in practice, the following results are obtained: During normal heart growth and in cardiac hypertrophy the number of *connective tissue cells* increases in parallel with the progressing heart weight (Fig. 2a). Immediately after birth we counted 1×10^9 connective tissue cells; at adult age this number has increased to fivefold this value, and in excessive cardiac hypertrophy 10×10^9 connective tissue cells are present. In addition to these results our findings revealed that the *number of heart muscle cells* increases during heart growth. Immediately after birth less than 1×10^9 cells are present, but this number duplicates rapidly (2×10^9). This duplication of the muscle cells is produced by a final post partum wave of mitosis (15) which can also be observed under the microscope. In cardiac hypertrophy a further increase of the cell number is observed which may reach the double value in excessive hypertrophy in hearts weighing 700 to 900 g showing 4×10^9 muscle cells (Fig. 2b). These findings confirm that numeric hyperplasia of the heart muscle cells occurs above the "critical heart weight". On the other hand, in the case of cardiac atrophy we observed a reduction of the individual heart muscle cells in addition to a decreased numer of myocardial cells. In hearts with a myocardium weight less than 100 g, the cell number will decrease down to less than 1×10^9.

B. Cardiac Insufficiency

In cardiac insufficiency macroscopically an extremely dilated heart along with an increased heart weight can be observed.

Dry Weight: Whereas in hearts with compensated myocardial hypertrophy the dry weight of the fibres increases to a maximum weight of about 420×10^{-12}g, the percentage concentration of the dry substance in hypertrophied heart muscle fibres is found to decrease

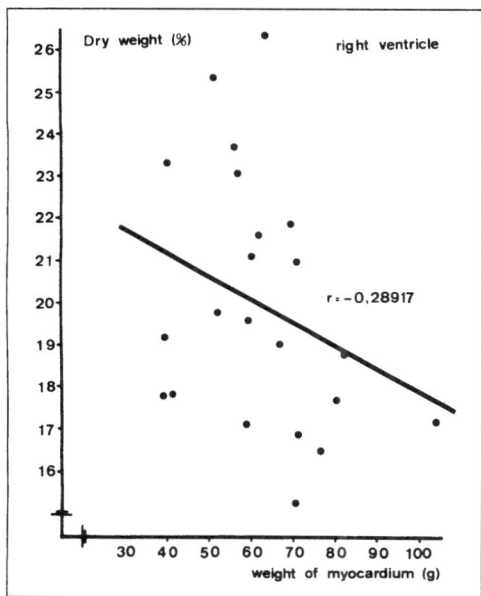

Fig. 3a.

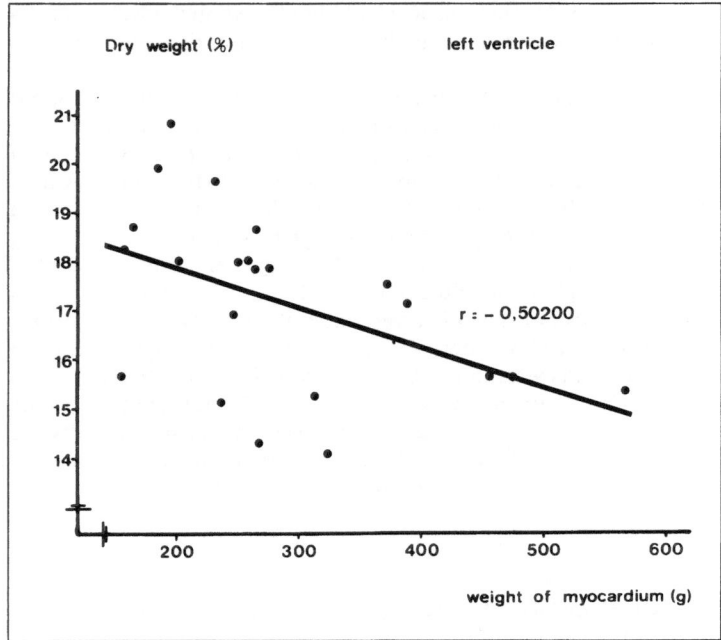

Fig. 3b.

Fig. 3. Medium percentage dry weight of heart muscle fibres in the right (a) and left heart ventricle (b) in relation to the pure myocardium weight. The amount of dry substances (below the regression line) is lower in insufficient hearts compared with non-insufficient hearts of the same weight of myocardium.

slightly. A significantly reduced content of the dry substances in heart muscle fibres of insufficient hearts showing a pronounced ventricular dilatation is remarkable (Fig. 3). Since the content of the dry weight of the heart muscle fibres is primarily determined by the contractile proteins, these measurements suggest that cardiac insufficiency results in a lack of contractile proteins.

DNA: The total amount of DNA of the myocardium increases with progressing heart weight. As a whole, the amount of DNA of insufficient hearts in comparison with non-insufficient hearts is insignificantly reduced. Particularly with respect to the higher weight ranges, in right-heart insufficiency more DNA is found to be present in the right than in the left ventricle. In the case of left-heart insufficiency, on the other hand, the amount of DNA shows the highest values in the stressed left ventricle.

Polyploidization: As in the case of cardiac hypertrophy due to hyperfunction, in insufficient hearts we also found – by means of cytophotometric measurements – an increased polyploidization of the heart muscle nuclei correlated with the pure weight of the myocardium: a comparison of the percentage distribution of the ploidy levels of the right and the left ventricle shows that polyploidization of the heart muscle nuclei of insufficient hearts begins at a low weight of the myocardium when a great number of various euploid and aneuploid DNA values are found to be present (Fig. 4). This "scattering of the ploidy levels" is not correlated with the cardiac weight. Whereas in non-insufficient hearts showing excessive hypertrophy of the myocardium no diploid and only 10–40% tetraploid cells are seen, in all insufficient hearts, including those with a high weight of the myocardium, both diploid and tetraploid cells are found to be present. The highest DNA values (16c, 24c, 32c) occur equally

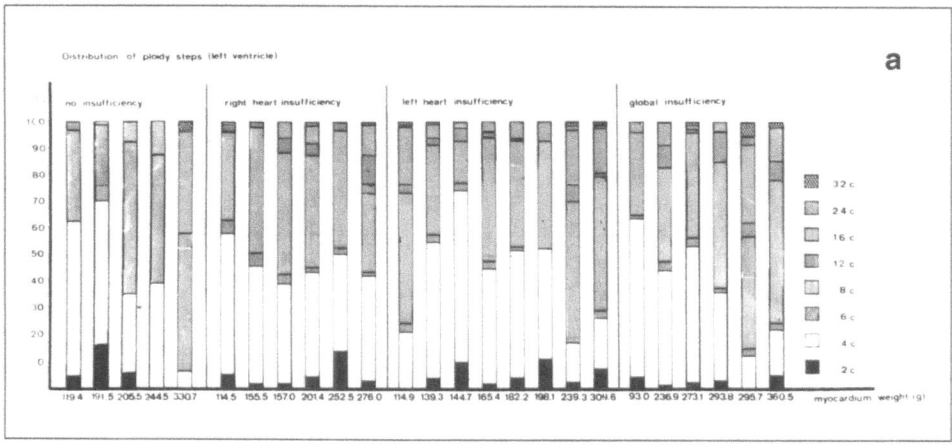

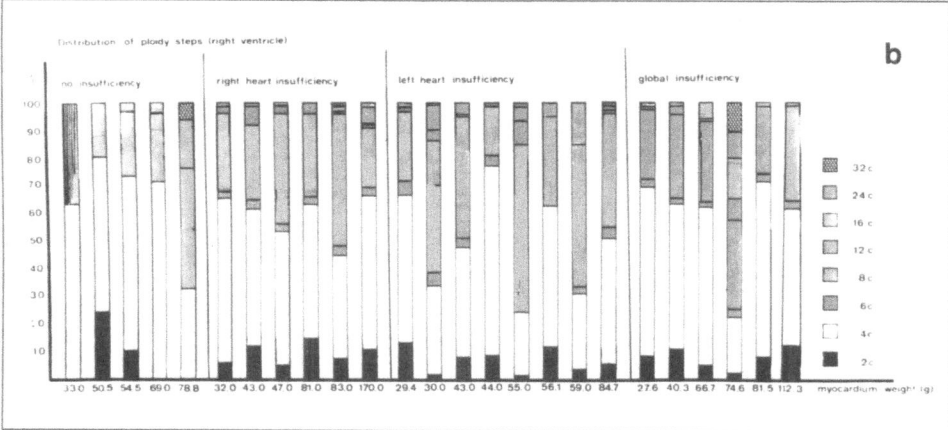

Fig. 4. Percentage distribution of the ploidy grades of heart muscle cell nuclei from the right (a) and left ventricle (b) of non-insufficient and insufficient human hearts. In hearts with different insufficiency an advanced polyploization with many aneuploid DNA values can be observed.

in most insufficient hearts, and, as a result, the heart muscle cells of insufficient hearts are also capable of producing a reactive synthesis of DNA. Usually, polyploidization is more pronounced in the left than in the right ventricle.

When comparing several insufficient hearts with non-insufficient hearts of the same weight, we made the following observations: A heart weighing 530 g of a 67-year-old man with a decompensated *cor pulmonale* showed an extremely high ploidy level in the insufficient right ventricle with 36 % tetraploid, 44 % octoploid and 6.7 % hexadekaploid cells which slightly exceeded that found in the left ventricle (Fig. 5b). In a heart of the same weight without insufficiency, about the same ploidy levels are seen to be present but in the right ventricle diploid cells are missing (Fig. 5a). A great many intermediate DNA values are noted in the insufficient heart in contrast to the normal control.

In *left-heart insufficiency* we were also able to show a polyploidization of the heart muscle

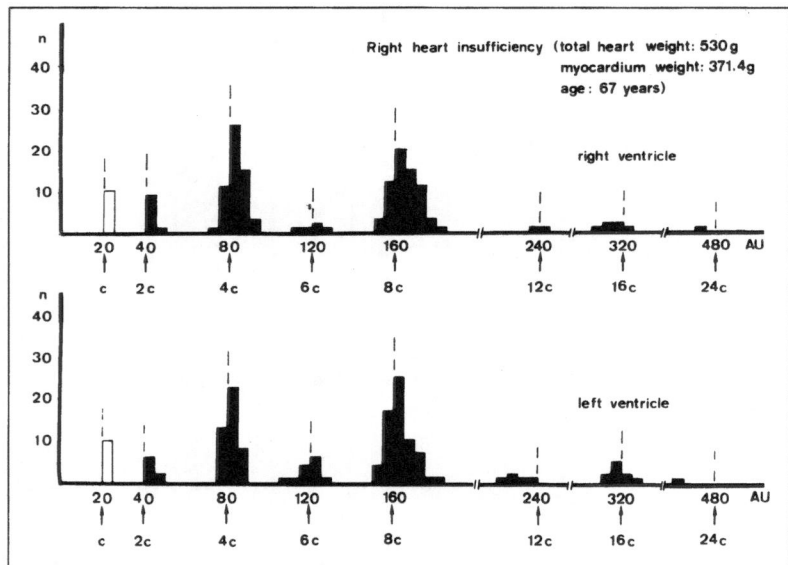

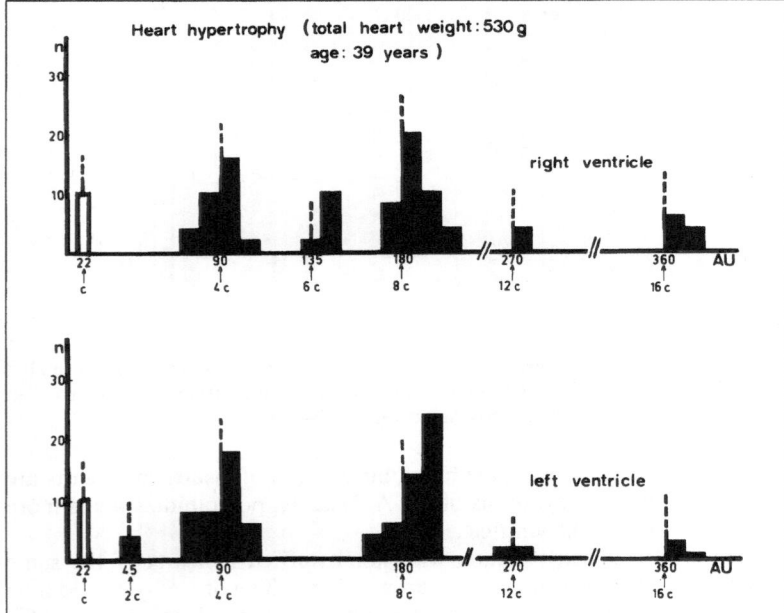

Fig. 5. a) DNA distribution of heart muscle cell nuclei in the right and left ventricle of a non-insufficient hypertrophied human heart weighing 530 g (c = haploid DNA content from bull spermatozoa, 2c = diploid DNA content of heart muscle cell nuclei, 4c = tetraploid etc. AU = DNA content in arbitrary units).

b) DNA distribution of heart muscle cell nuclei in the right and left ventricle of a human heart with right ventricular insufficiency weighing 371.4 g (myocardium weight).

nuclei correlated with the weight of the myocardium comparable to that found in hypertrophied hearts without insufficiency. In the left ventricle of an insufficient heart weighing 578.2 g, we detected 41.3 % tetraploid, 40.7 % octoploid and 5.3 % hexadekaploid cells. This chronic left-heart insufficiency must have involved the right ventricle which also showed an increased ploidy level (11.3 % 2c-, 50.7 % 4c-, 33.3 % 8c- and 4.7 % 16c-nuclei). In contrast to normal controls, in the insufficient heart 11.3 % (right) and 12.7 % (left) diploid cardiac muscle cells remain.

We observed the highest ploidy degrees in hearts suffering from *global insufficiency*. In this case even relatively low grade hypertrophy shows an extremely pronounced polyploidization. A heart weighing 500 g of a 37-year-old patient with endo-myocarditis revealed DNA values up to 32c levels in addition to numerous intermediate values in the left ventricle. The degree of polyploidization with predominatly tetraploid (63.3 %) and octoploid (25 %) cells is less pronounced in the right ventricle. The ploidy level is slightly higher than normal values seen in a non-insufficient heart.

In non-insufficient controls the *mean degreee of polyploidisation* of the heart muscle nuclei increases excessively in both ventricles in parallel with increasing weight of the myocardium. This increase is highly significant. Also in insufficient hearts an increase of the mean ploidy level correlated with the weight of the myocardium is observed. But this increase is very much reduced in both ventricles and only slightly significant. Moreover, in insufficient hearts with a low weight of the myocardium below the critical heart weight of 500 g, an increased mean ploidy level is noted which in this area is found to be above the mean ploidy level of non-insufficient hearts. Hearts suffering from global insufficiency or left-heart insufficiency show a significantly higher mean degree of polyploidization than hearts suffering from right-heart insufficiency.

Cell number: Our calculations of the cell number in insufficient hearts showed that a highly significant increase of the *connective tissue cells* in correlation with the pure weight of the myocardium occurs in chronic cardiac insufficiency in contrast to non-insufficient controls. Whereas in non-insufficient hearts, used as controls, an average of 4.094×10^9 connective tissue cells was found, the insufficient hearts showed a presence of 6.570×10^9 connective tissue cells indicating an increase of 60.5 %. In right-heart insufficiency the connective tissue cells are increased by 46.2 % as compared to controls whereas in left-heart insufficiency an increase of 42.6 % and in global insufficiency an increase of 92.5 % is observed. In cardiac insufficiency the most considerable increase of connective tissue cells is actually observed in the ventricle with a maximum stress. In hearts suffering from acute cardiac insufficiency, on the other hand, no considerable increase of the connective tissue cells was recognizable.

An increase of the absolute cell number in insufficient hearts by a total of 18.4 % as compared to non-insufficient controls is solely produced by a multiplication of the connective tissue cells in these hearts. Although in insufficient hearts an increase of the *heart muscle cells* is also observed, this increase is significantly reduced as compared to non-insufficient controls. While in controls an average of 3.070×10^9 heart muscle cells are found, in insufficient hearts as little as 1.920×10^9 heart muscle cells were seen showing a relative decrease of 37.5 % (Fig. 6). In right-heart insufficiency a decrease of 31.5 %, in left-heart insufficiency of 41.4 % and in global insufficiency of 39.5 % was observed. While the myocardium is growing in mass, a considerable insufficient increase of the heart muscle cells is seen mainly in the right ventricle, notably during left-heart and global insufficiency. But also in the left ventricle of insufficient hearts an increase of heart muscle cells related with the degree of hypertrophy of non-insufficient hearts will not be reached. Also in hearts suffering from acute cardiac insufficiency, we observed a significant reduction of the heart muscle cells.

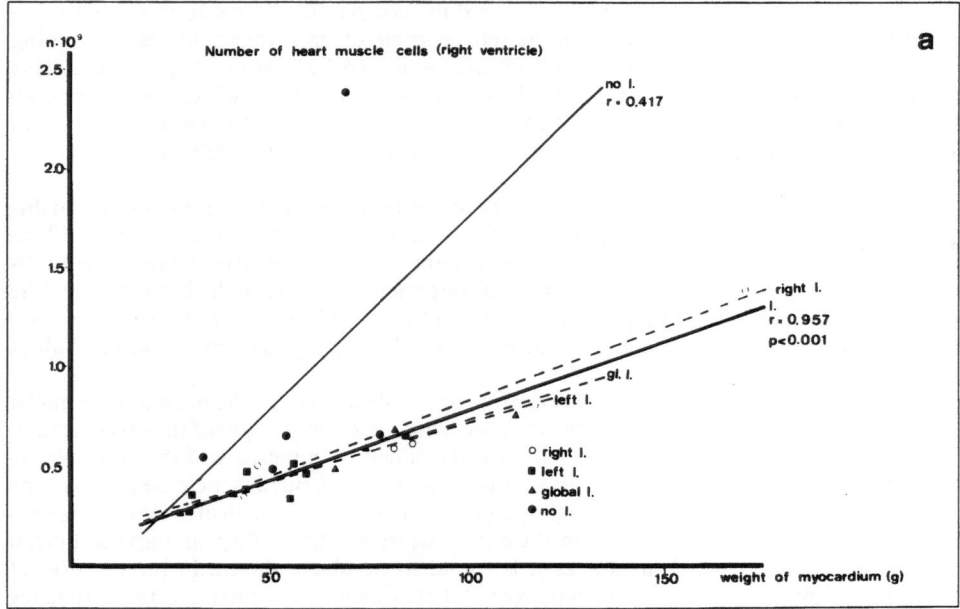

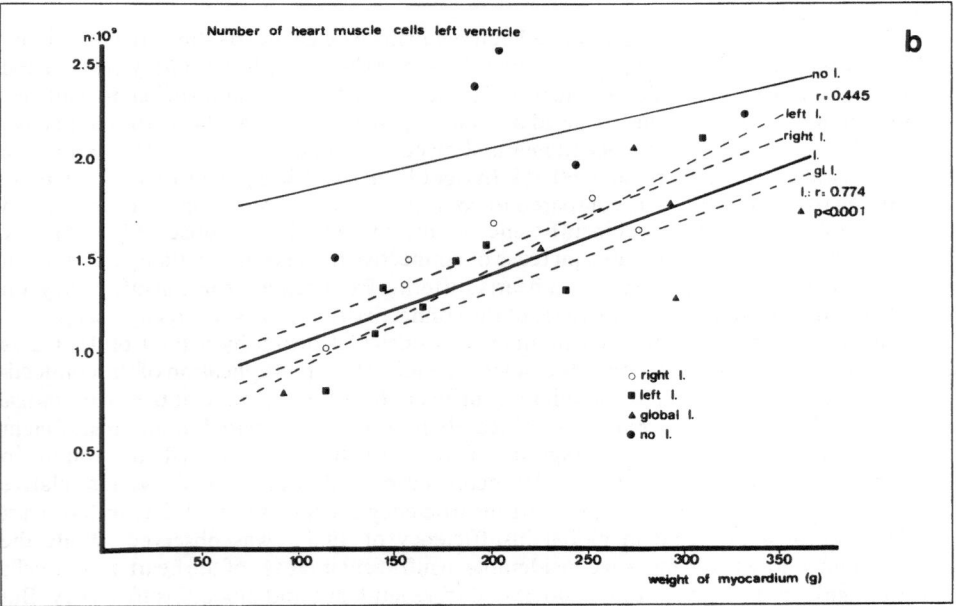

Fig. 6. Number of heart muscle cells in the right (a) and left ventricle (b) of human hearts with different types of insufficiency (I = regression line of all insufficient hearts; I = non-insufficient hearts; right I. = right-heart insufficiency; left I. = left-heart insufficiency; global I. = global insufficiency).

Conclusions

Summing up, our quantitative histochemical investigations revealed that in addition to structural changes in the macroscopic, microscopic and submicroscopic areas, in cardiac insufficiency quantitative changes of the substances of the myocardium are found which are of considerable functional significance. Within the heart muscle cells a lack of contractile proteins as well as a reduced DNA synthesis is observed. Due to a considerably advanced fibrozation of the myocardium in the insufficient heart and an increased number of connective tissue cells the total contraction of the myocardium may possibly be disturbed. A decisive factor, however, is the significantly reduced number of heart muscle cells in insufficient hearts which decreases the pumping action of the myocardium to such an extent with regard to the activity required that cardiac failure will finally be brought about.

References

1. Adler CP (1971) Polyploidisierung und Zellzahl im menschlichen Herzen. Habilitationsschrift, Freiburg i Br
2. Adler CP (1972) Morphologische Grundlagen der Herzhypertrophie und des Herzwachstums. Med Welt 23: 477–484
3. Adler CP (1972) Polyploidisierung und Zellzahl im menschlichen Herzen. Fortschr Med 90: 671–675
4. Adler CP (1972) Ultra-violet microspectrophotometric investigations on the cytoplasm in heart muscle cells. Folia Fac Med Unic Comenianae Bratisl X: 103–118
5. Adler CP (1973) Der Gehalt von Protein und Myoglobin in hypertrophierten Herzmuskelzellen. Mikrospektrophotometrische Untersuchungen an Menschenherzen. In: Roskamm H, Reindell H (eds) Das chronisch kranke Herz. Grundlagen der funktionellen Diagnostik und Therapie. Schattauer-Verlag, Stuttgart New York, pp 113–118
6. Adler CP (1976) DNS in Kinderherzen. Biochemische und zytophotometrische Untersuchungen. Beitr Path 158: 173–202
7. Adler CP (1983) Morphometric and cytophotometric investigations of myocardial diseases. In: Just H, Schuster HP (eds) Myocarditis – Cardiomyopathy. Springer Verlag, Berlin Heidelberg New York
8. Adler CP, Sandritter W (1977) Alterations of substances (DNA, myoglobin, myosin, protein) in experimentally induced cardiac hypertrophy and under the influence of drugs (isoproterenol, cytostatics, strophantin). Basic Res Cardiol 75: 342–362
9. Adler CP, Hartz A, Sandritter W (1977) Form and structure of cell nuclei in growing and hypertrophied human hearts. Beitr Path 161: 342–362
10. Aschoff L (1905) Zur Myokarditisfrage. Verh Dtsch Ges Path 8: 46–53
11. Burton K (1956) A study of the conditions and mechanism of diphenylamine reaction for the colorimetric estimation of deoxyribonucleic acid. Biochem J 62: 315–323
12. Dische Z (1930) Über einige neue charakteristische Farbreaktionen der Thymonukleinsäure und eine Mikromethode zur Bestimmung derselben in tierischen Organen mit Hilfe dieser Reaktionen. Mikrochemie 8: 4–32
13. Dische Z (1955) Color reactions of nucleic acid components. Academic Press Inc, New York
14. Ferrans VJ (1984) Cardiac hypertrophy: morphological aspects. In: Zak R (ed) Growth of the heart in health and disease. Raven Press Ltd, New York, pp 187–239
15. Klinge D (1967) Proliferation und Regeneration am Myokard. Ztschr Zellforsch 80: 488–517
16. Knieriem H-J (1972) Morphologische Grundlagen der Herzhypertrophie. Verh Dtsch Ges Kreisl Forsch 38: 1
17. Linzbach AJ (1960) Die pathologische Anatomie der Herzinsuffizienz. In: Hdb Inn Med Bd 9, Teil 1. Springer-Verlag, Berlin Göttingen Heidelberg, pp 706–800
18. Pannen F, Adler CP, Sandritter W (1973) Protein und Myoglobin in hypertrophierten und dilatierten Menschenherzen. Beitr Path 149: 70–83

19. Poche R (1958) Submikroskopischer Beitrag zur Pathologie des Herzmuskels. Verh Dtsch Ges Path 41:351
20. Poche R (1977) Die strukturellen Veränderungen des druck- und volumen-überlasteten Herzens. In: Reindell H, Roskamm H (eds) Herzkrankheiten. Springer-Verlag, Berlin Heidelberg New York
21. Poche R (1977) Die allgemeine Pathologie der myokardialen Herzinsuffizienz. In: Reindell H, Roskamm H (eds) Herzkrankheiten. Springer-Verlag, Berlin Heidelberg New York
22. Richter GW, Kellner A (1963) Hypertrophy of the human heart at the level of fine structure. J Cell Biol 18:195
23. Sandritter W (1958) Ultraviolett-Mikrospektrophotometrie. Hdb Histochemie Bd I/1. Fischer-Verlag, Stuttgart, pp 220–338
24. Sandritter W (1970) Funktionsstrukturen des Zellkerns. Eu- und Heterochromatin. Med Welt 21: 1–10
25. Sandritter W, Scomazzoni G (1964) Deoxyribonucleic acid content (Feulgen photometry) and dry weight (interference microscopy) of normal and hypertrophic heart muscle fibres. Nature 202: 100–101
26. Sandritter W, Adler CP (1971) Numerical hyperplasia in human heart hypertrophy. Experientia (Basel) 27: 1435–1437
27. Sandritter W, Adler CP (1972) A method for determining cell number on organs with polyploid cell nuclei. Beitr Path 146: 99–103
28. Sandritter W, Adler CP (1978) Polyploidisation of heart muscle nuclei as a prerequisite for heart growth and numerical hyperplasia in heart hypertrophy. In: Kobayashi T, Ito Y, Rona G (eds) Recent Advances in Studies on Cardiac Structure and Metabolism, Vol 12: Cardiac Adaptation. Univ Park Press, Baltimore
29. Sandritter W, Grosser KD, Schiemer HG (1960) Trockengewichtsbestimmung an normalen und pathologischen Herzmuskelfasern. Verh Dtsch Ges Path 44: 192–194
30. Sandritter W, Grosser KD, Rast D, Schlüter G, Beneke G (1971) Trockengewichtsbestimmung an Herzmuskelfasern bei experimenteller Herzhypertrophie (Röntgenhistographische Untersuchungen). Beitr Path 143: 261–270
31. Stegemann H (1958) Mikrobestimmung von Hydroxyprolin mit Chloramin-T und p-Dimethylaminobenzaldehyd. Z Physiol Chem 310: 41–45
32. Waldmann G (1968) Elektronenmikroskopische Untersuchungen an den eiweißproduzierenden Feinstrukturen in hypertrophierten menschlichen Herzmuskelzellen. Exp Path 2: 360

Author's address:

Prof. Dr. Claus-Peter Adler, Institute of Pathology, University of Freiburg, Albertstraße 19, D-7800 Freiburg i. Br. (F.R.G.)

Morphological reaction patterns in experimental cardiac hypertrophy – a quantitative stereological study

G. Mall, T. Mattfeldt, C. Hasslacher, and J. Mann

Pathologisches Institut und Medizinische Klinik der Universität Heidelberg (F. R. G.)

Summary

Four experimental models of myocardial hypertrophy were investigated in rats: 1. Mild hypertrophy induced by physical exercise, 2. mild hypertrophy induced by chronic pressure overload (24 weeks), 3. moderate hypertrophy induced by chronic pressure overload (8 weeks), 4. moderate hypertrophy in diabetes induced by chronic pressure overload (8 weeks). Stereological investigations on left ventricular papillary muscles disclosed different morphological reaction patterns: 1. The capillary bed of the myocardium responded differently in mild hypertrophy: physical training, but not mild chronic pressure overload, evoked neoformation of capillaries. 2. Mild hypertrophy and moderate hypertrophy induced by chronic pressure overload were not associated with quantitative structural reactions of myofibrils and mitochondria. Those alterations appeared, however, in hypertensive-diabetic rats with moderate hypertrophy. Our data provide further experimental evidence for the existence of a hypertensive-diabetic cardiomyopathy.

Key words: diabetes mellitus, myocardial hypertrophy, physical exercise, pressure overload, stereology

Introduction

A long series of quantitative morphological studies on experimental cardiac hypertrophy has been published during the past two decades. It is now generally accepted that the quantitative microstructural reaction pattern depends on degree and duration of hemodynamic overload (6, 19, 20, 21, 23, 25, 26, 29, 30). Furthermore, the hitherto published results indicate that the reaction is different in chronic pressure and volume overload, respectively (1, 2, 3, 6, 12, 14, 15, 22, 24).

Estimates of capillary-fiber ratios and capillary densities gave evidence of capillary neoformation (2, 22, 24) in mild hypertrophy induced by physical exercise, but not in hypertrophy induced by strenuous exercise (3, 5, 12, 15) and by chronic pressure overload (1, 5, 6, 7, 21, 25, 26). The coronary vasodilator reserve which may correlate with capillary vascularization is unchanged (or even augmented) in hypertrophy induced by physical exercise (22) and is depressed in hypertrophy induced by chronic pressure overload (6).

At the cellular level, a proportionate increase of mitochondrial and myofibrillar mass was found in hypertrophy induced by chronic physical training (2, 3, 15). In chronic pressure overload, however, a proportionate increase of organelles is restricted to the state of compensatory hyperfunction (6, 19), and many studies disclosed a disproportionate increase of the myofibrillar mass associated with a relative decrease of the mitochondrial mass. These quantitative ultrastructural alterations may promote decompensation of the hypertrophic heart (1, 6, 7, 19, 20, 25, 29, 30).

In later stages of hypertrophy induced by pressure overload a progressive myocardial fibrosis occurs which correlates with myocardial stiffness (23, 29). It is of particular interest that the fibrosis is more pronounced in hypertensive-diabetic rats as compared to hypertensive rats (9, 10, 11), which supports the concept of the hypertensive-diabetic cardiomyopathy in humans (8). An increased connective tissue content was not observed, however, in hypertrophy induced by training (2, 3, 15).

The available studies on hypertrophy induced by chronic pressure overload focused on moderate or even severe degrees of hypertrophy. In contrast, models of hypertrophy induced by physical exercise are frequently associated with a mild degree of hypertrophy. In the present paper we describe quantitative stereological studies on both models with comparable degrees of myocardial hypertrophy. In addition, our investigations on the myocardium of hypertensive-diabetic rats are reported.

Methods

Animal models of myocardial hypertrophy

Model I: Hypertrophy induced by physical training

Ten young female Sprague-Dawley rats performed an exercise program of 18 weeks duration with gradually increasing intensity on a motor-driven running decive. In the final phase the animals exercised 90 min/day at a speed of 32 m/min. 10 animals served as sedentary controls.

Model II: Mild hypertrophy induced by 24 weeks of hypertension

In seven young male Wistar rats slight renovascular hypertension was established by a slight surgical stenosis of the left renal artery. Seven rats served as sham-operated controls.

Model III: Moderate hypertrophy induced by 8 weeks of hypertension

In eleven young male Wistar rats a moderate renovascular hypertension was established by a surgical stenosis of the left renal artery. Twelve rats served as sham-operated controls.

Model IV: Moderate hypertrophy in diabetic rats induced by 8 weeks of hypertension

In eleven young male Wistar rats a moderate renovascular hypertension was established by a surgical stenosis of the left renal artery. Ten rats served as sham-operated controls. After four weeks all rats were treated with a single intraperitoneal injection of streptocotozin (75 mg/kg body weight) to evoke a diabetes mellitus in both groups. The average blood glucose concentration was ca. 16 mmol/l in both groups.

The animals were randomly assigned to the 4 groups of models III and IV.

Fixation technique

The viscera were fixed by retrograde vascular perfusion at a pressure of 110 mm Hg after catheterization of the abdominal aorta. Before fixation the vascular system was flushed with a dextran solution (Rheomacrodex) containing 0.5 g/l procaine-HCl for 2 minutes which improves the microcirculation and leads to cardiac arrest in diastole. The vena cava inferior was incised to drain the blood. The incision was performed 10 seconds after the start of the dextran infusion. This procedure may avoid the collapse of capillaries caused by low venous pressures. The vascular system was subsequently perfused with 0.2 mol phosphate buffer containing 3 % glutaraldehyde for 12 minutes.

Left ventricular papillary muscles were randomly cut either longitudinally or transversely with a tissue sectioner as described elsewhere (16, 18).

All specimens were postfixed in ice-cold 3 % glutaraldehyde for 24 hours and afterwards in 1 % OsO_4 for 30 minutes at room temperature, dehydrated in ethanol and embedded in Epon-Araldite. Semithin sections (1 μm) were stained with methylene blue and basic fuchsin (4) and examined by light microscopy using oil immersion and phase contrast. Ultrathin sections were stained with uranylacetate and lead citrate and examined with a Zeiss EM 10 electron microscope.

Morphometry

Volume densities (V_V) were obtained by the well established point counting procedure (28).

Length densities (L_V) of capillaries were calculated according to the following stereological equation (18, 27):

$$L_V = c_1(K_L, \alpha) * Q_A(\alpha) \text{ (capillaries)} \tag{1}$$

L_V is a model-based estimate of anisotropic tubular structures (based on a Dimroth-Watson orientation distribution [19, 27]). The c values depend on the sectioning angle α and the concentration parameter K (anisotropy constant). Estimates of K values are derived from the ratio of counts on transverse and longitudinal sections.

The stereological analysis was performed as a multistage sampling procedure.

Stage 1 (magnification 1,020 : 1, light microscopy): The volume densities of capillaries and myocardial cells and the length densities of capillaries were derived from counts at this stage. Reference volume was the total myocardial tissue of the left ventricular papillary muscles.

Stage 2 (magnification 32,500 : 1, electron microscopy): Two randomly selected ultrathin sections per animal were used to determine the volume density of components of the interstitial tissue. Reference volume was the myocardial tissue of the left ventricular papillary muscles. One randomly selected transverse ultrathin section per animal was used to determine the volume densities of mitochondria, myofibrils and sarcoplasmic matrix. Reference volume were the myocardial cells of the left ventricular papillary muscles.

Statistics

In all experimental models the quantitative parameters were compared with Student's t-test for unpaired data. A result was considered to be significant if $p < 0.05$.

Results and discussion

Discussion of methods

This is the first stereological investigation on capillaries in myocardial hypertrophy which is based on a Dimroth-Watson orientation distribution of capillaries. The assumptions of capillary orientations in space are hereby more adequate than in Krogh's cylinder model (18) and disclose "true" length densities of capillaries (mm/mm³) and "true" capillary-fiber ratios. With minor extra efforts, the method provides corrections for partial anisotropy and fixation in heterogeneous phases of the cardiac cycle.

Discussion of results

The mean systolic blood pressures showed a slight increase in model II and a moderate increase in models III and IV (Table 1). The body weights were unchanged in models I and II and slightly decreased in models III and IV (Table 2). In all experimental models cardiac

Table 1. Systolic blood pressure (mm Hg)

Experimental model	Experimental group $\overline{x} \pm SD$	Control group $\overline{x} \pm SD$	Change (%)	Level of statistical significance
Exercise-induced hypertrophy	–	–	–	–
Pressure overload hypertrophy (24 weeks)	154 ± 23	94 ± 16	+ 64%	p < 0.001
Pressure overload hypertrophy (8 weeks)	172 ± 21	91 ± 5	+ 89%	p < 0.001
Pressure overload hypertrophy + diabetes (8 weeks)	151 ± 23	79 ± 7	+ 91%	p < 0.001

Table 2. Final body weights (g)

Experimental model	Experimental group $\overline{x} \pm SD$	Control group $\overline{x} \pm SD$	Change (%)	Level of statistical significance
Exercise-induced hypertrophy	291 ± 16	284 ± 16	+ 2%	N. S.
Pressure overload hypertrophy (24 weeks)	503 ± 69	506 ± 49	– 1%	N. S.
Pressure overload hypertrophy (8 weeks)	267 ± 16	287 ± 25	– 7%	p < 0.05
Pressure overload hypertrophy + diabetes (8 weeks)	159 ± 18	178 ± 15	– 11%	p < 0.05

hypertrophy was observed. Increased left ventricular weights (Table 3) which are associated with unchanged or even increased volume densities of left ventricular myocardial cells (Table 6) are indicators of hypertrophy at unchanged or diminished body weights compared to controls. In addition, in models I, III and IV the mean cross sectional area of muscle cells was determined and was significantly increased (p < 0.01).

A mild hypertrophy was induced by physical exercise (model I) and by long-term pressure overload (model II) with a 20% change of the heart weight (Table 3). Female rats were employed in model I since male rats do not tend to augment their food intake during the exercise period. The unfavourable effect is frequently an unchanged left ventricular weight (2, 3, 15).

The stereological parameters show one basic microstructural difference between mild hypertrophy induced by long-term pressure overload and by long-term physical exercise,

Table 3. Heart weights (g)

Experimental model	Experimental group $\overline{x} \pm SD$	Control group $\overline{x} \pm SD$	Change (%)	Level of statistical significance
Exercise-induced hypertrophy	1.16 ± 0.07	0.97 ± 0.07	$+20\%$	$p < 0.001$
Pressure overload hypertrophy (24 weeks)	1.55 ± 0.19	1.29 ± 0.17	$+20\%$	$p < 0.05$
Pressure overload hypertrophy (8 weeks)	1.17 ± 0.14	0.88 ± 0.10	$+33\%$	$p < 0.001$
Pressure overload hypertrophy + diabetes (8 weeks)	0.75 ± 0.09	0.58 ± 0.06	$+29\%$	$p < 0.001$

Table 4. Length density (L_V) of capillaries (mm^2/mm^3)

Experimental model	Experimental group $\overline{x} \pm SD$	Control group $\overline{x} \pm SD$	Change (%)	Level of statistical significance
Exercise-induced hypertrophy	3803 ± 364	3744 ± 237	$+ 2\%$	N. S.
Pressure overload hypertrophy (24 weeks)	3297 ± 267	3577 ± 201	$- 8\%$	$p < 0.05$
Pressure overload hypertrophy (8 weeks)	2912 ± 284	3718 ± 237	-19%	$p < 0.001$
Pressure overload hypertrophy + diabetes (8 weeks)	4257 ± 509	5065 ± 365	-16%	$p < 0.001$

Table 5. Volume density (V_V) of non-capillary interstitial tissue (vol%)

Experimental model	Experimental group $\overline{x} \pm SD$	Control group $\overline{x} \pm SD$	Change (00)	Level of statistical significance
Exercise-induced hypertrophy	2.88 ± 1.38	2.63 ± 1.42	$+10\%$	N. S.
Pressure overload hypertrophy (24 weeks)	2.80 ± 1.04	3.22 ± 1.45	-13%	N. S.
Pressure overload hypertrophy (8 weeks)	2.99 ± 1.62	2.40 ± 1.04	$+25\%$	N. S.
Pressure overload hypertrophy + diabetes (8 weeks)	2.93 ± 1.42	1.80 ± 0.95	$+63\%$	N. S. ($p < 0.1$)

Table 6. Volume density (V_V) of myocardial cells (vol%)

Experimental model	Experimental group $\overline{x} \pm SD$	Control group $\overline{x} \pm SD$	Change (%)	Level of statistical significance
Exercise-induced hypertrophy	86.9 ± 1.6	86.8 ± 1.3	± 0%	N. S.
Pressure overload hypertrophy (24 wekks)	88.6 ± 2.1	85.4 ± 3.0	+ 4%	p < 0.05
Pressure overload hypertrophy (8 weeks)	91.0 ± 1.3	89.7 ± 1.4	+ 2%	p < 0.05
Pressure overload hypertrophy + diabetes (8 weeks)	90.6 ± 1.8	86.6 ± 1.1	+ 5%	p < 0.001

Table 7. Volume density (V_V) of mitochondria (vol%)

Experimental model	Experimental group $\overline{x} \pm SD$	Control group $\overline{x} \pm SD$	Change (%)	Level of statistical significance
Exercise-induced hypertrophy	27.3 ± 3.2	26.5 ± 3.5	+ 3%	N. S.
Pressure overload hypertrophy (24 weeks)	24.2 ± 1.8	21.7 ± 1.3	+ 12%	p < 0.05
Pressure overload hypertrophy (8 weeks)	24.9 ± 2.2	25.7 ± 2.1	− 3%	N. S.
Pressure overload hypertrophy + diabetes (8 weeks)	22.5 ± 1.2	25.8 ± 1.4	− 15%	p < 0.001

Table 8. Volume density (V_V) of myofibrils (vol%)

Experimental model	Experimental group $\overline{x} \pm SD$	Control group $\overline{x} \pm SD$	Change (%)	Level of statistical significance
Exercise-induced hypertrophy	65.2 ± 3.2	64.8 ± 6.0	+ 1%	N. S.
Pressure overload hypertrophy (24 weeks)	65.9 ± 2.7	68.1 ± 2.1	− 3%	N. S.
Pressure overlaod hypertrophy (8 weeks)	63.6 ± 2.3	64.2 ± 1.9	− 1%	N. S.
Pressure overload hypertrophy + diabetes (8 weeks)	64.5 ± 2.3	57.7 ± 1.5	+ 11%	p < 0.001

respectively: the length density of capillaries is decreased in chronic pressure overload, but not in physical exercise (Table 4). In other words, the intercapillary distance is increased or unchanged, respectively. Further stereological investigation of the exercised rats disclosed an increased three-dimensional capillary/fiber ratio (capillary length per fiber length) ($+19\%$, $p < 0.001$) which corresponds to neoformation of capillaries. It should be emphasized that the common model of capillary vascularity in hypertrophy (13) which is based on constant capillary-fiber ratios does not hold for mild hypertrophy induced by physical exercise, but evidently for the pressure overload model. The different reactions of capillaries are not correlated with different reactions of the myocardial cells and the non-capillary interstitium. The well-known effects of long-term pressure overload, i. e. increased volume densities of myofibrils (5, 6, 7, 19, 20, 25, 29, 30) and interstitial connective tissue (9, 10, 11, 23, 29) were not detected in model II (Tables 5 and 8). In contrast, the volume density of mitochondria was increased (Table 7) which was hitherto never observed in long-term pressure overload (17). The cause is, in all probability, the low degree of hypertrophy in our model. The result clearly demonstrates the dependence of chronic microstructural reactions on the serverity of hypertension.

In models III (8 weeks hypertension) and IV (8 weeks hypertension, 4 weeks diabetes mellitus) we found a moderate degree of hypertrophy (Table 3). The capillary bed responded identically as in model II. The three-dimensional "true" capillary-fiber ratio was not changed. The volume densities of the non-capillary interstitium were not altered in both models (Table 5). The lack of interstitial alterations may be explained with the short duration of the experiments and with only moderately enhanced blood pressures. In model IV the volume density of myofibrils was increased and the volume density of mitochondria was decreased, but neither were changed in model III (Tables 7 and 8). Duration and intensity of hypertension were obviously not adequate to evoke the typical reactions of pressure overload hypertrophy in model III, but the additional diabetes mellitus in model IV induced these reactions under similar hemodynamic conditions (Table 1). Recently, the concept of hypertensive-diabetic cardiomyopathy was experimentally established by the occurrence of a more severe fibrosis in hypertensive-diabetic rats (9, 10, 11). In addition to these experimental findings, our stereological data provide evidence that diabetes mellitus accelerates the appearance of chronic myofibrillar and mitochondrial reactions in the hypertrophic heart.

We conclude from our experimental studies:

1. The capillary bed of the myocardium responds differently to mild long-term physical exercise and to mild long-term hypertension: physical training, but not mild chronic pressure overload, evokes neoformation of capillaries.

2. Mild hypertrophy induced by mild long-term hypertension is not associated with quantitative structural reactions of myofibrils, mitochondria and the non-capillary interstitium.

3. The appearance of quantitative structural reactions of myofibrils and mitochondria in chronic hypertension is accelerated by diabetes mellitus. Thus, diabetes may facilitate the occurrence of heart insufficiency in chronic hypertension.

Acknowlededgments

The skilful technical assistance of Z. Antoni, H. Derks, and P. Rieger is gratefully acknowledged. The study was supported by a grant from the Deutsche Forschungsgemeinschaft (Ma 912/1–2).

References

1. Anversa P, Olivetti G, Melissari M, Loud AV (1980) Stereological measurement of cellular and subcellular hypertrophy and hyperplasia in the papillary muscle of adult rat. J Mol Cell Cardiol 12: 781–795
2. Anversa P, Levicky V, Beghi C, McDonald SL, Kikkawa Y (1983) Morphometry of exercise-induced right ventricular hypertrophy in the rat. Circ Res 52: 57–64
3. Anversa P, Beghi C, Levicky V (1985) Effects of strenuous exercise on quantitative morphology of left ventricular myocardium in the rat. J Mol Cell Cardiol 17: 587–595
4. Di Sant'Agnese PA, De Mesy Jensen KL (1984) Diabasic staining of large epoxy sections and applications to surgical pathology. Am J Clin Pathol 80: 25–29
5. Breisch EA, Houser SR, Carey RA, Spann JF, Bove AA (1980) Myocardial blood flow and capillary density in chronic pressure overload of the feline left ventricle. Cardiovasc Res 14: 469–475
6. Breisch EA, White C, Bloor CM (1984) Myocardial characteristics of pressure overload hypertrophy. Lab Invest 51: 333–341
7. Dämmrich J, Pfeifer U (1983) Cardiac hypertrophy in rats after supravalvular aortic constriction. Virchows Arch B 43: 265–307
8. Factor SM, Minase T, Sonnenblick EH (1980) Clinical and morphological features of human hypertensive-diabetic cardiomyopathy. Am Heart J 99: 446–458
9. Factor SM, Minase T, Bhan R, Wolinski H, Sonnenblick EH (1981) Hypertensive-diabetic cardiomyopathy in the rat. An experimental model of human disease. Am J Pathol 102: 219–317
10. Factor SM, Minase T, Bhan R, Wolinski H, Sonnenblick EH (1983) Hypertensive-diabetic cardiomyopathy in the rat: ultrastructural features. Virchows Arch A 398: 305–317
11. Fein SM, Minase T, Bhan R, Wolinski H, Sonnenblick EM (1984) Combined renovascular hypertension and diabetes in rats: a new preparation of congestive cardiomyopathy. Circulation 70: 318–330
12. Frenzel H (1985) Morphologische Befunde bei Rückbildung einer Herzhypertrophie. Z Kardiol 74 (Suppl 3): 91
13. Hort W (1955) Quantitative Untersuchungen über die Capillarisierung des Herzmuskels im Erwachsenen- und Greisenalter bei Hypertrophie und Hpyerplasie. Virchows Arch 327: 560–576
14. Hort W, Frenzel H, Lange P, Tezuka F (1985) Rückbildung der Herzhypertrophie. In: Mall G, Otto HF (eds) Herzhypertrophie. Springer-Verlag, Berlin, pp 43–47
15. Loud AV, Beghi C, Olivetti G, Anversa P (1984) Morphometry of right and left ventricular myocardium after strenuous exercise in preconditioned rats. Lab Invest 51: 104–111
16. Mall G, Reinhard H, Kayser K, Rossner JA (1978) An effective morphometric method for electron microscopic studies on papillary muscles. Virchows Arch A 379: 219–228
17. Mall G, Reinhard H, Stopp D, Rossner JA (1980) Morphometric observations on the rat heart after high-dose treatment with cortisol. Virchows Arch A 385: 169–180
18. Mattfeldt T, Mall G (1984) Estimation of length and surface of anisotropic capillaries. J Microsc 135: 181–190
19. Meerson FZ (1969) The myocardium in hyperfunction, hypertrophy and heart failure. Circ Res 25 (Suppl II): 1–163
20. Poche R, De Mello Mattos CM, Rembarz HW, Stoepel K (1968) Über das Verhältnis Mitochondrien: Myofibrillen in den Herzmuskelzellen der Ratte bei Druckhypertrophie des Herzens. Virchows Arch A 344: 100–110
21. Rakusan K, Hrdina PW, Turek Z, Lakatta EG (1984) Cell size and capillary supply of the hypertensive rat heart. Basic Res Cardiol 79: 389–395
22. Scheuer J (1981) Effects of physical training on myocardial vascularity and perfusion. Circulation 66: 491–495
23. Thiedemann KU, Holubarsch C, Medugorac I, Jacob R (1983) Connective tissue content and myocardial stiffness in pressure overload hypertrophy. A combined study of morphologic, morphometric, biochemical, and mechanical parameters. Basic Res Cardiol 78: 140–155
24. Tomanek RJ (1970) Effects of age and exercise on the extent of the myocardial capillary bed. Anat Rec 167: 55–62
25. Tomanek RJ, Hovanec JM (1981) The effects of long-term pressure-overload and aging on the

myocardium. J Mol Cell Cardiol 13: 471–488

26. Tomanek RJ, Searls JC, Lachenbruch PA (1982) Quantitative changes in the cpaillary bed during developing, peak, and stabilized cardiac hypertrophy in the spontaneously hypertensive rat. Circ Res 51: 295–304

27. Weibel ER (1980) Stereological Methods, Vol 2. Academic Press, London, pp 264–311

28. Weibel ER (1979) Stereological Methods, Vol 1. Academic Press, ondon, pp 26–36

29. Wendt-Gallitelli MF, Erbrecht G, Jacob R (1979) Morphological alterations and their functional interpretation n the hypertrophied myocardium of Goldblatt hypertensive rats. J Mol Cell Cardiol 11: 275–287

30. Wollenberger A, Schulze W (1962) Über das Volumenverhältnis von Mitochondrien zu Myofibrillen im chronisch überlasteten, hypertrophierten Herzen. Naturwissenschaften 49: 161–162

Authors' address:

Privat-Dozent Dr. G. Mall, Pathologisches Institut, Im Neuenheimer Feld 220–221, D-6900 Heidelberg (F.R.G.)

Pathophysiological mechanisms in cardiac insufficiency induced by chronic pressure overload – an attempt to analyze specific factors in animal experiment*

R. Jacob, M. Vogt, and H. Rupp

Physiologisches Institut II, Universität Tübingen (F.R.G.)

Summary

Experimental results obtained from studies on Goldblatt rats and spontaneously hypertensive rats as well as theoretical considerations render possible an approximate analysis and evaluation of the relative significance of specific factors at different levels of the heart for the manifestation of cardiac failure under chronic pressure overload.

In our experimental models congestive failure was never observed independently of structural dilatation. Thus, as a rule dilatation had already set in before symptoms of heart failure became manifest. However, at moderate dilatation of the ventricle, e. g., at double the end-diastolic volume, the geometrical state per se cannot be the cause of hydropic decompensation whereas extreme dilatation would, in principle, cause cardiac pumping failure even in the absence of any impairment of myocardial "contractility".

Generally, a more or less marked impairment of myocardial contractile capability was found, which exceeded the effects due to the altered isoenzyme pattern of myosin. As a rule, a reduction in myocardial "contractility" could be ascertained before a marked degree of dilatation was reached.

Diffuse fibrosis impairs the contractile capability of the myocardium and certainly contributes to the manifestation of heart insufficiency; although, as a rule, it should not be the main cause.

The adaptive transformation of myocardium towards a slower muscle (isoenzyme pattern of myosin; sarcoplasmatic reticulum) as such does not lead to resting insufficiency, not even under persisting pressure load. Further investigations on processes of excitation-mechanical coupling in the advanced stage of cardiac overload are indicated.

The absence of sympathetic support to the heart, e. g., following blockade of β-adrenergic receptors can, in the advanced stage, elicit a transition from the stage of pre-insufficiency to manifest failure. However, this was only observed when dilatation had already occurred.

A network of factors are responsible for cardiac insufficiency due to pressure overloading, whereby the respective significance of each component varies, depending on the experimental model used.

Key words: Goldblatt hypertension, spontaneous hypertension, congestive failure, structural dilatation, fibrosis, myosin isoenzyme pattern, β-receptor blockade

* This study was supported by the Deutsche Forschungsgemeinschaft (Ja 172/12-1)

Introduction

Chronic haemodynamic overloading of the heart leads to alterations at various levels of the organ; from changes in configuration and ventricular mass to structural changes at the level of cell organelles and macromolecules. Despite perennial clinical and experimental research it is still controversial today which factors or mechanisms, in the final analysis, are decisive for the terminal failure of the hypertrophied heart. Contemporary reviews as well as standard text- and handbooks of pathology, pathophysiology and cardiology reveal a variety of opinions stressing either structural dilatation due to exhaustion of protein synthesis and coronary insufficiency, impaired excitation-contraction coupling or, alternatively, biochemical changes at the level of contractile proteins as the cardinal factor conducive to cardiac insufficiency (for literature see [4, 6, 9, 11, 15, 19, 27, 31, 32, 38, 39, 42, 43, 45, 47, 48, 53]).

The following discussion is an attempt to ascertain the relative significance of specific factors for the manifestation of cardiac insufficiency on the basis of animal experimental results and theoretical deduction. The contribution is based on studies of our working group from previous years as well as on recent unpublished results derived from different methodological approaches. Male rats with Goldblatt hypertension and spontaneously hypertensive rats (SHR, Okamoto-Aoki) served as models. For methodological details see (5, 8, 12, 13, 17, 18, 23, 25, 26, 29, 30, 33, 40, 41, 50, 51, 52).

Concepts regarding the pathophysiological mechanisms of pressure-induced cardiac insufficiency

The scheme of Fig. 1 is an attempt to present a variety of controversial concepts that are regarded by certain authors as the predominant if not ecxlusive cause of cardiac failure in chronically overloaded heart. One is confronted firstly with two extreme views. One concept attributes the cause of failure to impaired myocardial performance. The other concept holds that the cause must predominantly lie in unfavourable geometrical states. Structural dilatation necessitates an increase in systolic wall stress thus reducing the degree of myocardial shortening and mechanical efficiency (31).

Other authors emphasize the functional significance of alterations at the tissue level: necrosis, fibrosis and scars imply loss of contractile material and thus impaired mechanical performance (6, 44). According to a contrary concept the cause lies mainly at the cellular level inclusive of the organelles. Aschoff (3) was among the first to postulate that the decisive myocardial alterations are not detectable by light microscopy. At the cellular level, an energy deficit ensuing from inadequate O_2 and substrate supply along with poor ATP production is held responsible by many authors (for literature see [4, 11, 43]). The converse states that a general energy deficit does not exist but rather the utilization of energy is reduced by defective activation processes or by changes in contractile proteins and/or regulatory proteins (9, 28, 53). The present discourse singles out various ascpects at the different levels of the organ (whole organ: structural dilatation; tissue level: collagen content; myofibrillar apparatus: myosin isoenzyme pattern).

The functional significance of structural dilatation.
Theoretical considerations

As is well known the pressure-hypertrophied ventricle has a concentric configuration while a more eccentric hypertrophy is characteristic of the volume-overloaded ventricle.

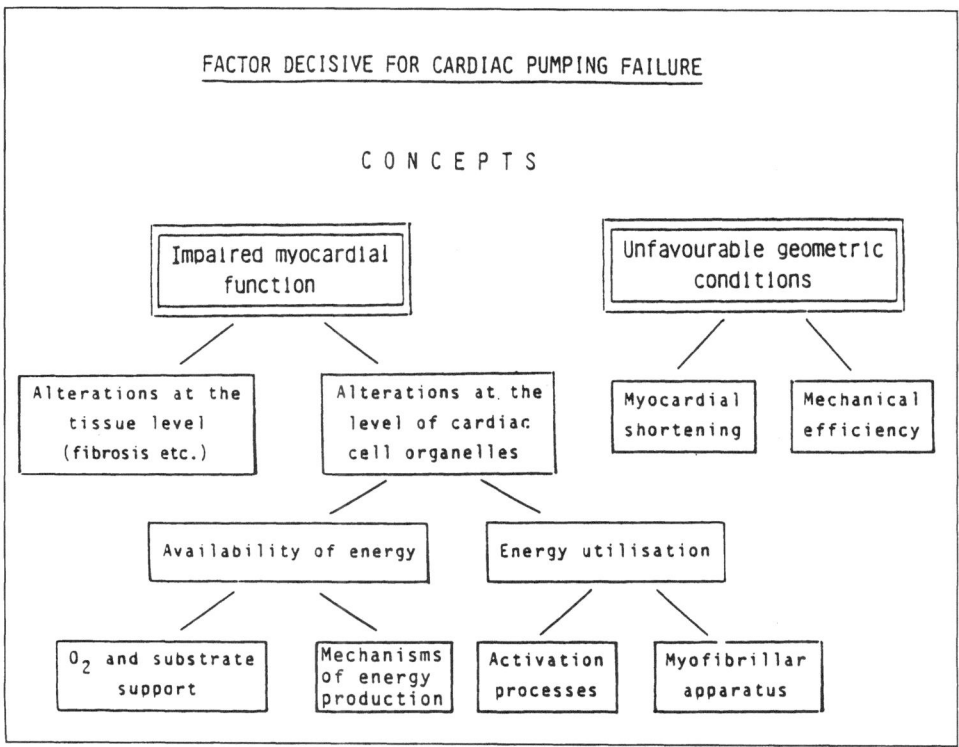

Fig. 1. Main concepts of factors responsible for cardiac failure under chronic pressure load.

Structural dilatation is characterized by insufficient increase in wall thickness relative to ventricular radius. Linzbach (31) emphasized the consequences of unfavourable geometric conditions; a decrease in contractility has virtually no bearing according to this concept. The increase in radius necessitates a corresponding increase in systolic wall stress development (La Place's relation). Based on the force-velocity relationship (and force-shortening relationship) diminution in external myocardium shortening must occur with increasing wall stress while O_2 consumption increases and cardiac efficiency decreases.

Obviously some aspects of this concept require additional analysis. The question arises 1. which of the two parameters is actually the decisive factor; the degree of shortening as such or the mechanical efficiency? and 2. at what degree of dilatation can detrimental effects on stroke volume be explained solely by the geometrical states?

An unfavourable relationship of external work to actual energy turnover cannot be the direct cause of heart failure. To cite an example in mechanics: a car with very high petrol consumption can theoretically still reach high driving speed. Of course, if the energy supply of the heart does not keep up with the requirements then the ensuing energy deficit would have functional and morphological consequences which in turn secondarily influence myocardial mechanics. In this case, however, a corresponding impairment of contractility should be demonstrable.

Regarding stress-induced diminution in fibre shortening, the following aspects should be considered:

Dilatation necessitates higher systolic stress development. Accordingly, both velocity and degree of shortening decrease. Assuming a sphere as the simplest model of a ventricle, the volume can be calculated using the formula $V = 4/3 \, r^3 \, \pi$.

In our studies ventricular midwall circumferential stress σ_R was calculated using the formula:

$$\sigma_R = \frac{P r_i^3}{r_o^3 - r_i^3} \left(\frac{r_o^3}{2R^3} + 1\right) = \frac{V \cdot P}{W} \cdot \left(1 + \frac{4(V + V)}{(V^{1/3} + (V + W)^{1/3})^3}\right) \quad (17, 34))$$

For preliminary considerations, however, it suffices to use the LaPlace formula: $\sigma_R = P \cdot r/2 \cdot h$ although the latter, strictly speaking, applies to a thin-walled sphere. Given constant values for 1. contractility, 2. diastolic wall thickness, and 3. aortic pressure and furthermore a stress reserve in early systole which under standard conditions is half of peak isovolumetric stress, a twofold increase in radius and thus stress would totally exhaust the systolic stress reserve. Since at high degrees of dilatation stress still has to rise considerably during the ejection period, shortening would be absolutely impossible. In other words, at high degrees of dilatation aortic blood pressure cannot be maintained. Even with the myocardium being fully intact, cardiac insufficiency would inevitably occur.

Yet, another very important viewpoint should be considered. At modest dilatation, only minimal fibre shortening is required to eject a given stroke volume for geometrical reasons: volume changes with the third power of the radius or circumference. Certainly ejection fraction and relative shortening decrease with increasing radius and wall stress. However, the absolute values of stroke volume as a function of ventricular radius would initially even increase despite rising wall stress and would drop below the starting value only when the radius has reached considerable dimensions, given that the parameters mentioned above are constant. In a thick-walled spherical model the critical inner radius would be 1.7 times that of control radius, the critical inner volume 4.8 times that of control volume.

Consequently, a decrease in stroke volume (and cardiac output) cannot be explained solely on the basis of geometrical states at modest degree of dilatation as e. g. at double end-diastolic volume. If, on the other hand, one postulates that myocardial exhaustion occurs due to elevated stress load, then a secondary impairment of myocardial contractility should be detectable accordingly.

Clinical observations and animal experimental results

Clinical observations support the concept that left ventricular mass/volume relationship plays an important role in the manifestation of pumping failure of the pressure hypertrophied heart. The diagrams of Grossman et al. (10) and Strauer (48) in particular could be interpreted to the effect that the diminution of ejection fraction is practically exclusively attributable to geometric states. Nevertheless, as already discussed in a previous chapter, a distinction must be made, in the given context, between ejection fraction on the one hand and the absolute value of stroke volume on the other. Furthermore, it seems justifiable to probe to what extent the relative significance of structural dilatation on the one hand and decreased myocardial contractile capability on the other is definable under conditions of clinical investigations.

Impaired cardiac performance and an inverse relationship between ejection fraction and ventricular systolic wall stress is also found in chronic animal experiments (7, 23, 36, 37). Mirsky et al. (35) reported reduced ejection fraction in 18 and 24 month old SHR although systolic wall stress was less than at the 6 and 12 month stage. Consequently, he postulated that reduced contractile state of the myocardium is the decisive determinant for development of "ventricular dysfunction" under chronic overload. However, the study does not reveal whether cardiac failure actually existed in these specimen.

Considering methodological aspects, it should finally be emphasized that in the case of substantial hypertrophy, ejection fraction is no longer a precise measure for midwall circumferential shortening, the latter being overestimated in ventricles with considerable increase in wall thickness.

Animals with definite congestive failure (pleural effusion, ascites, skin edema) were

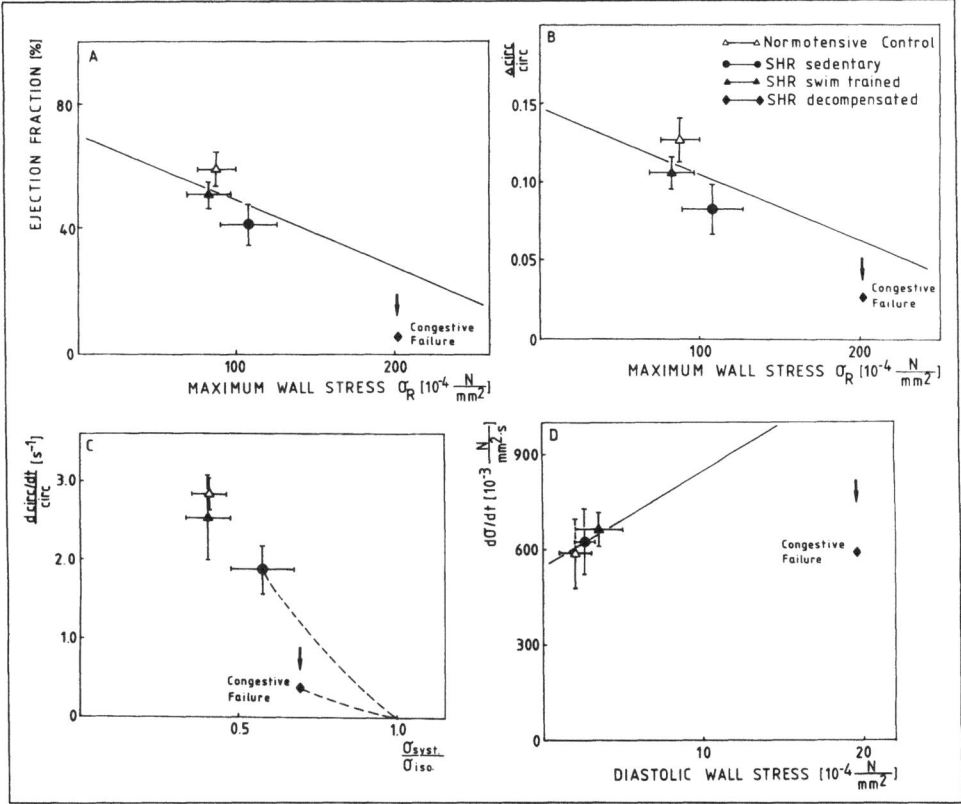

Fig. 2. Myocardial function in SHR in the compensated stage (sedentary rats and swim-trained rats) and in the stage of congestive failure as compared to normotensive Wistar rats. Correlation of left ventricular ejection fraction (A) and relative circumferential shortening (B) with maximum systolic midwall circumferential wall stress; normalized circumferential shortening velocity as related to the ratio of developed stress to isovolumetric stress (C); maximum rate of stress development as a function of end-diastolic stress (D).

Age of (male) animals: Compensated groups, 10 months; cardiac failure, 15 months. Average degree of hypertrophy (evaluated on the basis of the ratio ventricular weight/tibia length, referred to normotensive rats of the same age): SHR: $+73\%$; swim-trained SHR: $+91\%$, congestive failure: $+125\%$ (Vogt M, Jacob R, unpublished results).

included in our investigations. Ventricular dynamics and calculated muscle physiological parameters were compared with those of normotensive Wistar rats, 10 month old SHR (with mainly concentric left ventricular hypertrophy) and swim-trained SHR (showing a slight tendency towards eccentric hypertrophy).

Due to structural dilatation, insufficient hearts reveal the highest values of wall stress as shown in Fig. 2. Ejection fraction, relative fibre shortening and shortening velocity and rate of isovolumic rise of stress were also significantly reduced, compared to non-insufficient rats. (Although this is evident, strictly speaking the regression lines should be calculated for each group after experimental manipulation of systolic wall stress and should be related to common diastolic stress.)

The essential alterations are impressively demonstrated using pressure-volume diagrams (Fig. 3). The left ventricular end-diastolic volume of SHR with manifest cardiac failure is

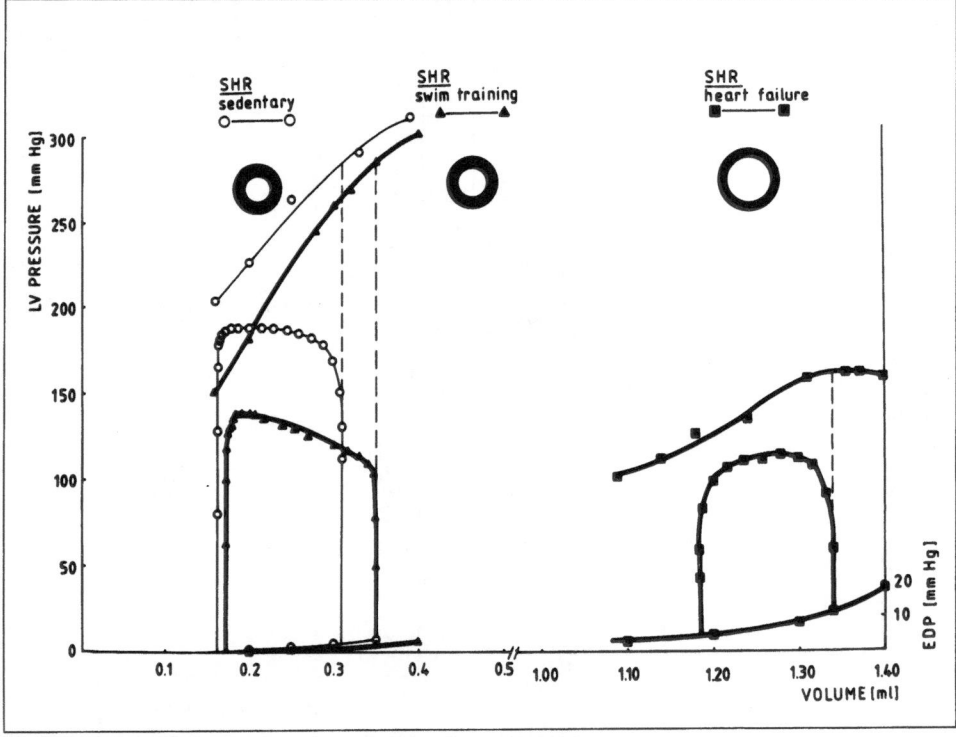

Fig. 3. Representative left ventricular pressure-volume relations in the state of structural dilatation compared with compensated sedentary SHR as well as SHR after 6 week swimming training. Degree of hypertrophy: see Fig. 2.

extremely increased. Ventricular working capacity (potential work under defined mechanical conditions) is decreased, the isovolumetric pressure-volume relationship showing a flat course. End-diastolic left ventricular pressure exceeds normal value significantly while systemic hypertension cannot be maintained.

Calculated length-stress diagrams (Fig. 4) make evident the decreased myocardial shorte-

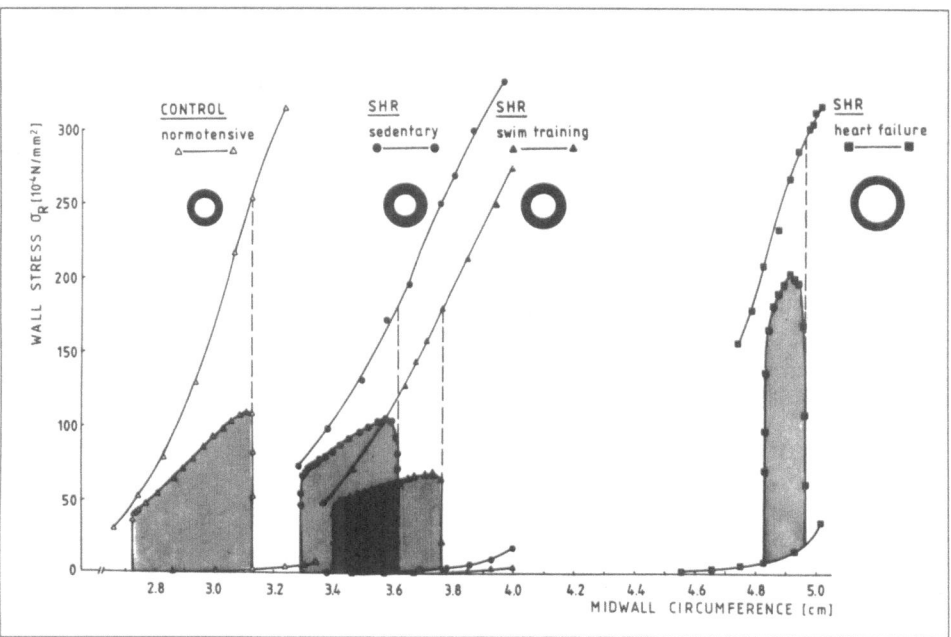

Fig. 4. Left ventricular length-stress diagrams calculated from pressure-volume relations of Fig. 3. The diagram of a younger normotensive Wistar rat is also included.

ning capability and reduced myocardial working capacity of insufficient hearts. The area between isovolumic and end-diastolic length-stress curve is considerably reduced, even more when related to diastolic muscle length (ventricular circumference). Stress development is extremely increased with marked additional rise during the ejection period. Stress reserve – although markedly curtailed – is never completely utilized in such cases, despite stroke volume and systemic pressure being reduced.

Based on investigations on Goldblatt rats, we were able to demonstrate that structural dilatation occurs before cardiac failure becomes manifest (23). In some of the animals, the left ventricular volume loop is shifted to the right and systolic wall stress is increased already at the 6 month stage of renal hypertension, while end-diastolic pressure is only insignificantly elevated and signs of congestive decompensation are absent.

Furthermore, at this stage moderate impairment of myocardial contractile properties is demonstrable in isolated muscle preparations. In earlier stages (4–8 week after unilateral renal artery coarctation) unloaded shortening velocity (and myofibrillar ATPase activity) is already reduced whereas isometric tension development is even increased (21, 23, 24, 26). The reasons for this discrepancy are discussed elsewhere (22, 24). In the subsequent weeks, both mechanical parameters decrease so that maximum myocardial power (represented by the greatest rectangle under the tension-velocity curve) is significantly reduced at the 24 week stage (21, 26).

From these results, it can be deduced that both impaired myocardial contractility and structural dilatation are involved in final insufficiency of the chronically overloaded heart, at least in the models of chronic pressure overload we studied – although it must be assumed that the consequences of moderate dilatation are indirect via energy deficit and ensuing impairment of contractility.

Functional significance of fibrosis versus alterations at the cellular and subcellular level

Marked fibrosis which occurs in Goldblatt rats myocardium at an earlier stage than in SHR (18, 23, 33, 50) leads to impairment of cardiac mechanics. Fibrosis, being a diffusion barrier, has further detrimental consequences on the myocardial cells causing the latter to become literally walled-in by collagen in the late stages of overload (50).

Fibrotic ventricles reveal impaired myocardial distensibility. Apparently not only collagen concentration but also its arrangement influences the myocardial stiffness constant (slope of the relation between differential elastic modulus E and wall stress σ) (50). Shortening velocity and isometric tension development are significantly reduced in fibrotic preparations. As expected, control values of non-fibrotic preparations are not reached by experimentally optimizing the conditions for excitation contraction coupling in both groups (21, 23). Thus, fibrosis undoubtedly contributes to manifestation of cardiac failure although some insufficient ventricles of SHR showed only moderate fibrosis in the region of subendocardial muscle layers.

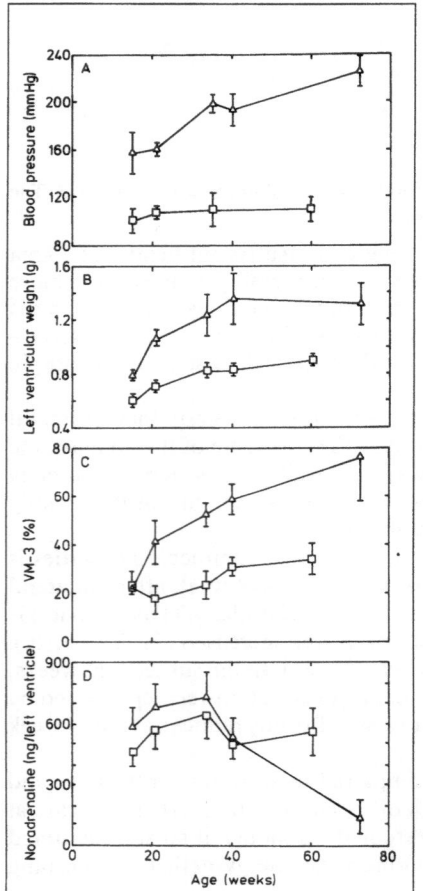

Fig. 5. Age-dependent changes in blood pressure (A), left ventricular weight (C), noradrenaline (B) and VM-3 (D) content in normotensive rats and SHR. The data are represented as means ± S. D.

Noradrenaline was determined by HPLC using electrochemical detection (Rupp et al., unpublished results).

Among the alterations at the subcellular level, reduced myofibrillar ATPase activity plays a big role in the discussion of the cause of chronic heart failure (1, 32, 53). Some authors regard these alterations or the underlying redistribution of myosin isoenzyme pattern (Fig. 5) as the substantial cause of chronic cardiac failure (53).

Our experimental results contradict the assumption that cardiac insufficiency could be solely due to a redistribution of myosin isoenzyme pattern. Young normotensive rats (5–8 week old) show a fairly homogeneous VM-1 isoenzyme pattern of ventricular myosin; rats after thyreostatic treatment show a fairly homogeneous VM-3 pattern. The difference between myofibrillar ATPase activity of both groups is about 40%. The same is true for the maximum unloaded shortening velocity of chemically skinned fibres. However, isometric tension development is not significantly reduced after extreme isoenzyme redistribution. Influences of excitation and excitation-contraction coupling are superimposed in native preparations so that isometric tension can even increase despite a prevalence of VM-3 (22).

Also in the whole heart, maximum transformation of the myocardium towards a "slow" muscle by thyreostatic treatment has little effect on isovolumetric pressure development and ejection fraction (25) although rate of pressure and stress rise as well as other velocity parameters are considerably decreased (Fig. 6).

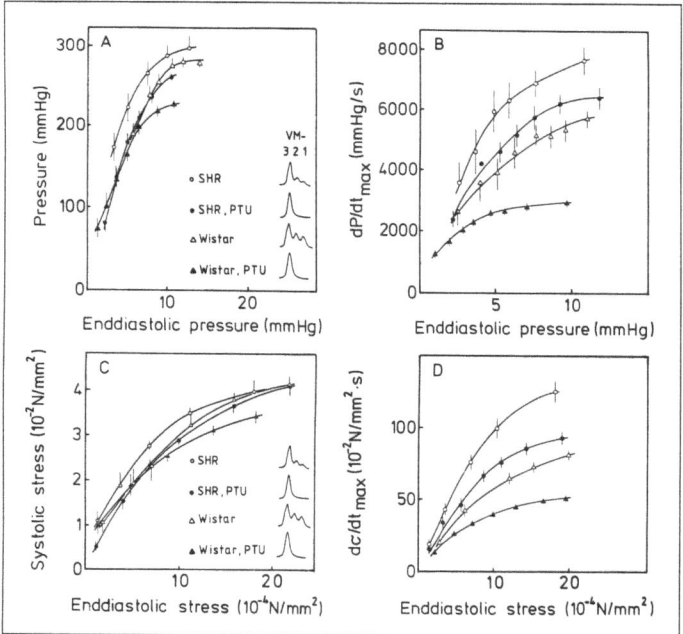

Fig. 6. Isovolumetric peak pressure (A) and maximum rate of pressure rise (B) as a function of end-diastolic pressure in SHR and Wistar rats (both 40 weeks old).

Calculated stress (C) and maximum rate of stress development (D) as a function of end-diastolic stress corresponding to the pressure values of A and B.

In both groups homogeneous VM_3 was induced by administration of 0.8 g/l propylthiouracil (PTU) in drinking water for 4 weeks (cf. inset) (Jörg E and Jacob R, unpublished results).

Systemic blood pressure of the SHR is reduced after thyreostatic treatment but still lies ca. 30 mm Hg above control values of normotensive Wistar rats. Despite persistent pressure overload, no signs of congestion – at least at rest – are detectable after extreme transformation towards a slow myocardium (25). This holds for an observation period of ca. 4 weeks. Thus, the functional significance of myocardial transformation of the pressure overloaded heart for manifestation of cardiac failure seems to be rather overestimated in literature. Although retardation of the contractile process, in combination with additional unfavourable factors, should contribute to final decompensation it must be emphasized that the process of the transformation in itself also involves favourable effects, heat release (2) and oxygen consumption (30) related to tension-time integral being reduced in the pressure hypertrophied myocardium.

Factors contributing to pumping failure of the chronically pressure overloaded heart. – Attempt at a synopsis

In literature it is often attempted on the basis of myocardial ATP content to distinguish between cardiac insufficiency due to energy deficit on the one hand and "utilisation failure" on the other (9, 19, 43, 45). The limitation of such an approach lies mainly in the fact that O_2 and substrate deficit in themselves also influence the activation processes. Obviously one should distinguish more precisely between primary causes conducive to specific functional and structural alterations on the one hand, and those factors finally responsible for pumping failure on the other. This postulation may seem trivial, however, the consequences are substantial, as already discussed for the geometrical conditions.

In contrast to a popular opinion, ATP deficit of the contractile apparatus does not, in itself, induce a decrease in total isometric tension; rather it leads to rigor-bindings with corresponding impairment of relaxation. However, O_2 deficiency causes a number of acute and chronic alterations in action potential, Ca^{++} transport mechanisms, myoplasmic pH, phosphate concentration – and finally, at its worst, degenerative changes including cellular necrosis – all being changes that in themselves are detrimental for myocardial contractile properties.

Even in the initial stage of acute hypoxia, ATP deficit of the contractile apparatus itself does not seem decisive for decreased "contractility". This can be demonstrated by improving excitation-contraction coupling: paired-pulse stimulation (post-extrasystolic potentiation) of hypoxic guinea-pig papillary muscle, e. g., leads to an increase in contraction amplitude despite persisting O_2 deficiency, The latter can significantly exceed the control amplitude recorded before onset of hypoxia (Fig. 7). Thus, even in acute O_2 deficiency, the prototype of "deficiency failure", energy deficit in the contractile apparatus itself is not necessarily the limiting factor. This is an incentive to reconsider conceptions like "deficiency failure" and "utilization failure", respectively.

Certainly, alterations, in excitation-contraction coupling play a role in decreased contractility of the pressure overloaded heart (9, 28). These alterations have in part an adaptive character (20, 24, 27), at least as far as they involve the sarcoplasmic reticulum (16, 49). In the rat model, an increase in the proportion of VM-3, the myosin isoenzyme with lowest ATPase activity is accompanied by reduced Ca^{++} uptake of the SR. This concerted change which suggests common trigger mechanisms was observed during maturation and aging as well as following pressure overload (Rupp H and Jacob R, unpublished results). However, in later stages of Goldblatt hypertension we could show that optimal conditions for excitation contraction coupling (by lowering Na^+ concentration and raising Ca^{++} concentration) did not lead to the same level of isometric contraction amplitude observed in equally treated

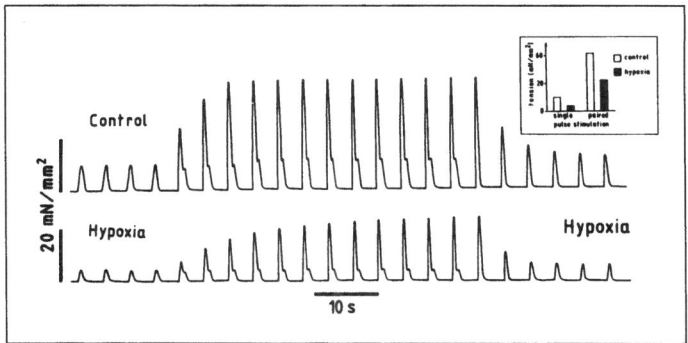

Fig. 7. Postextrasystolic potentiation under hypoxic conditions. Under paired stimulation the isometric tension of the hypoxic preparation even exceeds the control amplitude (recorded under normoxic conditions and stimulation with single impulses).

Isolated left ventricular papillary muscle of the guinea-pig. Tyrode solution, [Ca++] 2.2 mmol/l, [Mg++] 1.2 mmol/l; temperature 30° C (Gülch RW and Jacob R, unpublished results).

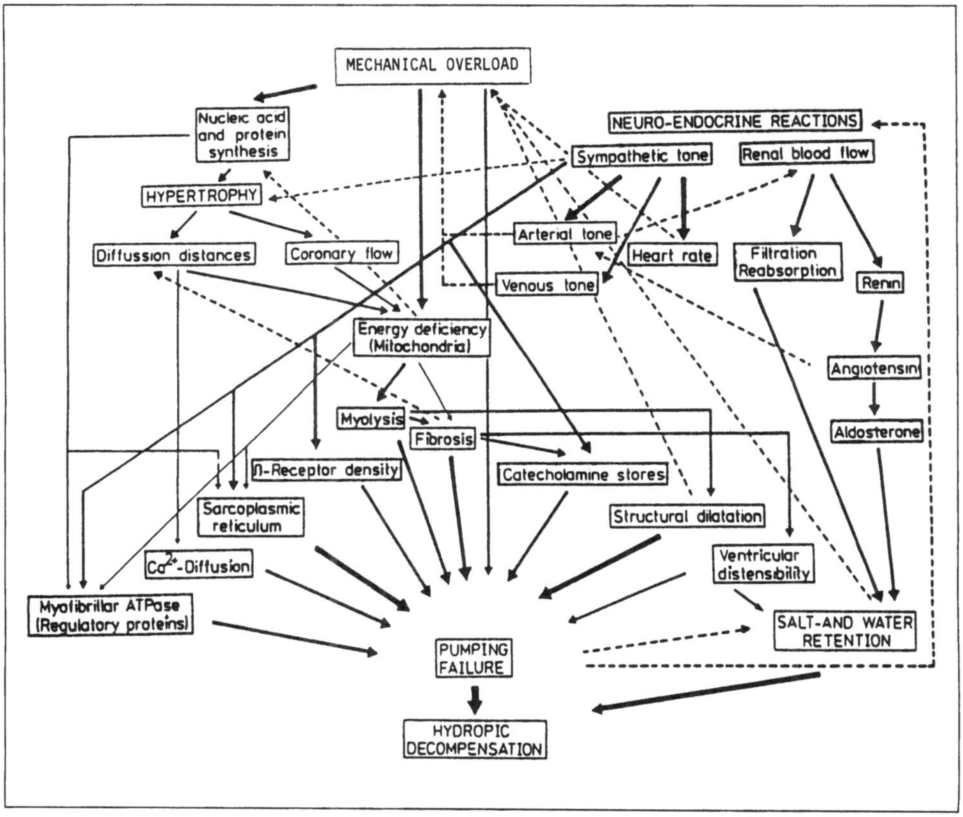

Fig. 8. Schematic of factors leading to congestive cardiac insufficiency, arranged in their hypothetical hierarchy and interactions.

non-hypertrophied control preparations. Furthermore, neither model of pressure overload (renal and spontaneous hypertension) ever revealed congestive failure in the absence of structural dilatation.

An attempt has been made in Fig. 8 to present the essential pathogentic mechanisms that contribute to the manifestation of cardiac failure and to define their position within the framework of multifactorial causes. The lowest row of factors in the scheme are assumed to be the potential direct causes for insufficient cardiac pumping function. In order to emphasize the significance of neuroendocrine reactions (14) a distinction is made between impaired ventricular pumping function on the one hand, and congestive failure on the other. In this context, mention must be made of the progressive depletion of catecholamine stores (Fig. 5) which is mainly due to persistent sympathetic drive. The former as well as the adaptive decrease in β-receptor density limit the compensatory adrenergic support of cardiac function maintained in the stage of preinsufficiency. In 10 month old SHR, in the compensatory stage of left ventricular hypertrophy, blockade of the β-adrenergic receptors by atenolol alone did not produce cardiac failure. However, β-receptor blockade was the final trigger for pumping failure in a section of Goldblatt rats (12 months after unilateral renal artery coarctation) with structural dilatation of the left ventricle (Vogt M, Onegi B, and Jacob R, unpublished results).

Our results confirm that, as a rule, multifactorial events are involved in chronic cardiac insufficiency. However, the respective significance of individual components at the level of whole heart, tissue and myocardial cell varies, depending on the experimental model used.

Acknowledgement

The authors express their gratitude to Prof. Dr. A. Bohle, Institute of Pathology, University of Tübingen, for histologic investigations.

References

1. Alpert NR, Gordon MS (1962) Myofibrillar adenosine triphosphatase activity in congestive heart failure. Am J Physiol 202: 940–946
2. Alpert NR, Mulieri LA (1982) Increased myothermal economy of isometric force generation in compensated cardiac hypertrophy induced by pulmonary artery constriction in the rabbit. Circ Res 50: 491–500
3. Aschoff L (1934) Über die nicht gefäßbedingten Schädigungen des Herzmuskels. In: Hrsg Vereinigung der Bad Nauheimer Ärzte (eds), Klinik der Erkrankungen des Herzmuskels. Steinkopff Verlag, Dresden, pp 14–28
4. Braunwald E, Ross J, Sonnenblick EH (1967) Mechanisms of contraction of the normal and failing heart. Little, Brown and Company, Boston
5. Brenner B, Jacob R (1980) Calcium activation and maximum unloaded shortening velocity. Investigations on glycerinated skeletal and heart muscle preparations. Basic Res Cardiol 75: 40–46
6. Büchner F, Weyland R (1968) Die Insuffizienz des hypertrophierten Herzmuskels im Lichte seiner Narbenbilder. Urban & Schwarzenberg, München Berlin Wien
7. Bürger SB, Strauer BE (1981) Left ventricular hypertrophy in chronic pressure load due to spontaneous essential hypertension. I. Left ventricular function, left ventricular geometry and wall stress. In: Strauer BE (ed) The Heart in Hypertension. Springer-Verlag, Berlin Heidelberg New York, pp 13–35
8. Ebrecht G, Rupp H, Jacob R (1982) Alterations of mechanical parameters in chemically skinned preparations of rat myocardium as a function of isoenzyme pattern of myosin. Basic Res Cardiol 77: 220–234
9. Fleckenstein A (1968) Experimentelle Pathologie der akuten und chronischen Herzinsuffizienz. Verh dtsch Ges Kreisl Forsch 34: 15–34
10. Grossman W, Carabello BA, Ganther S, Fifer MA (1983) Ventricular wall stress and the development of cardiac hypertrophy and failure. In: Alpert NR (ed) Myocardial hypertrophy and failure. Raven Press, New York, pp 1–18

11. Grothe J, Schömerich P (1985) Herzinsuffizienz. In: Bock HE, Kaufmann W, Löhr GW (eds) Pathophysiologie. Thieme, Stuttgart, pp 326–337
12. Gülch RW (1980) The effect of elevated chronic loading on the action potential of mammalian myocardium. J Mol Cell Cardiol 12: 415–520
13. Gülch RW, Jacob R (1975) Length-tension diagram and force-velocity relations of mammalian cardiac muscle under steady-state conditions. Pflügers Arch 355: 331–346
14. Harris P (1983) Evolution and the cardiac patient. Cardiovasc Res 17 (No 6): 313–319; 17 (No 7): 373–378; 17 (No 8): 437–445
15. Hatt PY, Jouannot P, Moravec J, Swynghedauw B (1974) Current trends in heart hypertrophy. Basic Res Cardiol 69: 479–483
16. Heilmann C, Lindl T, Müller W, Pette D (1980) Characterization of cardiac microsomes from spontaneously hypertonic rats. Basic Res Cardiol 75: 92–96
17. Hepp A, Hansis M, Gülch R, Jacob R (1974) Left ventricular isovolumetric pressure volume relations, "diastolic tone", and contractility in the rat heart after physical training. Basic Res Cardiol 69: 516–532
18. Holubarsch Ch, Holubarsch T, Jacob R, Medugorac I, Thiedemann KU (1983) Passive elastic properties of myocardium in different models and stages of hypertrophy: A study comparing mechanical, chemical, and morphometric parameters. In: Alpert NR (ed) Myocardial Hypertrophy and Failure, Vol 7. Raven Press New York, pp 323–336
19. Hort W (1977) Spezielle Pathologie und Anatomie. Kreislauforgane. In: Eder M, Gedigk P (eds) Lehrbuch der Allgemeinen Pathologie und der Pathologischen Anatomie. Springer-Verlag, Berlin Heidelberg New York, pp 314–360
20. Jacob R (1983) Chronic reactions of myocardium at the myofibrillar level. Reflections on "adaptation" and "disease" based on the biology of long-term cardiac overload. In: Jacob R, Gülch RW, Kissling G (eds) Cardiac adaptation to hemodynamic overload, training and stress. Steinkopff Verlag Darmstadt, pp 3–24
21. Jacob R, Ebrecht G, Kämmereit A, Medugorac I, Wendt-Gallitelli MF (1977) Myocardial function in different models of cardiac hypertrophy. An attempt at correlating mechanical, biochemical and morophological parameters. Basic Res Cardiol 72: 160–167
22. Jacob R, Ebrecht G, Holubarsch Ch, Rupp H, Kissling G (1983) Mechanics and energetics in cardiac hypertrophy as related to the isoenzyme pattern of myosin. In: Alpert NR (ed) Myocardial Hypertrophy and Failure. Raven Press, New York, pp 553–569
23. Jacob R, Kissling G (1981) Left ventricular dynamics and myocardial function in Goldblatt hypertension of the rat. Biochemical, morphological and electrophysiological correlates. In: Strauer BE (ed) The Heart in Hypertension. Springer-Verlag, Berlin Heidelberg New York, pp 89–106
24. Jacob R, Kissling G, Ebrecht G, Holubarsch Ch, Medugorac I, Rupp H (1983) Adaptive and pathological alterations in experimental cardiac hypertrophy. In: Chazov E, Saks V, Rona G (eds) Advan Myocardiol 4: 55–77 Plen Publish Corporation
25. Jacob R, Kissling G, Ebrecht G, Jörg E, Rupp H, Takeda N (1984) Cardiac alterations at the myofibrillar level: Is a redistribution of the myosin isoenzyme pattern decisive for cardiac failure in hemodynamic overload? Eur Heart J 5: (Suppl F)
26. Kämmereit A, Jacob R (1979) Alterations in rat myocardial mechanics under Goldblatt hypertension and experimental aortic stenosis. Basic Res Cardiol 74: 389–405
27. Katz AM (1977) Physiology of the heart. Raven Press, New York
28. Kaufmann RL, Homburger H, Wirth H (1971) Disorder in excitation-contraction coupling of cardiac muscle from cats with experimentally produced right ventricular hypertrophy. Circ Res 28: 346–357
29. Kissling G, Gassenmaier T, Wendt-Gallitelli MF, Jacob R (1977) Pressure-volume relations, elastic modulus, and contractile behaviour of the hypertrophied left ventricle of rats with Goldblatt II hypertension. Pflügers Arch 369: 213
30. Kissling G, Rupp H, Malloy L, Jacob R (1982) Alterations in cardiac oxygen consumption under chronic pressure overload. Significance of the isoenzyme pattern of myosin. Basic Res Cardiol 77: 255–269
31. Linzbach AJ (1960) Heart failure from the point of view of quantitative anatomy. Amer J Cardiol 5: 370–382

216

32. Meerson FS (1976) Insufficiency of hypertrophied heart. Basic Res Cardiol 71: 343–354
33. Medugorac I (1980) Collagen content in different areas of normal and hypertrophied rat myocardium. Cardiovasc Res 14: 551–554
34. Mirsky I (1974) Review of various theories for the evaluation of left ventricular wall stress. In: Mirsky I, Ghista DN, Sandler H (eds) Cardiac Mechanics. John Wiley & Sons Inc, New York London Sydney Toronto, pp 381–409
35. Mirsky I, Pfeffer JM, Pfeffer MA, Braunwald E (1983) The contractile state as the major determinant in the evolution of left ventricular dysfunction in the spontaneously hypertensive rat. Circ Res 53: 767–778
36. Pfeffer JM, Pfeffer MA, Braundwald E (1983) Development of left ventricular dysfunction in the female spontaneously hypertensive rat. In: Alpert NR (ed) Myocardial hypertrophy and failure. Raven Press, New York, pp 73–84
37. Pfeffer JM, Pfeffer MA, Fletcher P, Braunwald E (1981) Impaired cardiac performance in rats with long-term spontaneous hypertension. In: Strauer BE (ed) The Heart in Hypertension. Springer-Verlag, Berlin Heidelberg New York, pp 389–399
38. Poche W (1982) Strukturelle Veränderungen des druck- und volumenüberbelasteten Herzens. In: Roskamm H, Rendell H (eds) Herzkrankheiten. Pathophysiologie, Diagnostik, Therapie. Springer-Verlag Berlin Heidelberg New York, pp 487–494
39. Riecker G (1975) Klinische Kardiologie. Springer-Verlag, Berlin Heidelberg New York
40. Rupp H (1981) The adaptive changes in the isoenzyme pattern of myosin from hypertrophied rat myocardium as a result of pressure overload and physical training. Basic Res Cardiol 76: 79–88
41. Rupp H, Kissling G, Jacob R (1983) The hormonal and hemodynamic determinants of polymorphic myosin. In: Alpert NR (ed) Myocardial Hypertrophy and Failure, Vol 7. Raven Press, New York, pp 373–383
42. Rutishauser W, Krayenbühl HP (1983) Herz. In: Siegenthaler W (ed) Klinische Pathophysiologie. Thieme, Stuttgart, pp 606–677
43. Sandritter W, Beneke G (1974) Allgemeine Pathologie. Schattauer, Stuttgart New York
44. Schaper J (1983) Morphometry of cardiac muscle. The relationship between structure and function in human hypertrophied hearts. An ultrastructural morphometric study. In: Alpert NR (ed) Myocardial hypertrophy and failure, Vol 7. Raven Press, New York, pp 177–196
45. Schölmerich P (1972) Anpassungserscheinungen des Herzens, Herzinsuffizienz. In: Bock HE (ed) Pathophysiologie. Bd II. Thieme, Stuttgart, pp 96–104
46. Schwartz K, Lecarpentier Y, Martin JL, Lompré AM, Mercadier JJ, Swynghedauw B (1981) Myosin isoenzyme distribution correlated with speed of myocardial contraction. J Mol Cell Cardiol 13: 1071–1075
47. Sodeman WA, Sodeman TM (1979) Pathologic Physiology. Mechanisms of Disease. WB Saunders Comp, Philadelphia London Toronto
48. Strauer BE (1980) Hypertensive Heart Disease. Springer-Verlag Berlin Heidelberg New York
49. Suko J, Ito Y, Chidsey A (1973) Intracellular metabolism of calcium in the hypertrophied and failing heart. In: Roskamm H, Reindell H (eds) Das chronisch kranke Herz. Schattauer Verlag, Stuttgart New York, pp 183–189
50. Thiedemann KU, Holubarsch Ch, Medugorac I, Jacob R (1983) Connective tissue content and myocardial stiffness in pressure induced cardiac hypertrophy. Basic Res Cardiol 78: 140–155
51. Vogt M, Jacob R (1985) Myocardial elasticity and left ventricular distensibility as related to oxygen deficiency and right ventricular filling. Analysis in a rat heart model. Basic Res Cardiol 80: 537–547
52. Wendt-Gallitelli MF, Ebrecht G, Jacob R (1979) Morphological alterations and their functional interpretation in the hypertrophied myocardium of Goldblatt hypertensive rats. J Mol Cell Cardiol 11: 275–287
53. Wikman-Coffelt J, Parmley WW, Mason DT (1979) The cardiac hypertrophy process: Analyses of factors determining pathological vs physiological development. Circ Res 45: 679–707

Authors' address:

Prof. Dr. R. Jacob, Physiologisches Institut II, Universität Tübingen, Gmelinstraße 5, D-7400 Tübingen (F.R.G.)

Immunologic regulator and effector functions in perimyocarditis, postmyocarditic heart muscle disease and dilated cardiomyopathy

B. Maisch

University Hospital of Internal Medicine, Würzburg (F. R. G.)

Summary

In acute perimyocarditis we found that OKIAI-positive cells were increased, and in dilated cardiomyopathy OKMI-positive cells were increased. No significant alteration in suppressor T cell activity was observed in our patients with either disease. The characteristic immunofluorescent pattern in carditis and postmyocarditic heart disease is the presence of antimyolemmal antibodies with intact rat and human cardiocytes in titers of 1 : 40 – 1 : 320 as antigens. The antimyolemmal fluorescence can be absorbed with the respective causative virus in Coxsackie B, influenza, mumps and EBV-myocarditis, indicating that the antibodies are a cross-reactive. AMLA-positive sera induce cytolysis of vital rat cardiocytes in vitro, suggesting that the antibodies are of pathogenetic relevance. Cytolytic serum activity could be absorbed out with the respective virus.

Immunohistologic specimens obtained from patients with carditis demonstrate the fixation of IgG and IgM antibodies; IgG antibodies also occur in dilated cardiomyopathy and coronary artery disease. In dilated postmyocarditic heart disease both antimyolemmal fluorescence and cytolytic activity are preserved at a lower level when compared to carditis. These antibodies can also fix complement. In the acute phase of carditis circulating immune complexes can be demonstrated. Cellular effector mechanisms against vital cardiocytes were maintained or even slightly enhanced in carditis, postmyocarditic and primary dilated cardiomyopathy. In vitro NK cell activity against K 562, however, was decreased. This is compatible with a sustained target-specific cytotoxicity whereas reduced NK cell activity may indicate impairment of this effector organ.

Key words: perimyocarditis, dilated cardiomyopathy, cell-mediated immunity, suppressor T cell activity, antiheart and antisarcolommal antibodies, NK cell activity

Introduction

Myocarditis and dilated cardiomyopathy are still unresolved and controversial problems, since diagnosis, etiology and pathogenesis are difficult to ascertain in carditis and in dilated cardiomyopathy are by definition (WHO-ISCF task force) unknown (55). In myocarditis this is partly due to nonuniform clinical criteria (21, 32), controversial histomorphologic definitions (2, 9, 10, 13, 14, 16, 21, 32) and the speculative viral etiology (6, 7, 17, 20, 28, 34, 35, 36, 50, 58, 62, 65). It has became the medical equivalent of Churchill's "riddle wrapped in a mystery inside of an enigma" (26).

This can also be exemplified by statements from different periods of research in myocarditis: Whereas in 1899 von Schroetter (60) postulated "the most important role in heart failure is played by inflammatory processes of the myocardium", a recent medical text book (33) stated in likewise controversial manner "from a clinical point of view myocarditis is a very rare cardiac disease".

In histomorphologic investigations from biopsies and necropsies, a variable incidence of the possible immunologic effector organs, the polymorphs or mononuclear cells, in the heart ranged from 0.1 % to more than 90 % (9, 13, 14, 16, 21, 43, 51, 63, 64, 65), depending either on the patients studied or the individual pathologist and his own interpretation of myocarditis (14). It seems clear, however, that myocarditis can be detected more often, the earlier biopsy samples are acquired in the course of the disease, and the greater the number of biopsy specimens that are available for histomorphological evaluation. In patients with acute cardiomegaly infiltrates are seen more often than in cases of dilated cardiomyopathy lasting some years (13). Nor are infiltrates bound to cardiomegaly (43). Complex tachycardias may indicate myocarditis as may sudden death (25). From a panoramic point of view acute inflammatory heart muscle disease and dilated cardiomyopathy can be seen as different stages of the same disease on the road of time. So the WHO definition of dilated cardiomyopathy (55) as "heart muscle disease of unknown cause" most likely describes more our lack of knowledge than a disease entity. The investigation of immunologic regulator (5, 15, 18, 29, 59) and effector mechanisms (1, 3, 8, 12, 23, 24, 27, 37, 38, 40, 41, 42, 44, 45, 46, 47, 50, 61, 66, 67) has both broadened our understanding of the pathogenesis, etiology and prognosis of carditis and of dilated cardiomyopathy and raised new questions.

Diagnostic criteria, patients and methods

Diagnosis of myocarditis was based on the criteria of Daly et al. (9) or the almost identical histological definitions of the Dallas panel of pathologists (10). In the cases of perimyocarditis, pericardial effusion or pericardial rubs were detected together with histologically proven myocarditis changes or segmental wall motion abnormalities, assessed by TM- and two-dimensional echocardiography or angiography (Table 1) (39). Viral etiology was ascertained when a change in titer of more than two-fold occurred within 2–4 weeks in complement fixation or neutralization tests.

Table 1 a. Criteria of myocarditis and perimyocarditis

Essential criteria
1) Inflammation of the myocardium determined by biopsy/necropsy (infiltrate, focal necrosis, interstitial swelling) with or without fibrosis.
   Classification according to Daly et al. (9) and the Dallas criteria (10) as
   – acute (prominent infiltrate, necrosis ± little fibrosis)
   – healing (little infiltrate, fibrosis, little or no necrosis)
   – healed myocarditis (focal fibrosis, sparse or no infiltrate)
   or
2) Pericardial rubs or pericardial effusion with segmental wall motion abnormality and dysrhythmia after exclusion of coronary artery disease by coronary angiography

Additional helpful criteria
A more than threefold alteration of titer in complement-fixation or neutralization tests against cardiotropic viruses for more than 2 weeks

Table 1 b. Criteria of dilated cardiomyopathy

Essential criteria
- Cardiomegaly in laevocardiography (left ventricular end-diastolic volume index > 100 ml/m²) and reduced ejection fraction ($< 55\%$)
- exclusion of coronary artery disease
- exclusion of valvular heart disease
- exclusion of hypertension
- exclusion of other forms of secondary heart muscle disease (e. g. diabetes mellitus, neuroendocrine disorders, extraordinary alcohol consumption)

Additional helpful criteria
Indicative histomorphology (hypertrophy with branching of myocytes, intestitial fibrosis (diffus/focal).

Table 1 c. Criteria for postmyocarditic heart muscle disease

1) Biopsy proven cellular infiltrate in first biopsy and missing infiltrate in second biopsy
   or
2) perimyocarditis proven by clinical criteria (Table 1 a) during first examination, no infiltrate in second biopsy but cardiomegaly with reduced ejection fraction at the second examination.

Patients

Analysis of humoral effector mechanisms was derived from more than 11,500 sera of patients with different forms of heart disease and from 200 healthy controls of both sexes and all ages without heart disease. Coxsackie B (n = 10), influenza A (n = 4), mumps (n = 4), cytomegalovirus (n = 2), herpes simplex (n = 2), Epstein Barr virus myocarditis (n = 2) and perimyocarditis of unknown origin (n = 144) were established according to the above mentioned criteria. Immunohistology was carried out in 605 biopsied patients (including immediate post-mortem biopsy in 16 non cardiac death and biopsies from 96 patients with coronary artery disease). The respective numbers of patients are for acute or healing myocarditis 13, acute or healing perimyocarditis 19, pericardial effusion 24, healed myocarditis 17, healed perimyocarditis 14, postmyocarditic cardiomyopathy 43, primary dilated cardiomyopathy 35. There was a male preponderance (3 : 2) in all forms of viral carditis but not for the undefined group (1 : 1). Mean age of the patients with carditis was 32 ± 6 years. The number of patients analyzed for cellular immune reactions can be derived from the respective figures and tables.

Methods

Analysis of lymphocyte subpopulations was carried out with monoclonal antisera from Ortho (OKT 3, OKT 4, OKT 8, OKT 11, OKIa1, OKMI) and Becton and Dickinson (Leu 7) as described (5).

Spontaneous T-cell suppressor activity was assessed according to Breshnihan and Jasin (4) as described (59).

Con A generated T suppressor cell activity was determined as described by Hallgren and Yunis (22), which is modified only slightly when compared to Anderson et al. (1), Eckstein et al. (15) and Fowles et al. (18) as previously described (59). The calculation of the indices of suppressor T cell activity was carried out according to (4) and (22).

Immunohistologic investigations were carried out using the direct technique as described (43). In addition a double sandwich technique was used for the demonstration of circulating antiheart antibodies to bind on the same cryostat section at the same antibody binding site using TRITC- and FITC-labelled antisera (43).

Circulating antiheart and non organ specific antibodies were determined on cryostat sections of human, rat and bovine heart and skeletal muscle, thyroid gland, stomach, kidney and liver (42, 45, 50).

Circulating heterologous *antimyolemmal antibodies* were determined on intact rat cardiocytes isolated by Percoll gradient centrifugation after perfusion with a collagenase (Worthington)-Ringer perfusate (49).

Circulating homologous antimyolemmal antibodies were assessed on intact myocytes from human atrial appendages removed during open heart surgery, minced and incubated in a calcium-free Ringer collagenase solution (composition according to medium 2 in 49) at 37° C, sedimented by centrifugation (80 g) after addition of EDTA. Fixation was accomplished by acetone given to the Ringer solution in equal volume used for centrifugation.

Antibody mediated cardiocytolysis was assessed on adult living rat heart cells as described previously (44, 48, 50).

Lymphocytotoxicity (LC) and *antibody dependent cellular cytototxicity (ADCC)* with normal and the patients own lymphocytes (analysis for blocking factors) was carried out as described (44, 48, 50). NK-cell activity against the human erythroblast cell line K 562 was carried out according to Perlman et al. (54).

Enriched sarcolemma was prepared according to Paris et al. (53). Contamination of microsomes or mitochondria as judged by electron microscopy was <70%. SDS-polyacrylamide electrophorsis of the preparation was carried out and followed by a Western Blot. Patients' sera were incubated with the blotted bands and stained with antiperoxidase labelled anti human immunoglobulin (Medac 1 : 100) according to standard procedures. Circulating immune complexes were assessed by a newly developed Cl_q-fluorometric assay according to (48).

Statistical analysis included a parametric Student t-test preceded by a Fisher test, testing the homogeneity of variances or non parametric Welch test, the U-test according 003014n and Whitney, rang correlation and chi-square analysis, whenever appropriate, on a TR 440 Computer (Telefunken) of the center of statistics, Würzburg University (in collaboration with Dr. I. Haubitz).

Results

Lymphocyte subpopulations in myocarditis and dilated heart disease

White cell blood count did not show significant differences between patients with myocarditis (7300 ± 2400), perimyocarditis (8600 ± 2200), pericardial effusion (6900 ± 1600), dilated cardiomyopathy (5900 ± 1700) postmyocarditic heart disease (7230 ± 2300) and non cardiac controls (6800 ± 1700). Although in one fourth of patients with acute carditis lymphocytosis was observed this was not a consistent finding. By the enumeration of circulating T-lymphocyte subpopulations in patients with carditis a significant difference in pan-T (OKT3-positive, OKT11-positive), T-helper (OKT4-positive), T suppressor (OKT8-positive), NK cells (Leu 7/II-11-positive) and monocytes (OKMI-positive) was not demonstrated, although in individual patients divergent results may be present. In perimyocarditis the OKIa1-positive B cells and activated T lymphocytes were significantly increased (Table 2), in postmyocarditic heart disease a tendency for a decrease in T-suppressor cells was demonstrated (Table 3). In contrast in primary dilated cardiomyopathy circulating OKMI-positive monocytes were increased (Table 2). The T_4/T_8-ratio did not differ from that of age- and sex-matched controls.

T-suppressor cell activity

Spontaneous in vivo and ConA generated T suppressor cell activity did not differ from sex- and age-matched controls without heart disease (59). In postmyocarditic dilated heart disease in selected indicator systems such as the autologous irradiated mixed lymphocyte reaction and the allogenic mitogen stimulation a significant reduction in T suppressor cell

Table 2. Incidence of T cell subpopulations and mononuclear cells (peripheral blood) in (peri) myocarditis and dilated heart muscle disease ($\bar{x} \pm S\bar{x}$)

	(Peri) myocarditis (n = 19)	Postmyoc. cardiomegaly (n = 5)	Primary DC++ (n = 19)	Healthy and non cardiac controls (n = 56)
Pan T-cells (OKT3)	74.3 ± 6.1	75.6 ± 3.5	71.1 ± 1.4	72.6 ± 7.0
Helper/induces (OKT4)	48.6 ± 4.7	50.0 ± 2.8	50.4 ± 1.9	48.7 ± 7.3
Suppressor/cytotoxic (OKT8)	23.2 ± 5.3	17.8 ± 2.8*	21.2 ± 1.8	22.9 ± 5.7
B-lymphocyte (+ activated T-cells) OKIa1	28.3 ± 8.5*	19.8 ± 3.2	22.7 ± 1.7	23.6 ± 7.6
Monocytes + NK-cells (OKMI)	14.5 ± 4.3	10.8 ± 2.4	19.1 ± 1.9*	13.2 ± 5.6

* $p < 0.05$ by chi-square analysis, when compared to controls
++ dilated cardiomyopathy

Table 3. Evidence for and against a disorder of humoral and cellular immunity in perimyocarditis (PM), primary dilated cardiomyopathy (DC) and postmyocarditic cardiomegaly (PMDC)

Disorder/mechanism	Arguments		Comment
	For	Against	
Regulator cells			
T suppressor cells (OKT8)	–	PM; DC, PMDC unchanged (5)	
B cells (OKT8)	increased in PM (5, here)	–	
Monocytes, NK-cells	increased in DC (5, 7, here)	–	
T suppressor cell activity	increased (15, 18)	normal (1, 38, here)	nonuniform results, global, not tissue-specific activity tested
T helper cells	no assays done;	subpopulation (normal)	
Cellular immunity			
PHA stimulation of peripheral lymphocytes	decreased in DC (12, 19)	but also in other heart diseases (CAD); inadequate controls	sensitive for cardiac disorder but not specific of myocarditis or DC
Lymph. stimulation with heart antigen	slightly increased in DC (12)	–	–
Migration inhibition Factor (MIF)	positive (12)	–	–
Natural killer (NK) cell activity	decreased in PM (here) PMDC (here)	NK-cell activity is not cardiospecific	uniform results, disease characteristic, but not cardioselective

Disorder/mechanism	Arguments		Comment
	For	Against	
Lymphocytotoxicity against heart cells (non MHC-restricted)	sustained or increased in PM and PMDC (50) increased in $1/3$ of pts in DC (27, 48)	also in 24% of other heart diseases (27)	uniform results, cardio-specific, but not disease specific results for PM or DC
Antibody dependent cellular cytotoxicity (ADCC)	in few patients positive (44, 50)	nonuniform for groups of PM, DC, PMDC	cardiospecific but not very sensitive
Humoral immunity			
a) Antisarcolemmal ab (ASA)	present in PM (3, 31, 37, 39, 40, 44, 50), PMDC (here and	except for IgM-subtype and complement fixation	in serum not cardio-selective due to similar staining by anticollagen and antilaminin etc.
b) Bound ASA (immunohistology of biopsy)	in 11, 30, 31, 37, 43, 50; diagnostic if of IgM-type or if complement fixation present	also found in coronary artery disease and cardiac controls	if bound cardio-selective, heart not disease specific (diagnostic for IgM, and complement fixation)
c) Circulating AMLA (ho/he)	diagnostic if IgM (+ IgA-type) (here)	not diagnostic if IgG-type; since also present in cardiac controls	
d) Circulating antibodies (31) circulating	diagnostic for part of PM and DC		membrane expression of the equivalent antigen has to be proven for biological relevance
e) Anti-nucleotide transferase ab (61)			
f) Circulating immune complexes	present in most cases (47)	not cardiospecific since antigen of complex is not characterized	monitors disease activity
g) Antibody mediated cytolysis (AMC) – in vitro –	diagnostic in Coxs. B, influenza + EBV + mumps and a large part of undefined PM, M and PMDC (40, 50)		in vivo relevance is yet to be proven

activity was seen when compared to patients with acute myocarditis, who themselves demonstrated a significantly enhanced, but not a decreased suppressor cell activity when compared to non cardiac controls (Fig. 1). Furthermore it can be concluded:

1. There is broad variance in T suppressor cell activity, both in controls and in patients with acute inflammatory heart disease.
2. The different indicator systems for the assessment of T suppressor cell activity may be particularly sensitive in expressing changes in some of the T suppressor cell subpopulations but most are not altered in myocarditis and dilated cardiomyopathy.
3. Even though a global reduction of T suppressor cell activity is not evident from our data, it cannot be ruled out that the antigen (= heart)-specific suppressor cell activity may have been changed. The assessment of antigen-specific T suppressor cell activity would need cloned T cell subpopulations elicited by specific cardiac membrane antigens (or other molecules), a prerequisite which is not yet available.

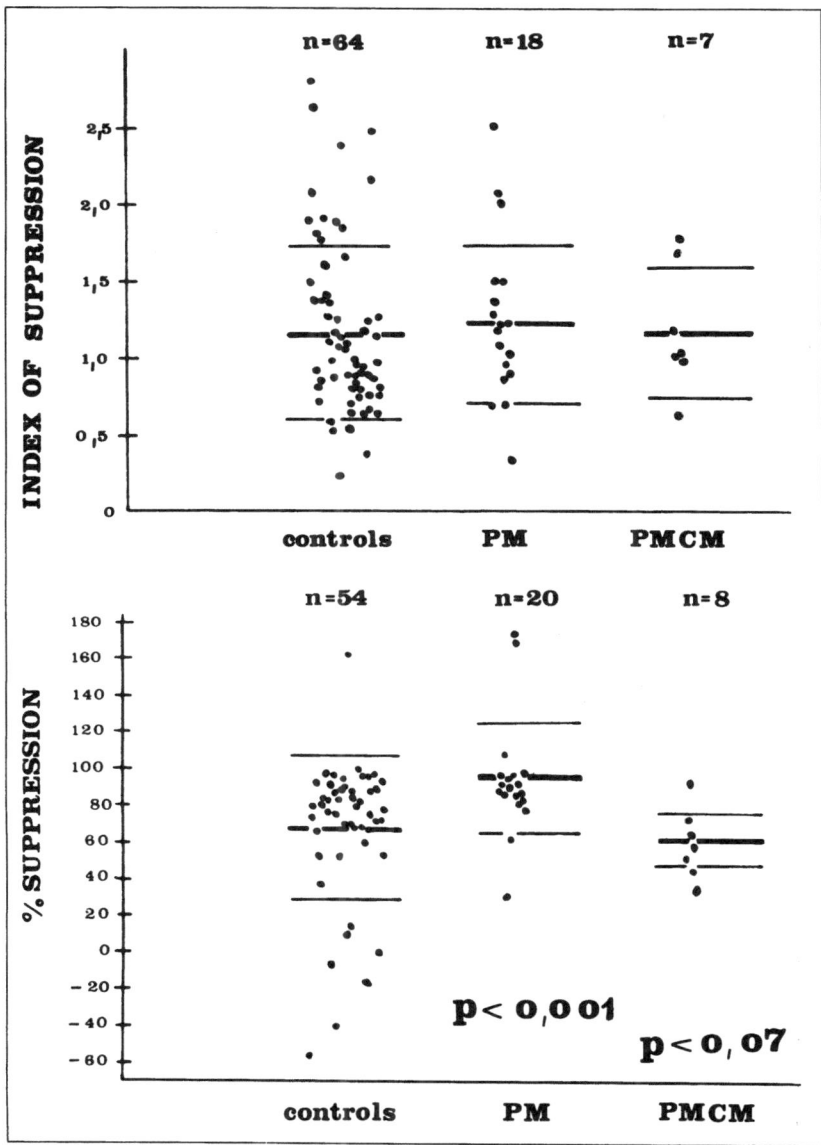

Fig. 1. Spontaneous in vivo activated and Con-A-induced b. T-suppressor cell activity in carditis and primary as well as secondary postmyocarditic cardiomyopathy was intact when compared with age-matched controls. A tendency toward a reduction in T suppressor cell activity was demonstrated, e. g. in the indicator system of the autologous mixed lymphocyte reaction with irradiated bystander, suppressor, and stimulator cells. This reduction was in contrast to enhanced suppression in acute perimyocarditis (p < 0.001) in patients with postmyocarditic heart disease (p < 0.001, when compared with perimyocarditis, p ≤ 0.07 when compared with controls). All other systems used did not show a significant deviation of suppressor cell activity (59). PM perimyocarditis, PMCM = postmyocarditic cardiomyopathy.

Assessment of cellular effector mechanisms in man

In patients with perimyocarditis peripheral blood analysis of lymphocyte subpopulations demonstrated an increase in the OKIa1-positive cells which may be either B- and/or activated T-lymphocytes. An increase in B cells could explain the increased antibody response found in carditis, an increase in activated Tcells would explain the strong activity of cytolytic T cells as demonstrated in mice (23, 24, 66, 67), for which no adequate assay system in man is yet available.

Natural killer cell activity

Natural killer cell activity in patients with carditis was markedly decreased in the acute state in all three lymphocyte/target cell ratios examined (Fig. 2 a). In postmyocarditic dilated

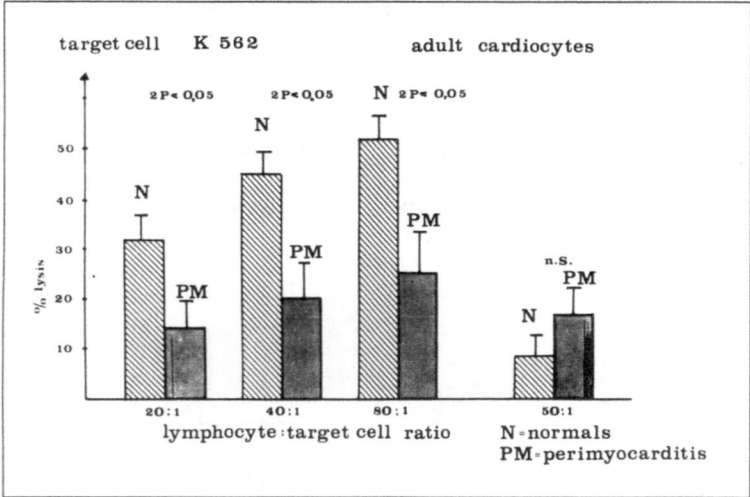

Fig. 2a. Natural killer (NK) activity (left), target cell-erythroblast cell line K 562, and specific cytotoxicity (right) target cell-adult rat cardiocyte, of peripheral blood lymphocytes in acute perimyocarditis (PM). Whereas NK-cell activity is reduced in all three lymphocyte to target cell ratios, target cell-specific cytotoxicity remains sustained or even slightly increased. Different lymphocyte to target cell ratios were used for both assays. For target cell-specific MHC non restricted cardiocytotoxicity (47) the index was not used but instead the percent age lysis was calculated from data already published (44, 50) to allow a direct comparison with NK cell activity.

muscle heart disease, NK cell activity had almost returned to normal (Fig. 2b). In primary dilated cardiomyopathy however, a significantly decreased NK-cell activity was observed again (Fig. 2b).

Target cell specific non MHC restricted lymphocytotoxicity

In contrast in myocarditis target cell specific non MHC restricted lysis against living adult allogeneic rat myocytes is sustained or slightly enhanced (Fig. 2a). This also applies to postmyocarditic dilated heart disease (Fig. 2b) and primary dilated cardiomyopathy (Fig. 2c), in which one third of patients demonstrated a significant increase of target cell

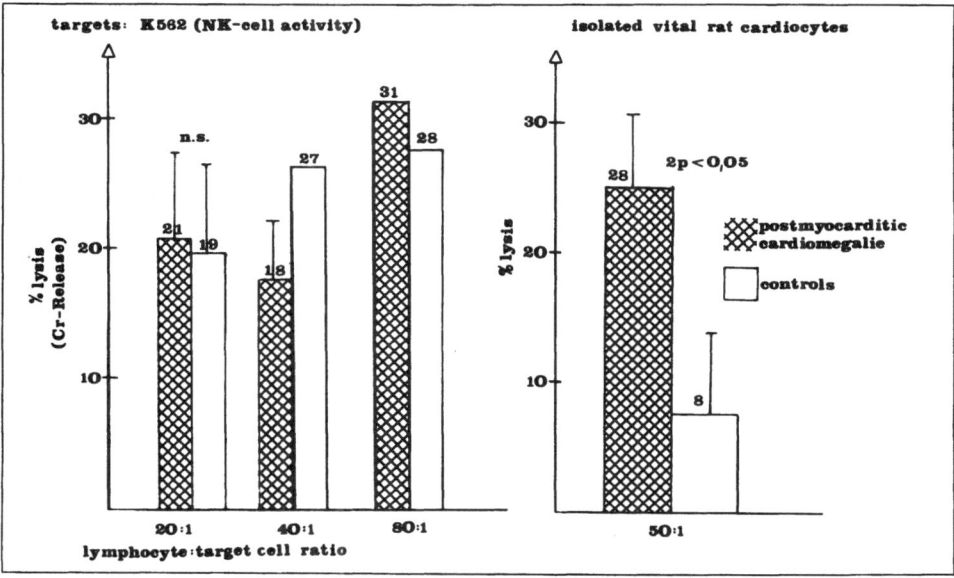

Fig. 2b. NK cell activity (left) and cardiocytotoxicity (right) in postmyocarditic dilated heart disease. NK cell activity is only slightly reduced, whereas target cell-specific cytotoxicity is sustained.

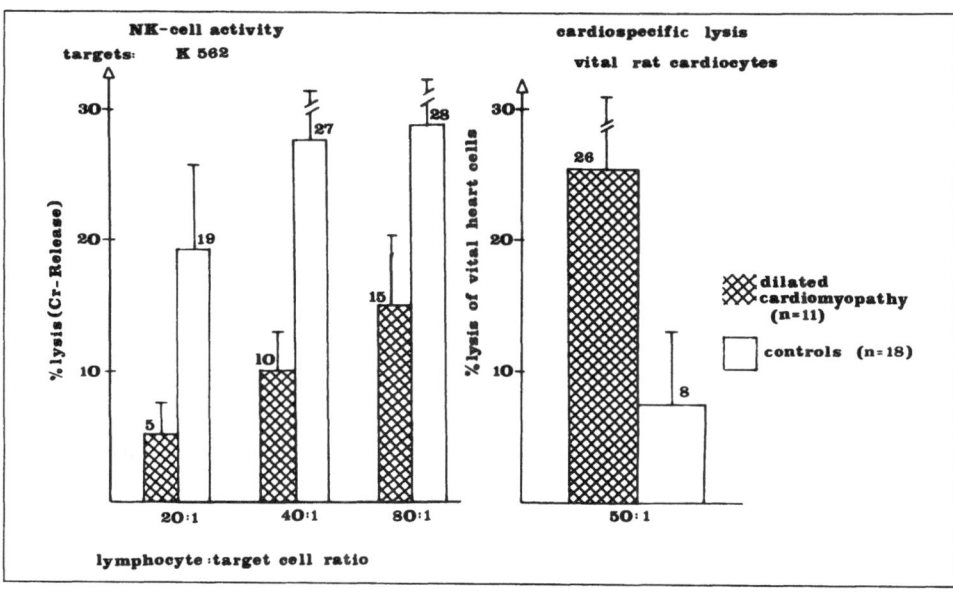

Fig. 2c. In primary dilated cardiomyopathy NK cell activity is also reduced. One third of these patients demonstrated significant target cell specific lysis, giving a slightly increased mean of percent lysis after 9 hours of incubation when compared to controls. This indicates that the patients with dilated cardiomyopathy are not a homogenous group.

specific cytotoxicity. Other than a sporadic increase in cell lysis, analysis of antibody-dependent cellular cytotoxicity (ADCC) showed little variation from normal in perimyocarditis, primary and secondary postmyocarditic heart muscle disease. In the myocardial biopsy, the infiltrating cell populations operating at the site of lesion were mostly round cells, particularly lymphocytes (Fig. 3). Subtyping as in the case of Fig. 3 demonstrated the presence of T-cells

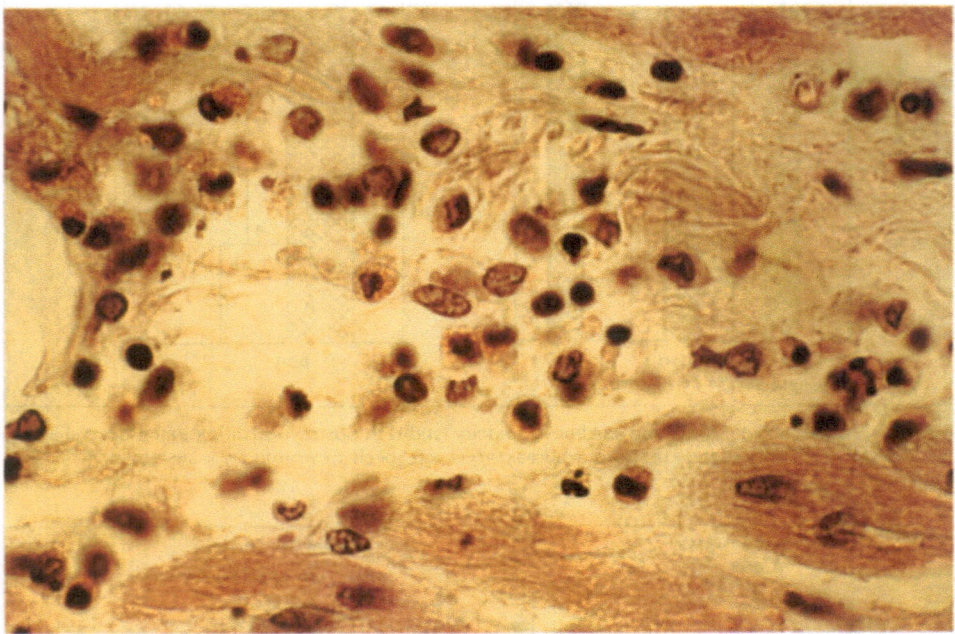

Fig. 3. Myocarditis in a 17 year old girl who demonstrated concomitant pleuritis and pericarditis (effusion of 100 ml in 2D-echocardiography) and normal to hypercontractile left ventricular function in levocardiography. Left ventricular biopsy revealed a mixed focal infiltrate including polymorphs and mononuclear cells (lymphocytes). Fraying or necrosis can be observed as well as interstitial edema. According to (9), (10) this is classified as active myocarditis. Due to normal left ventricular function and histomorphology immunosuppressive therapy was not started. Analysis of the mononuclear cell infiltrates revealed a positive staining for OKT3-, partly also for OKT4- and OKMI-positive cells (the example gives a OKT3-positive staining).

(OKT 3-positive), and partly OKT4-positive. The infiltrates so far analysed have been too small and occurred too sporadicaly to allow a quantification of subpopulations or specific pattern to be derived yet.

Humoral effector mechanisms:
The role of circulating antimyocardial antibodies

Antimyocardial antibodies are classified according to the corresponding cardiac antigens (Fig. 4).

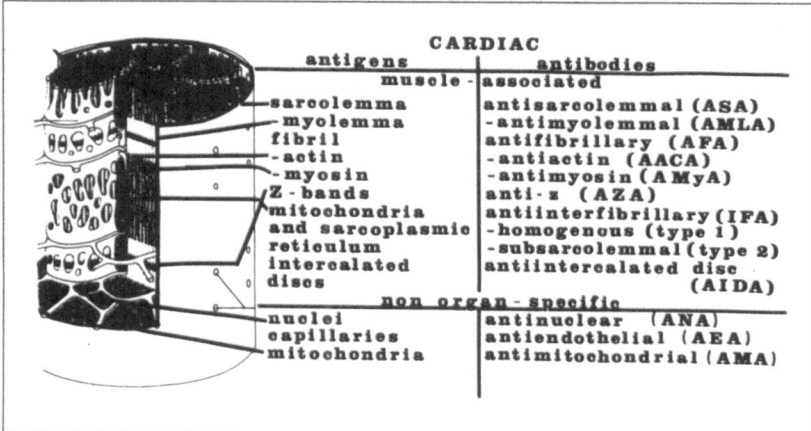

Fig. 4. Classification of antibodies according to the epitope to which they are bound in the direct and indirect immunofluorescence test.
Antimyolemmal antibodies are detected only with isolated intact human atrial (homologous type) or ventricular rat cardiocytes (heterologous type).

Antisarcolemmal and antimyolemmal antibodies

The greatest diagnostic relevance can be attributed to antimyolemmal antibodies (AMLA; Fig. 5 b/c) or antisarcolemmal antibodies (ASA) directed against autologous myocardium (Fig. 5 a). AMLA are a subtype of ASA which can be demonstrated only with isolated heart muscle cells; the collagen part of the membrane and the external perimysium of which were digested by crude collagenase during the isolation procedure. In this study, we were also able to use for the first time adult intact human atrial myocytes as antigen for the indirect immunofluorescence test (Fig. 5 c). The typical immunoserologic pattern in patients with carditis following Coxsackie B, influenza, mumps, and Epstein-Barr (EB) virus infections is antimyolemmal antibodies with a linear membrane fluorescence (Fig. 5 b/c) sometimes associated with a staining of the Z-bands (Fig. 5 b), which may give a pattern indistinguishable from antibodies against cytoskeletal antigens and intermediate filaments. Results obtained with human atrial and rat cardiocytes are comparable (Fig. 5 d) and differ significantly from controls. In EBV- and CMV-myocarditis homologous human myocoytes were more sensitive for AMLA, however. In postmyocarditic dilated heart disease circulating AMLA are also a sensitive diagnostic marker. In the time course of myocarditis AMLA of the IgM subclass (Table below Fig. 6) and complement fixation (Fig. 6) of the antibodies are diagnostic, since neither the IgM antibody nor complement fixation were observed to a significant extent in coronary artery disease (CAD) or in patients with precordial discomfort without coronary artery disease. Six to 8 weeks later incidence of IgM antibodies decreased whereas those of the IgG subclass increased. Complement fixation was not seen in status post myocarditis any longer but could still be demonstrated in part of the patients with postmyocarditic cardiomyopathy. Preliminary electron microscopic investigations indicate that AMLA preferably bind to the subsarcolemmal part of the cardiac membrane.

In primary dilated cardiomyopathy AMLA of the IgM class or complement fixation were seen only rarely. Incidence of AMLA of the IgG-type was present in 49% (homologous type) and 46% (heterologous type).For the incidence of antimyosin, antiactin, antiinterfibrillary and antiendothelial antibodies see Table 4.

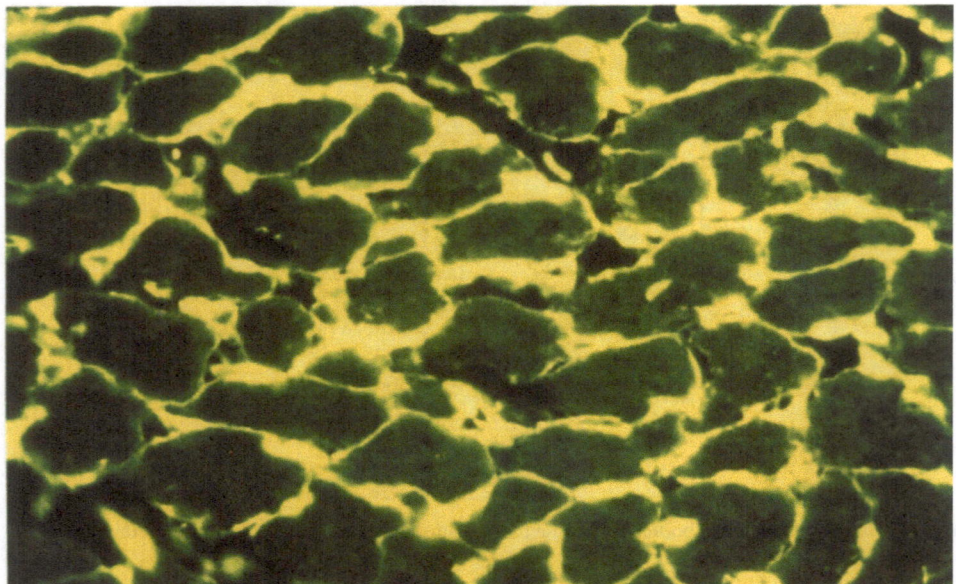

Fig. 5a. Circulating antisarcolemmal antibodies demonstrated by indirect immunofluorescence test on homologous human myocardium. A distinct fluorescence of perimysium internum and of capillaries is present.

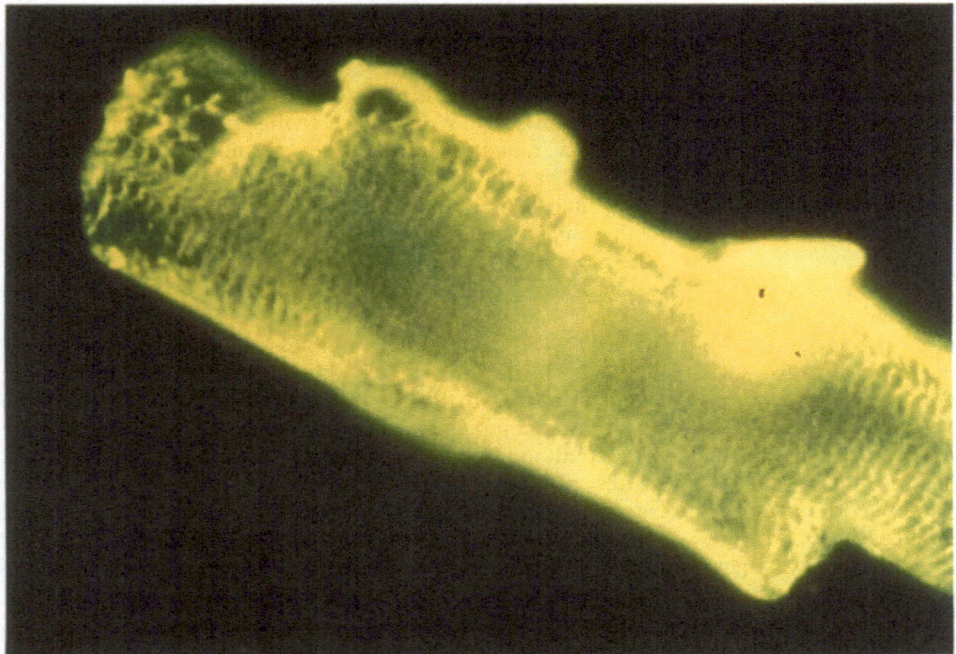

Fig. 5b. Antimyolemmal antibodies demonstrated with isolated rat cardiocytes by the indirect fluorescence test (titer 1 : 320 by serial dilution, FITC-labeled antihuman antiserum, F(ab)$_2$-fragments from goat (Medac, dilution 1 : 100).

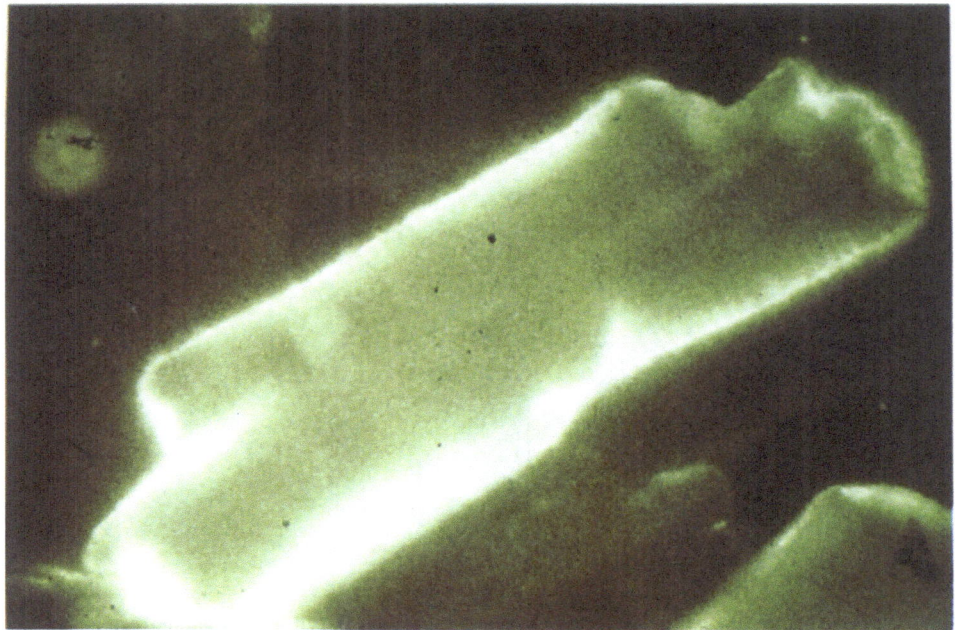

Fig. 5 c. Antimyolemmal antibodies demonstrated by an indirect FITC-labeled antihuman antiserum (trivalent, F(ab)$_2$-fragments, dilution 1 : 100). The antigen used is an intact human atrial cardiocyte.

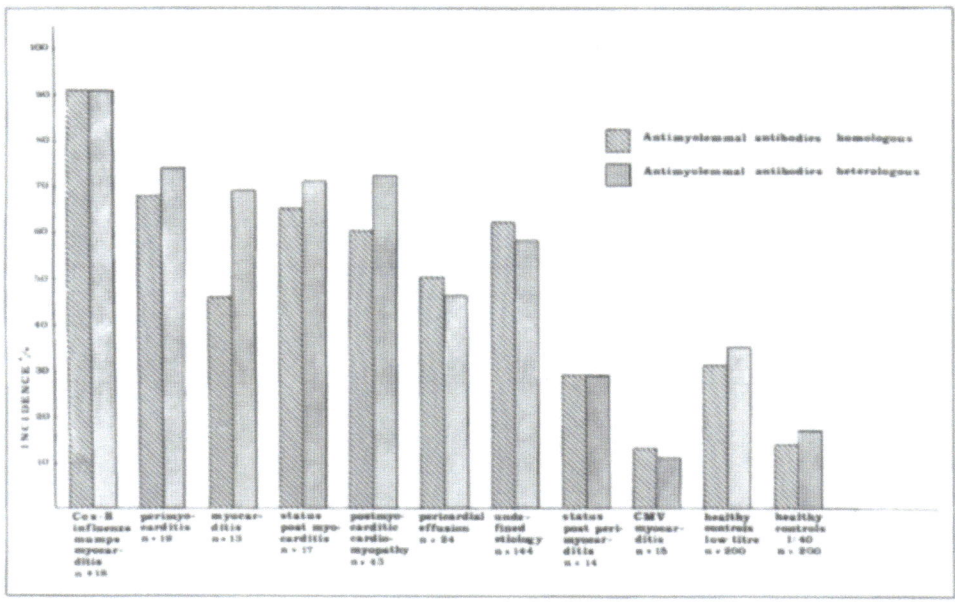

Fig. 5 d. Comparison between circulating homologous (left column) and heterologous (right column of each group analyzed) antimyolemmal antibodies on intact human and rat cardiocytes. These data are from biopsied patients only with histologically proven myocarditis and were aquired with a trivalent antiserum. For immunoglobulin class analysis see Fig. 6.

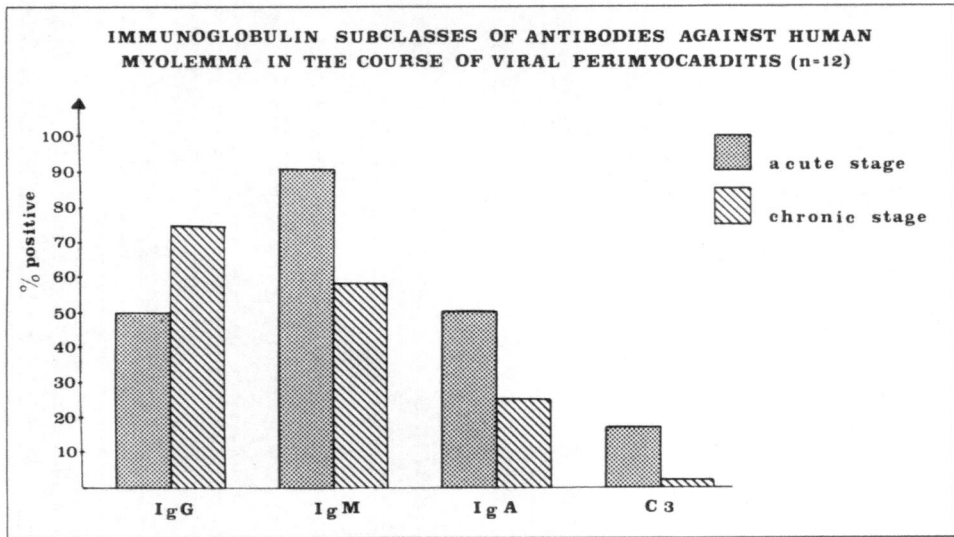

Fig. 6. Time course of appearance of AMLA (homologous type) of different immunoglobulin subclasses and complement fixation in viral carditis (Coxsackie B (n = 8), influenza (n = 2), Epstein-Barr virus (n = 3), cytomegalovirus (n = 3)). Incidence of IgM in the acute stage reaches 90%, complement fixation (C3) 20%. In the chronic stage incidence of IgM-antibodies decreased whereas incidence of IgG-antibody increased instead. In healthy non cardiac controls (n = 50), in coronary artery disease (n = 30) incidence of AMLA of the IgM-type is < 5% of complement fixation < 3%.

Analysis of immunoglobulin subclasses of the antibodies directed against the human myolemma (isolated adult human atrial myocytes) revealed the predominance of IgG- and IgM-subtype in Coxsackie B EBV, influenza myocarditis and the predominance of IgM-subtype alone in cytomegalovirus myocarditis:

	IgG	IgM	IgA	C3
Coxsackie B (n = 8)	7	6	4	1
Influenza A/B (n = 2)	2	2	1	0
Epstein-Barr virus (n = 3)	3	3	2	1
Cytomegalovirus (n = 3)	1	3	1	1

Table 4. Autoantibodies in perimyocarditis, postmyocarditic cardiomegaly, primary dilated cardiomyopathy and controls

	Coxsackie B (n = 10) Influenza A/B (n = 4) Mumps (n = 4)	Cytomegalovirus (n = 15)	Undefined etiology (n = 144)	Tuberculous pericarditis (n = 12)	Postmyocarditic cardiomegaly (n = 18)	Healthy controls (n = 200)	CAD[c] (n = 51)
Muscle-specific antibodies							
Antimyolemmal (AMLA$_a$) (autologous, human cardiocyte)	91[a]	13	62[b]	ND	89[b]	31 (low titer) 14 (> 1 : 40)	43
Antimyolemmal (AMLA$_h$) (heterologous, rat cardiocyte)	91[a]	6	58[b]	100[b]	89[b]	35 (low titer) 17 (> 1 : 40)	40
Antisarcolemmal (ASA) (homologous)	100a	6	45	100	94	32 (low titer) 20 (> 1 : 40)	34
Antifibrillary (AFA)	9	16	31	67[b]	16	4	4
Anti-interfibrillary (IFA)	18	100a	16	12	39	3	6
Nonorgan-specific antibodies:							
Anti-endothelial (AEA)	82a	0	73	42	13	25	19
Anti-smooth muscle (ASMA)	18	5	16	27	11	7	12

[a] p < 0.001 in $\hat{X}^2$-test, when compared to controls (titer > 1 : 40)
[b] p < 0.01 in $\hat{X}^2$-test, when compared to controls (titer > 1 : 40)
[c] CAD = coronary artery disease

Further characterization of ASA and AMLA with the Western Blot

With enriched human and rat sarcolemmal preparations, which were contaminated by less than 7% with other organelles according to electromicroscopy and were negative for mitochondrial enzymes (Malat dehydrogenase), it could be demonstrated that antisarcolemmal and antimyolemmal antibodies form a microheterogeneity. Since low affinity binding to some bands may also occur in controls Table 5 summarizes the incidence of binding of serum antibodies to different bands in those cases only, in wich either no binding was present in the control sera, or the binding of the patients serum superceded that of the low affinity binding at least two-fold. Molecular candidates for binding of AMLA or ASA are therefore the bands of molecular weights of 90 KD, 78 KD, 72 KD, 67 KD, 62 KD, 48 KD, 29 KD, and 26 KD.

Table 5. Western Blot analysis of circulating antisarco- and antimyolemmal antibodies with human and rat sarcolemma in myocarditis (n = 14)

Bands	MW (KD)	Sarcolemma Rat	Sarcolemma Human
	78	6	9
	72	7	9
	67	6	8
	58	7	–
	48	10	10
	38	5	5
	31	4	–
	28	9	2
	26	9	7

Low affinity binding of healthy controls was observed to some of the same bands. For a positive staining an intensity of twice as much as the control was required.

Bound antisarcolemmal antibodies

AMLA or ASA not only circulate in the peripheral blood, they also bind to the autologous biopsy specimens. Bound IgG is observed in up to 100% of cases in perimyocarditis (Table 5), but IgA- or IgM-binding is less frequent, the latter being a fair marker for discriminating between acute and chronic heart disease (Fig. 7 b.). The simulataneous demonstration of bound and circulating ASA was accomplished by a double-sandwich technique: bound IgG is visualized by rhodamin-labeled antihuman IgG (F(ab)-fragment) (Fig. 7 a left side). After a second incubation with autologous serum, circulating antimyocardial antibodies are labeled with an FITC-antihuman immunoglobulin (F[ab]$_s$-fragment) (Fig. 7 a right side).

Out of 605 myocardial biopsies analyzed all 3 immunoglobulin subclasses and complement fixation occurred significantly more ofter in myocarditis, perimyocarditis, pericardial effusion, dilated cardiomyopathy and postmyocarditic heart disease than in healthy controls. However, patients with coronary artery disease and those who underwent coronary angiography due to "angina" but had no significant stenosis (precordial discomfort) also demonstrated bound antisarcolemmal antibodies particularly of the IgG-type. Most specific for perimyocarditis and myocarditis, however, were bound ASA of the IgM-type. Complement fixation was highest in perimyocarditis and postmyocarditic cardiomyopathy, thus differing significantly from controls (p < 0.05). It is remarkable that one third of the patients with dilated cardiomyopathy also had complement fixing ASA, whereas none occurred in non cardiac controls.

Pathogenetic relevance of antibodies directed against the cardiac membrane

The pathogenetic key role of AMLA can be assessed by incubating a patient's sera with isolated vital heart cells in the presence of complement. In Coxsackie B, influenza, mumps, and to some extent, in EB virus myocarditis, cytolytic activity as expressed by an index < 0.75, correlated roughly with the AMLA titer (Fig. 8 a). This also applied to sera of patients with carditis of unknown etiology (Fig. 8 b). In postmyocarditic cardiomegaly, AMLA titers are less prominent and cytolytic serum activity, though present, is not as pronounced (44). In Coxsackie B, influenza, and mumps virus myocarditis, both the cytolytic serum activity and the AMLA staining could be absorbed with the respective causative virus (50). The cytolytic

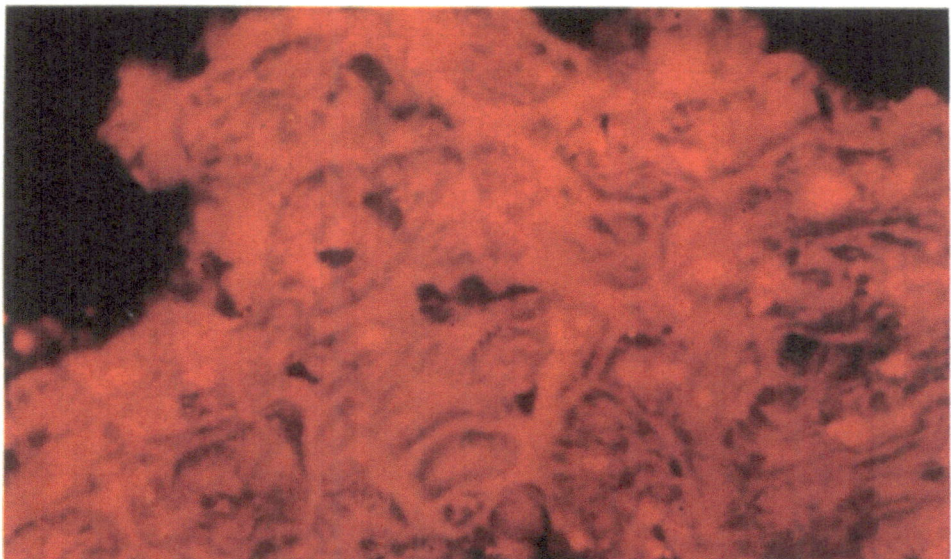

Fig. 7a. Demonstration of bound immunoglobulin on a cryostat section from a biopsy of a patient with histologically proven myocarditis. In this section, immunoglobulin (anti-IgG- and anti-IgM-positive and complement-fixing) bound to the sarcolemma and the interstitial space was demonstrated focally using a TRITC (rhodamin)-labeled antiserum (Medac, dilution 1 : 50 left side). After incubation with unlabeled antihuman-immunoglobulin (rabbit) patient sera (dilution 1 : 10) was added. After washing, FITC-labeled goat antihuman immunoglobulin (F(ab$_2$)-fragments, dilution 1 : 100, Medac) was added and circulating antimyocardial antibodies directed against the autologous heart tissue were also demonstrated (right side).

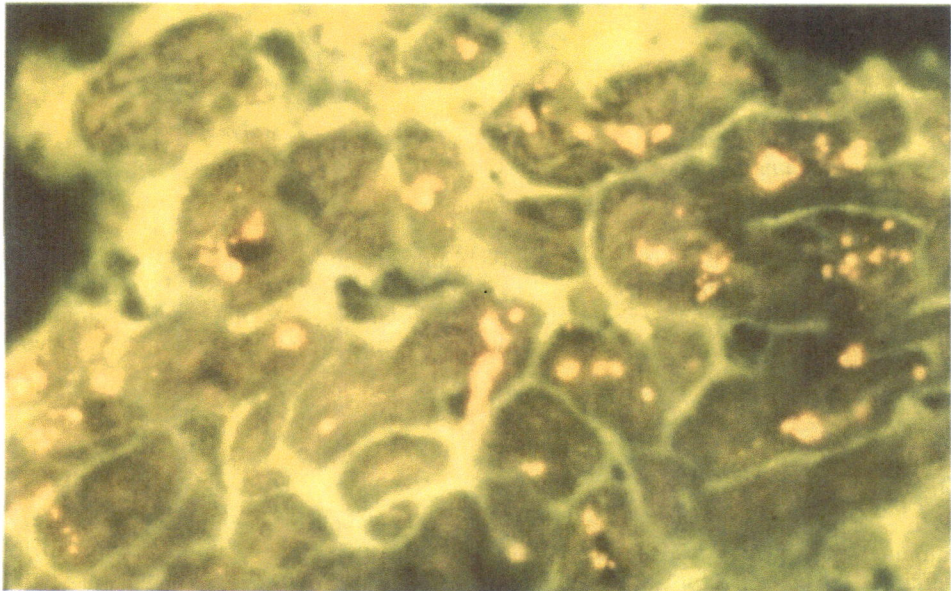

Fig. 7b. Immunoglobulin classes of bound antisarcolemmal/antimyolemmal antibodies in patients with carditis, cardiomyopathy and controls.

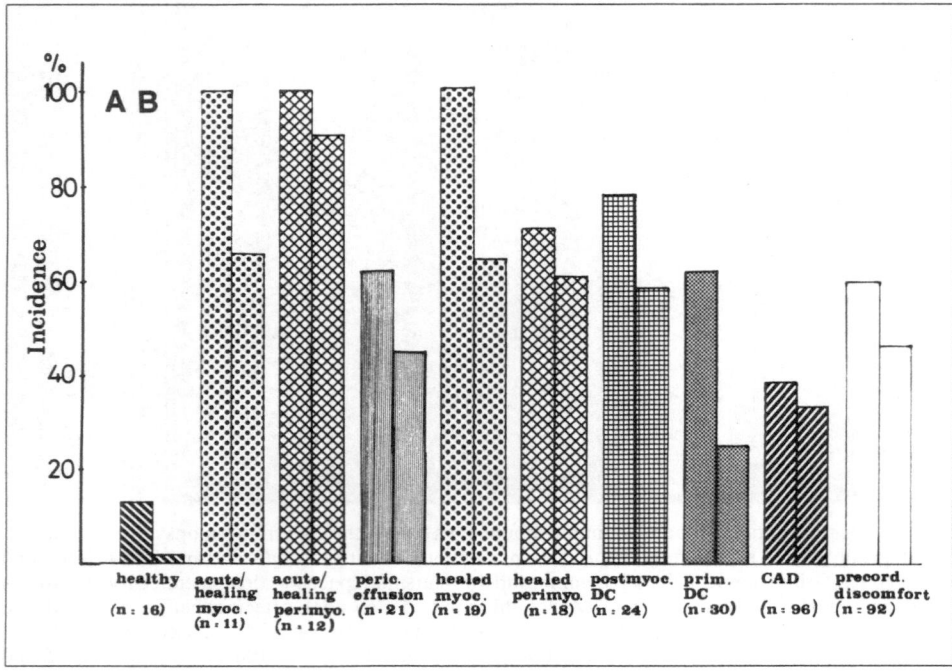

Fig. 7c. Comparison of circulating (B = indirect test second column) and bound antisarcolemmal antibodies (A = direct test first column) as assessed by a double sandwich technique.

activity was complement-dependent and could not be abolished by pre- and co-incubation with the proteinase inhibitor aprotinin.

Circulating immune complexes in myocarditis

For the monitoring of inflammatory cardiac diseases, e. g., in endocarditis (48) and myocarditis, the follow-up of the concentration of circulating immune complexes is helpful. In almost all patients with carditis of viral and undetermined origin, circulating immune complexes were demonstrated by Cl_q-FIAX (47). Both concentration and incidence of immune complexes decreased remarkably 4–6 weeks later (Fig. 9). Since only the immunoglobulin part of the complex can be determined, it remains unresolved, as to which the bound antigens may be.

Discussion

In carditis, as in other inflammatory diseases, it is one of the essential functions of the immune system to recognize the antigen, induce an immune response, amplify it, and finally eliminate the antigen. Only complete elimination of the antigen – be it a viral or bacterial agent or a neoantigen – will lead to the suppression of cellular and humoral effector mechanisms and the resolution of the disease. Effector organs of the immune response are: 1)

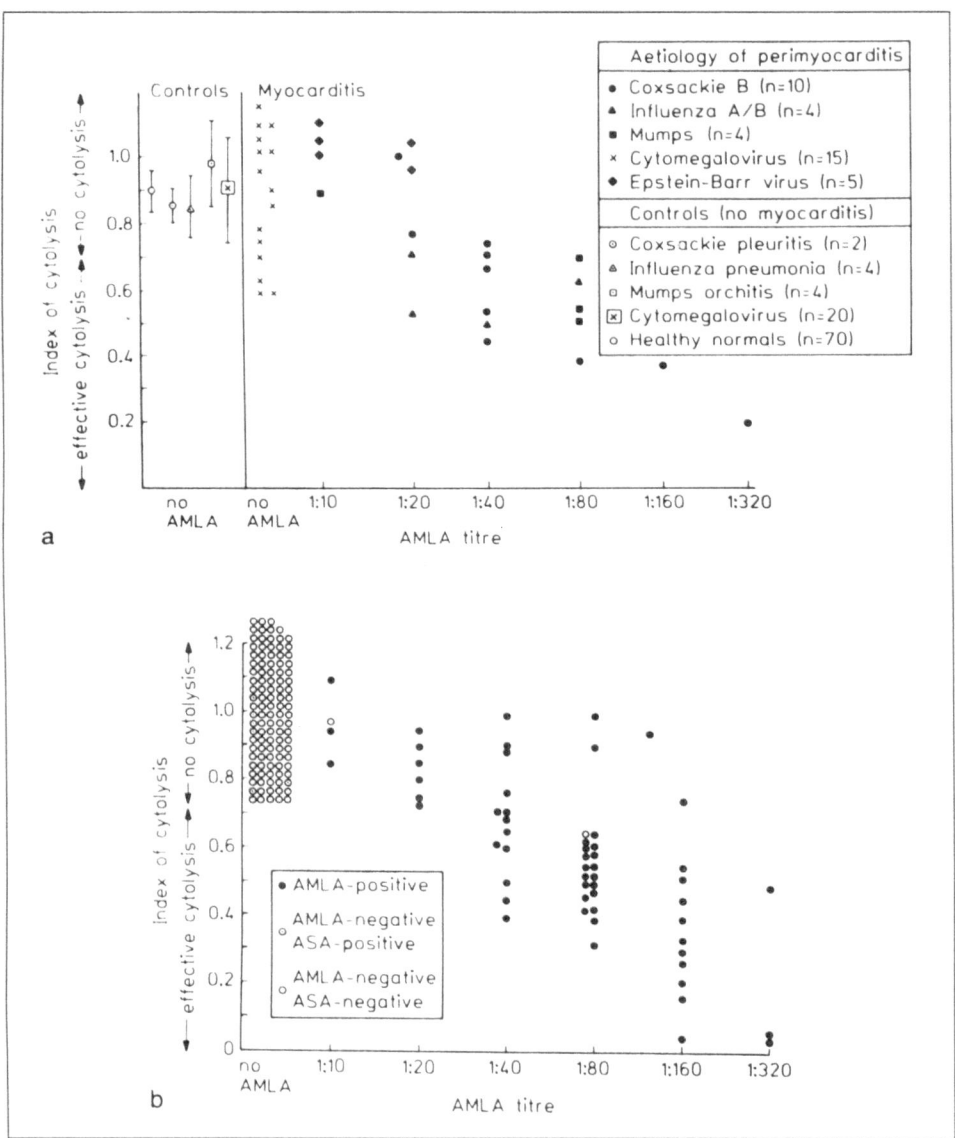

Fig. 8. Antibody- and complement-dependent cardiocytolysis with AMLA-positive sera in acute carditis. No cytolysis is present in healthy and non-cardiac viral controls (index < 0.75), whereas cytolytic serum activity roughly correlating to the AMLA-titer was demonstrated both in viral carditis (a) and myocarditis of unknown etiology (b).

the thymus-derived T lymphocytes and their subpopulations, e. g. the T helper, T suppressor and the cytotoxic T cells; 2) the B lymphocytes, which may differentiate either into memory cells or secreting plasma cells; 3) cytotoxic cells with broader specificity (e. g. NK-cells, macrophages), which do not underly the restriction of the major histocompatibility complex (MHC). In murine Coxsackie B myocarditis, it has been demonstrated that the primary

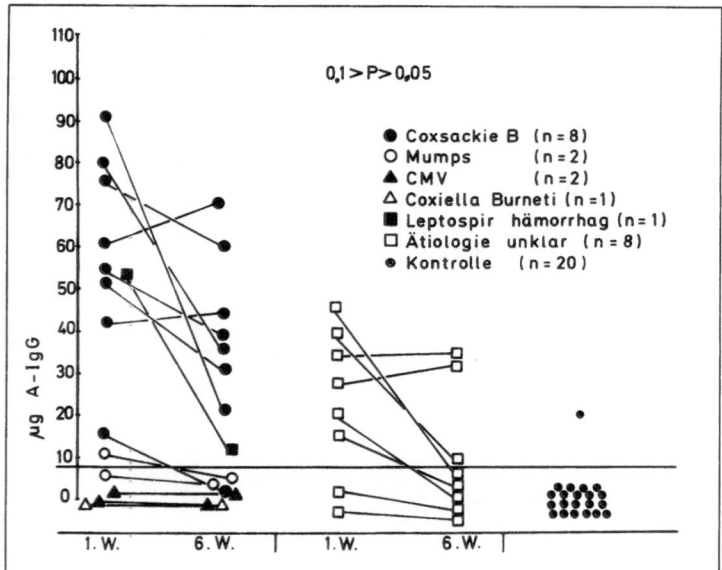

Fig. 9. Demonstration of circulating immune complexes (IC) in the acute phase of carditis and during follow-up. In the resolving or resolved state of carditis a decrease in immune complex concentration can be observed (A-IgG = aggregated IgG; W = week).

immune reaction – after an initial episode of increased NK-cell activity – is controlled by cytolytic T lymphocytes (23, 24, 66, 67) which underly the H_2 (in mice) or human leukocyte antigen (HLA) major histocompatiblity complex (MHC) restriction (68). The T lymphocytes can be specifically stimulated only after antigen-processing, in which the participation of antigen presenting cells (e. g. macrophages) or a second signal such as interleukin 2 and/or its receptor inducing factor and/or the T cell growth factor are essential. Simultaneously mediators and lymphokines are secreted which activate, inactivate, or amplify the cytotoxic reaction. Serum inhibition factors which decrease the proliferation of normal lymphocytes are examples of mediators that we previously demonstrated in carditis (42).

In contrast to carditis in which immunocompetent cells are by definition to play a role, although in man data on humoral and cellular effector mechanisms are rare, in dilated cardiomyopathy the evidence of an immunopathogenesis, that is a humoral or cellular disorder, is only suggestive in some patients.

It is crucial therefore to distinguish patients with a history highly suggestive of myocarditis or with biopsy proven carditis from those without, as has been done in this study. By clear criteria patients with postmyocarditic cardiomegaly were distinguished from those with primary dilated heart disease. A critical overview of the evidence in literature for and against a secondary immunopathogenesis in both myocarditis and primary dilated heart muscle disease can be derived from Table 3.

T cell subpopulations and cellular regulator mechanisms

Enumeration of peripheral T cells revealed an increase in OKTal-positive B cells in myocarditis and OKMI-positive monocytes and NK cells in dilated cardiomyopathy. The first observation is well compatible with a polyclonal antibody production including anti-heart antibodies, the latter with increased cardiospecific, non MHC restricted lymphocytotoxicity in dilated cardiomyopathy and myocarditis, although from the mere number of cells one can and should not readily extrapolate to function. But global regulator mechanisms, such as spontaneous and Con A-induced T suppressor cell activity remained unchanged in our patients with myocarditis, postmyocarditic cardiomegaly or dilated cardiomyopathy in agreement with careful studies by Anderson et al. (1) and sporadic investigations by others (38) but contrasting to Fowles et al. (18) and Eckstein et al. (15).

It may well be, that the different results come from slightly different methods, different patient populations with different treatment and different disease stages. The non uniform results (Table 3) call for testing with cloned cardiospecific suppressor T cells. Only then, if no alteration in specific T suppressor cell activity is present, would an increased T helper function be the most logical interpretation for the elicited effector function in myocarditis and in some patients with dilated cardiomyopathy.

Cellular effector mechanisms

Uniform results were obtained when compared to others (1, 8) as to the decrease in NK-cell activity in myocarditis and dilated cardiomyopathy, although Cambridge et al. (8), found decreased NK-activity only in assays supplemented with interferon. Decreased NK cell activity, however, is not cardioselective, since it is observed in various infections and also in neoplastic disease. This also applies to decreased proliferation of patients' lymphocytes after PHA stimulation (12, 19) or the demonstration of migration inhibition (12) or of serum inhibition factors (42). Despite reduced NK cell activity, however, sustained or increased cellular cytotoxicity against heterologous cardiocytes was present in both perimyocarditis and dilated cardiomyopathy (Table 3). This is compatible with experiments by Jacobs et al. (27) with fetal heart cells and may indicate a switch of the immune system to target specific effector mechanisms. Although being heart specific, since no lysis of hepatocytes occurred in an control assay (44, 50), the test is not specific for myocarditis or dilated cardiomyopathy, since target cell specific lysis occurs at least in fetal target systems (27) in other heart diseases as well (Table 3).

Humoral effector mechanism

Although data on circulating (3, 11, 30, 31, 37, 38, 39, 40, 41, 42, 44, 46, 48, 56, 61) and bound (3, 11, 30, 37, 39, 40, 43) antiheart antibodies (Table 3) were published, some of the studies have not been performed in a blind manner (3, 11) or lacked adequate control groups (11). In both biopsies and the analysis of circulating antisarcolemmal antibodies only cryostat sections of heterologous of homologous cardiac tissue have been available to date in which non organ-specific antibodies against capillaries or external (collagenous) perimysium could not be early distinguished from antisarcolemmal antibodies. Only when using heterologous (44, 49, 50) isolated rat cardiocytes could this disadvantage be overcome and heart specifity established. For the first time also species specifity could be attained by the use of intact adult human atrial myocytes as antigens in the immunofluorescence test. It could be clearly established that homologous AMLA are the characteristic marker of myocarditis of the Coxsackie B, influenza, mumps and EBV type. Sera from patients with cytomegalo virus myocarditis also demonstrated homologous AMLA of the IgM subtype which was not detected when using rat cardiocytes as antigen. These antibodies are cross-reactive to the virus itself, since they can be absorbed by the virus (50). They are cytolytic to heterologous heart cells in vitro as well, thus indicating their pathogenetic relevance. In the early stage of disease both circulating AMLA of the homologous or heterologous subtype and bound ASA are the IgM and IgG class and may fix complement. The demonstration of either circulating AMLA or bound ASA that fulfill both criteria (IgM class and complement fixation) are, although not sensitive, highly diagnostic for acute perimyocarditis. Lytic activity vanishes in sera from patients with status post myocarditis without cardiomegaly, and diminishes but is still present in postmyocarditic dilated heart disease. Western Blot analyses of ASA and AMLA are highly indicative that a microheterogeneity of these antibodies exists. The attribution of the lytic activity to one or more of the antibodies specifically directed against one or more bands of the sarcolemma in polyacrylamide gel electrophoresis will further clarify the binding sites of the antibodies and their pathogenetic role.

Conclusions

The investigation of immunologic regulator and effector systems in carditis and dilated cardiomyopathy has demonstrated that altered effector reactivity is present both with the cellular and antibody mediated reactions, suggesting a secondary immunopathogenesis in protracted forms of carditis in patients with postmyocarditic cardiomegaly, and in some patients with dilated cardiomyopathy. The analysis and interpretation of immunologic effector mechanisms will be an important prerequisitive or an immunosuppressive for immunostimulatory therapy (2, 51, 64).

Acknowledgements:

The excellent technical assistance of C. Dienesch, I. Wendel, T. Thometzek, Ph. D. and M. Cirsi is gratefully acknowledged. Parts of the work were performed by D. Klopf, M. D., K. Schmier, M. D., U. Schmier, M. D., and D. Koper.

Histological examination (light microscopy) was performed by Prof. U. Pfeiffer, M. D. (Department of Pathology Würzburg), and Prof. E. Olson, M. D. (London, Kings College Hospital), and compared with histological data on our cryostat sections. Part of the sera and biopsies were obtained from the German Heart Center Munich, in close collaboration with R. Regitz, M. D., the University Hospital of Pediatrics, Tübingen, in close collaboration with Prof. A. Schmaltz, M. D., and the Deegenberg Sanatorium (Priv. Doz. P. Deeg MD). This work was supported by grants of the Deutsche Forschungsgemeinschaft Ma 780/1–5.

References

1. Anderson JL, Carlquist JF, Hammond EH (1982) Deficient natural killer cell activity in patients with idiopathic dilated cardiomyopathy. Lancet II: 1124–1127
2. Billingham ME, Mason JW (1984) Endomyocardial biopsy changes in myocarditis treated with immunosuppressives. In: Bolte H-D (ed) Viral heart disease. Springer-Verlag, Berlin Heidelberg New York Tokyo, pp 200–210
3. Bolte HD, Schultheiss P, Cyran J, Goss F (1980) Binding of immunoglobulins in the myocardium (biopsy). In: Bolte H-D (ed) Myocardial Biopsy, Springer-Verlag Berlin Heidelberg New York, pp 85–92
4. Bresnihan B, Jasin ME (1977) Suppressor function of peripheral blood mononuclear cells in normal individuals and in patients with systemic lupus erythematosus. J Clin Invest 59: 106–116
5. Bülowius H, Maisch B, Klopf D, Schmier K, Hiby A, Schunk D, Kochsiek K (1983) Lymphozytensubpopulationen bei akuter Perimyokarditis, sekundären und primären dilatativen Herzmuskelerkrankungen. Z Kardiol 72 (Suppl 1): 16
6. Burch GE, Giles TD (1972) The role of viruses in the production of heart disease. Am J Cardiol 29: 231–240

7. Cambridge G, MacArthur CGC, Waterson AP, Goodwin JF, Oakley C (1979) Antibodies to Coxsackie B viruses in congestive cardiomyopathy. Br Heart J 16: 692–696
8. Cambridge G, Campbell-Blay G, Wilmhurst P, Coltart DJ, Stern CMM (1983) Deficient 'natural' cytotoxicity in patients with congestive cardiomyopathy (Abstr) Br Heart J 49, 623
9. Daly K, Richardson PJ, Olsen EFJ, Morgan-Capner P, McSorley C, Jackson G, Jewitt DE (1984) Acute myocarditis – Role of histological and virological examination in the diagnosis and assessment of immunosuppressive treatment. Br Heart J 51: 30–35
10. Dallas criteria for myocarditis (according to a summary from ME Billingham at AHA congress, Miami Beach, 1984)
11. Das SK, Callen JP, Dodson VN, Cassidy JT (1971) Immunoglobulin binding in cardiomyopathic hearts. Circulation 44: 612–621
12. Das SK, Petty RE, Meengs WA, Tubergen DG (1980) Studies of cell-mediated immunity in cardiomyopathy. In: Sekiguchi M, Olsen EGJ (eds) Cardiomyopathy. University of Tokyo Press, Tokyo Baltimore, pp 375–377
13. Deck WG, Palacios IF, Fallon JT, Aretz HT, Mills J, Lee DCS, Johnson RA (1985) Active myocarditis in the spectrum of acute dilated cardiomyopathies. Engl J Med 342, 885–897
14. Doerr W (1971) Morphologie der Myokarditis. Verh Dtsch Ges Inn Med 77: 301–335
15. Eckstein R, Mempel W, Bolte H-D (1982) Reduced suppressor cell activity in congestive cardiomyopathy and in myocarditis. Circulation 65: 1224–1229
16. Fenoglio JJ Jr, Ursell PC, Kellogg CF, Drusin RE, Wiss MB (1983) Diagnosis and classification of myocarditis by endomyocardial biopsy. N Engl J Med 308: 12–18
17. Fletcher GF, Coleman MT, Feorius PM, Marine WM, Wenger NK (1968) Viral antibodies in patients with primary myocardial disease. Am J Cardiol 21, 6–14
18. Fowles KE, Bieber CP, Stinson EB (1978) Defective in vitro suppressor cell function in idiopathic congestive cardiomyopathy. Circulation 59: 483–491
19. Francesini R, Petillo A, Corazza M, Nizzo MC, Azzolini A, Gianrossi R (1983) Lymphocyte response in dilated cardiomyopathy. IRCS Med Sci 11: 1019
20. Grist NR, Boll EJ (1974) A six year study of Coxsackie virus B infections in heart disease. J Hyg 73, 165–174
21. Gore I, Kline IK (1968) Pericarditis and myocarditis. In: Gould SE (ed) Phatology of the heart and blood vessels 3 rd ed Thomas, Springfield Ill, pp 731–759
22. Hallgren HM, Yunis EJ (1977) Suppressor lymphocytes in young and aged humans. J Immunol 118: 2004–2008
23. Huber SA, Jod LP, Woodruff JF (1980) Lysis of infected myofibers by Coxsackie virus B$_3$ immune T-lymphocytes. Am J Pathol 98: 681–694
24. Huber SA, Lodge PA (1984) Coxsackie virus B-3 myocarditis in Balb/c mice. Am J Pathol 116: 21–29
25. James TM, Umamura K (1981) Virus-like particles associated with intracardiac ganglionitis in two cases of sudden unexpected death. Jpn Heart J 22, 447–454
26. James TN (1983) Myocarditis and cardiomyopathy. N Engl J Med 308: 39–41
27. Jacobs B, Matsuda Y, Deodhar S, Shirey S (1979) Cell-mediated cytotoxicity to cardiac cells of lymphocytes from patients with primary myocardial disease. Am J Clin Pathol 72: 1–4
28. Kawai C, Matsumori A, Kitaura Y, Takatsu T (1978) Viruses and the heart: Viral myocarditis and cardiomyopathy. In: Yu PN, Goodwin JF (eds) Progress in Cardiology. Lea and Febiger, Philadelphia, pp 141–162
29. Kipshidze NN (1983) Some problems of etiology and pathogenesis of cardiomyopathies. Abstracts, Wissenschaftliches Symposium "Kardiomyopathie". Jena, p 18
30. Kirsner AB, Hess EV, Fowler NO (1973) Immunologic findings in idiopathic cardiomyopathy. Am Heart J 86: 625–630
31. Klein R, Maisch B, Kochsiek K, Berg PA (1984) Demonstration of organ specific antibodies against heart mitochondria (anti-M7) in sera from patients with some forms of heart disease. Clin Exp Immunol 58: 283–292
32. Kline IK, Saphir O (1960) Chronic pernicious myocarditis. Am Heart J 59: 681–684
33. Kuhn H, Loogen F (1981) Erkrankungen des Myokards. In: Krayenbühl HP, Kübler W (eds) Kardiologie in Klinik und Praxis Voll II. Thieme Stuttgart, pp 48.1–48.13

34. Lerner AM, Wilson FM (1973) Virus myocardiopathy. Progr Med Virol 15: 63–91
35. Longson M, Cole FM, Davies D (1969) Isolation of a Coxsackie virus group B, type 5, from the heart of a fatal case of myocarditis in an adult. J. Clin Pathol 22: 654–658
36. Lowry PJ, Edwards CW, Nagle RE (1982) Herpes-like virus particles in myocardium of patient progressing to congestive cardiomyopathy. Br Heart J 48: 501–504
37. Lowry PJ, Thompson RA, Littler WA (1983) Humoral immunity in cardiomyopathy. Br Heart J 50: 390–394
38. Lowry PJ, Thompson RA, Littler WA (1984) Humoral and cellular mechanisms in congestive cardiomyopathy (Abstr) Br Heart J 51: 109
39. Maisch B (1984) Humorale immunologische Effektormechanismen bei Perimyokarditis. Internist 25: 155–164
40. Maisch B (1984) Diagnostic relevance of humoral and cell-mediated immune reactions in patients with acute myocarditis and congestive cardiomyopathy. In: Chazov EL, Smirnov VN, Organov RG (eds) Cardiology. Plenum Press, London, pp 1327–1338
41. Maisch B (1984) Cytolytic serum activity in patients with carditis. In: Bolte HD (ed) Viral heart disease. Springer-Verlag, Berlin Heidelberg New York Tokyo, pp 121–130
42. Maisch B, Berg PA, Kochsiek K (1980) Autoantibodies and serum inhibition factors (sif) in patients with myocarditis. Klin Wochenschr 58: 219–225
43. Maisch B, Büschel G, Izumi T, Eigel P, Regitz V, Deeg P, Pfeifer U, Schmaltz A, Herzum M, Kochsiek K (1985) Four years of experience in endomyocardial biopsy. An immunohistologic approach. Heart and Vessels, Heart and Vessels, Suppl 1, 59–67
44. Maisch B, Deeg P, Liebau G, Kochsiek K (1983) Diagnostic relevance of humoral and cytotoxic immune reactions in patients with primary and secondary heart muscle disease. Am J Cardiol 52: 1072–1078
45. Maisch B, Eichstädt H, Kochsiek K (1983) Immune reactions in infective endocarditis. Part I: Clinical data and diagnostic relevance of antimyocardial antibodies. Am Heart J 106: 329–337
46. Maisch B, Maisch St, Kochsiek K (1982) Immune reactions in tuberculous and chronic constrictive pericarditis. Am J Cardiol 50: 1007–1013
47. Maisch B, Mayer E, Kochsiek K (1982) Nachweis zirkulierender Immunkomplexe bei kardialen Erkrankungen. Verh Dtsch Ges Inn Med 88: 624–627
48. Maisch B, Mayer E, Schubert U, Berg PA, Kochsiek K (1983) Immune reactions in infective endocarditis part 2: Relevance of circulating immune complexes, of serum inhibition factors, of lymphocytotoxic reactions, and of antibody dependent cellular cytotoxicity against cardiac target cells. Am Heart J 106: 338–344
49. Maisch B, Trostel-Soeder R, Berg PA, Kochsiek K (1981) Assessment of antibody mediated cytolysis of adult cardiocytes isolated by centrifugation in a continuous gradient of Percoll™ in patients with acute myocarditis. J Immunol Methods 44: 159–169
50. Maisch B, Trostel-Soeder R, Stechemesser E, Berg PA, Kochsiek K (1982) Diagnostic relevance of humoral and cell-mediated immune reactions in patients with acute viral myocarditis. Clin Exp Immunol 48: 533–545
51. Mason JW, Billingham ME, Ricci DR (1980) Treatment of acute inflammatory myocarditis assisted by endomyocardial biopsy. Am J Cardiol 45: 1037–1044
52. Mills AS, Hastillo A, Hess ML (1984) Lymphocytic infection of the myocardium in idiopathic dilated cardiomyopathy: Underestimation of myocarditis with endomyocardial biopsy. Circulation 70 (Suppl II): 401 (Abstr)
53. Paris S, Fosset M, Samuel D, Ailhaud G (1977) Chick embryo plasma membrane from cardiac muscle and cultured heart cells: isolation procedures and absence of fatty acid-activating enzymes. J Mol Cell Cardiol 9: 161–173
54. Perlmann P, Perlamnn H (1971) Cytotoxic lymphocytes. Mechanisms of activation and target cell destruction. Int Arch Allergy 41, 36–39
55. Report of the WHO/ISCF Task force on the definition and classification of cardiomyopathies (1980) Br Heart J 44: 672
56. Sack W, Scheuring H, Wachsmuth ED (1975) Antikörper gegen Herzmuskelsarkolemm im Serum von Patienten mit primärer Cardiomyopathie. Clin Wochenschr 53: 103–111

57. Sainani GS, Krompotic E, Slodki SJ (1968) Adult heart disease due to the Coxsackie virus B infection. Medicine 47, 133–137
58. Saphir O (1971) Myocarditis. Arch Pathol 32: 1000–1007
59. Schmier K, Klopf D, Maisch B, Schunk D, Hiby A, Bülowius U, Röder A, Auer I (1983) Suppressorzellaktivität bei Perimyokarditis und dilatativen Herzerkrankungen. Z. Kardiol 72 (suppl I): 17
60. Schroetter P von (1899) Die Insuffizienz des Herzmuskels. Verh Congr Inn Med L, pp 17–23
61. Schultheiß HP, Bolte HD, Schwimmbeck P (1984) Autoantibodies against the adenine nucleotide translocator in myocarditis and dilated cardiomyopathy. In: Bolte HD (ed) Viral Heart Disease. Springer-Verlag, Berlin, pp 131–143
62. Waterson AP (1978) Virology investigation in congestive cardiomyopathy. Postgrad Med J 54: 505–509
63. Weiland DS, Donaldson KP, Isner JM (1984) How well does the endomyocardial biopsy represent the state of the heart. Circulation 70 (Suppl II): 501 (Abstr)
64. Weiss MB, Ursell PC, Scala F, Drusin R, Fenoglio JJ Jr (1982) Immunosuppression therapy in chronic forms of myocarditis. Circulation 66 (Suppl II): 215 (Abstr)
65. Woodruff JF (1980) Viral myocarditis. A review article. Am J Pathol 101: 425–484
66. Wong Y, Woodruff JJ, Woodruff JF (1977) Generation of cytolytic T-lymphocytes during Coxsackie virus B_3 infection. I. Model and viral specificity. J Immunol 118: 1159–1164
67. Wong Y, Woodruff JJ, Woodruff JF (1977) Generation of cytolytic T-lymphocytes during Coxsackie virus B_3 infections. II. Characterization of effector cells, and demonstration of cytotoxicity against viral infected myofibers. J Immunol 118: 1165–1169
68. Zinkernagel RM, Doherty PC (1974) Restriction of in vitro T cell-mediated cytotoxicity in lymphocytic choriomeningitis within a syngeneic or semiallogeneic system. Nature 248: 701–702

Author's address:

Prof. Dr. Bernhard Maisch, Medizinische Universitätsklinik, Josef-Schneider-Straße 2, D-8700 Würzburg (F. R. G.)

Alterations of β-adrenoceptors subsequent to myocardial infarction

P. Dominiak and D. Türck

Physiologisches Institut der Universität München (F.R.G.)

Summary

Elevations and reductions of the number of β-adrenoceptor binding sites are dependent on the strength and the duration of receptor interaction with respective agonists. – In the paper presented here, results obtained by the authors concerning biosynthesis, storage and release of catecholamines following experimentally induced infarction of the myocardium in rats are compared with those of other authors for other species.

Principally, storage and release of noradrenaline from ischemic hearts do not differ with the mode of inducing tissue hypoxia (stopped-flow ischemia, coronary artery ligation, occlusion of the great cardiac vein), nor for various species (rat, dog, guinea-pig).

Differences are, however, present in the results of several β-adrenoceptor binding studies performed after experimental myocardial infarction. Following acute infarction, an increase in the number of β-adrenoceptor binding sites is generally observed, which is explained on the basis of an externalization of receptors from the cytoplasm ot the sarcolemmal membrane. Results pertaining to 2–3 days after infarction are not uniform: in guinea-pig hearts a marked drop in the number of β-adrenoceptors has been reported, a mild rise in the number has been detected in the left and right ventricle of rat hearts.

These divergent observations could arise from the experimental protocol employed, for instance in the binding assay and in the pretreatment given to the hearts prior to assay.

Key words: myocardial infarction, changes in β-adrenoceptor binding sites, catecholamines, translocation of β-adrenoceptors

Introduction

The "up- and down-regulation" of peripheral β-adrenoceptors can be induced by alterations of the sympathetic tone, i. e. via local modulation of the release of noradrenaline, and by the way of the sympatho-adrenal release of adrenaline from the adrenal medulla. Numerous investigations have demonstrated that the enhanced release of noradrenaline (NA) and/or adrenaline (A) causes a reduction in the number of β-adrenoceptor binding sites (for review see [20]). Similar observations were made following the application of synthetic β-adrenergic agents such as isoproterenol (4, 10).

As shown in studies on intact cardiomyocytes, the up- and down-regulation is a relatively rapid process, which has been explained on the basis of a respective ex- and internalization of β-adrenoceptors from and into the cytosol (10, 19). Cytosolic (internalized) β-adrenoceptors, however, cannot elicit β-adrenergic effects in the target organ. Thus, the process of translocation of β-adrenoceptors seems well suited for a rapid adaptation of tissue response to an altered sympathetic tone. Prolonged exposure to catecholamines, on the other hand, can initiate a change in the rate of protein biosynthesis leading to additional formation of the corresponding membrane proteins (24, for review see [20]).

Heart and circulatory disorders, such as coronary artery disease and essential hypertension, are associated with heightened sympathetic tone, evidenced, for example, by increased levels of circulating catecholamines (NA and A) (6, 8).

In contrast to the above cited β-adrenoceptor desensitization during high levels of catecholamines, there are some references to an increased number of β-adrenoceptor binding sites in lymphocytes of patients with essential hypertension (3, 16).

However, the β-adrenoceptors only respond to changes of the plasma concentrations of catecholamines. Since sympathetic innervation is lacking, studies on blood cells obviously cannot yield precise information concerning the alterations of β-adrenocpetors in individual organs such as the heart.

For this reason, the results of adrenoceptor binding studies performed on hearts subjected to experimental myocardial infarction are of particular interest. Both reduced and elevated numbers of β-adrenoceptor binding sites in the myocardium have however been reported (1, 12), apparently depending on the animal species and the time elapsed after coronary occlusion.

Regulation of catecholamines in myocardial ischemia

A) Plasma catecholamines:

Coronary heart disease, the chronic narrowing of the coronary arteries, leads to an elevation of cardiac noradrenaline (NA) release at rest as well as under physical exercise which is expressed in a rise in the coronary arterio-venous difference of the NA-concentration (7, 8).

Following an acute myocardial infarction, very high plasma levels of catecholamines are observed after 1 h, becoming gradually less only after 24–32 hours (14). Especially important (because of the arrhythmogenic potential) are the changes in plasma catecholamine concentrations occurring within the first 60 min subsequent to coronary artery occlusion. However, this time interval is hardly ever accessible to measurement in man.

Owing to this practical infringement, we have investigated the time courses of noradrenaline and adrenaline in the plasma of rats (Sprague-Dawley, IVANOVAS, strain SIV 50) subjected to acute myocardial infarction (total occlusion of the great cardiacvein).

Plasma noradrenaline was considered as a measure of the liberation of NA from the heart, plasma adrenaline as an indicator of the sympatho-adrenal reactions. Both catecholamines were determined radioenzymatically (adapted from the methods of [5] and [17]).

Only after 30 min could an increased liberation of NA and A be ascertained. After 60 min, the plasma concentrations of both catecholamines were significantly elevated, particularly in the case of A (Fig. 1). The haemodynamic parameters (dP/dt_{max} and blood pressure) were reduced at this time (Table 1).

The observed time dependent rises in plasma concentrations of the catecholamines are in accordance with results of Schömig et al. (18), obtained from studies on isolated hearts of rats undergoing stopped-flow ischemia. In these in vitro experiments a similar time course of NA release into the coronary effluent is described.

Our results with rats are indicative of an enhanced sympatho-neuronal and sympatho-adrenal activity after experimentally induced myocardial infarction.

B) Synthesis and storage:

In an infarction study on dogs, in which the left anterior descending coronary artery (LAD) was occluded, Mukherjee and coworkers (12) detected a progressive loss of noradrenaline in

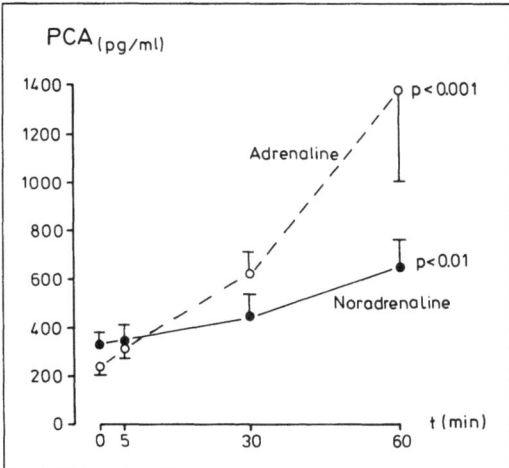

Fig. 1. Circulating plasma catecholamine concentrations (PCA, blood samples were collected from the left carotid artery) of rats after acute experimental myocardial infarction (occlusion of the great cardiac vein). Black circles and solid line = noradrenaline, open circles and broken line = adrenaline.

Values are given as mean ($\overline{X}$) ± SEM (n = 12). Significance was calculated by ANOVA.

Table 1. Haemodynamic parameters and plasma catecholamine concentrations in rats (n = 12) after myocardial infarction.

Time:	0	5	30	60	(min)
BP:	$130/108 \pm 7/6$	$91/73 \pm 5/5*$	$75/51 \pm 3/4**$	$65/40 \pm 4/3***$	(mm Hg)
dp/dt_{max}:	7130 ± 1018	6460 ± 1120	6340 ± 710	$5280 \pm 690*$	(mm Hg/sec)
NA:	332 ± 71	346 ± 74	439 ± 95	$648 \pm 112*$	(pg/ml)
A:	234 ± 51	311 ± 41	$618 \pm 89**$	$1381 \pm 385**$	(pg/ml)

Results are given as mean ($\overline{X} \pm$ SEM. Significance levels: * = $p < 0.05$, ** = $p < 0.01$, *** = $p < 0.001$ (Student's t-test).
Abbreviations: BP = blood pressure, NA = circulating noradrenaline, A = circulating adrenaline.

the ischemic area as compared to the non-infarcted regions. At 15 min there was no significant difference between the infarcted and the non-infarcted areas. The NA content of the infarction zone was reduced by 30% after 1 hour, by 50% after 3 hours and by 80% at 8 hours.

We have determined the noradrenaline content of hearts from rats subjected to myocardial infarction two days previously (occlusion of the left coronary artery) or to sham operation. The catecholamine was quantified by means of high pressure liquid chromatography (HPLC) in association with electrochemical detection (ELCD [9]). A 48 hour wait was chosen, because investigations of plasma catecholamine levels in man by Nadeau and deChamplain (14) have shown that the concentrations of catecholamines circulating freely only begin to gradually fall on the 2nd day post infarction.

As depicted in Fig. 5 the NA content of the infarcted left free wall was reduced by about 80% in comparison to the shams, whilst only slight differences were evident for the right ventricle and for the interventricular septum. The residual content of NA in the left free wall may probably be ascribed to the border zone of the infarction area and to a remainder of intact myocardial tissue. The slight depletion of the right ventricle and the septum could be an expression of the increased release of NA accompanying infarction.

Since experimentally induced myocardial infarction can lead to changes in heart performance (1) and thus also to altered circulatory conditions, a secondary stimulation of sympatho-adrenal activity is very likely. To investigate this possibility, we assessed the sympatho-adrenal activity in rats 2 hours and 2, 7 and 21 days subsequent to ligation of the left coronary artery. The parameters chosen were the activity of tyrosine hydroxylase, the rate limiting enzyme for the biosynthesis of NA (method adapted from [15]), and the adrenaline content of the adrenal medulla (9).

It is evident from Figs. 2 and 3 that tyrosine hydroxylase (TH) attains the highest activity around the 2nd day after infarction, and the A content is also at its peak at this time.

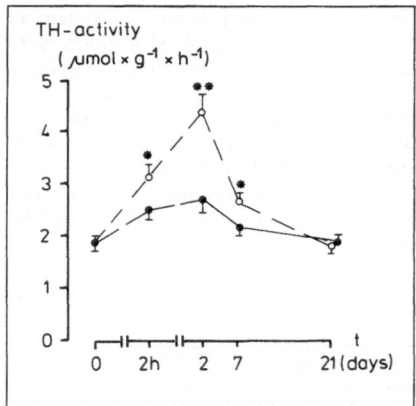

Fig. 2. Tyrosine hydroxylase activity (TH) in the adrenal medulla of rats at different times after experimental myocardial infarction (occlusion of the left coronary artery) or sham operation.

Black circles and solid line = sham operated rats, open circles and broken line = rats with myocardial infarction.

Significance was calculated between sham operated and coronary artery occluded rats, * = $p < 0.05$, ** = $p < 0.01$. (Student's t-test). Values are the mean ± SEM ($n = 8$ animals for each point).

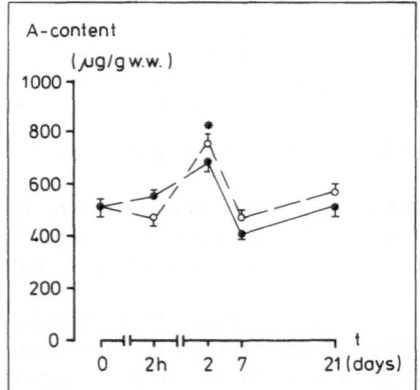

Fig. 3. Adrenaline content (A) in the adrenal medulla of rats at different times after experimental myocardial infarction (occlusion of the left coronary artery) or sham operation.

Black circles and solid line = sham operated animals, open circles and broken line = rats with myocardial infarction.

For significance see Fig. 2. $n = 8$ animals for each point.

Increased activity of TH is already evident 2 hours after infarction – a consequence of the enhanced release of A from the adrenal medulla. TH activity is still elevated after 7 days, but after 21 days no difference exists to sham operated controls. The comparison of the two parameters (TH activity and A content) reveals, furthermore, that the determination of TH yields more information concerning an altered activity of the adrenal medulla, than does the measurement of adrenaline content. In retrospect, this result is not surprising.

Changes in β-adrenoceptors

With respect to the alteration of the number of β-adrenoceptors, two processes can be distinguished. One is relatively rapid and involves the translocation of the adrenoceptors between the plasmalemmal and intracellular compartments. A slow process is based on the biosynthesis or degradation of receptor molecules (see review in [20]).

The number of β-adrenoceptors in the membrane can be regulated homologously, i. e., by catecholamines or corresponding antagonists (β-adrenoceptor blockers), or heterologously, i. e., by hormones (thyroid and adrenal cortex hormones) and by agents directed at reactions or intermediates formed subsequent to receptor stimulation (e. g. at adenylate cyclase [20]).

The rapid "down-regulation" (desensitization) of β-adrenoceptors following exposition to β-agonists is explained by an internalization of the receptors into the cytoplasm (4). Using intact cardiomyocytes, Limas and Limas (10) have demonstrated the fast internalization under the influence of isoproterenol, and the rapid externalization upon washout of the agonist.

Alterations after myocardial infarction:

As already mentioned above, myocardial infarction leads to liberations of NA and A into the synaptic cleft and the plasma respectively, a release which can attain massive proportions and is the expression of a reflex (compensatory?) elevation of sympathetic tone. On the basis of the previously described regulatory characteristics of β-adrenoceptors, this rise in circulating catecholamine levels should be expected to induce a reduction of β-adrenoceptor density in the heart and other organs innervated by the sympathetic nervous system after infarction.

In binding studies with ^{3}H-dihydroalprenolol Mukherjee et al. (12, 13) therefore examined the behaviour of cardiac β-adrenoceptors in the dog at different times subsequent to occlusion of the LAD.

Just 1 hour after infarction, the number of β-adrenoceptor binding sites in the ischemic tissue was twice that of sham operated animals (Table 2), and at 3 and 8 hours there was still

Table 2. β-adrenoceptor binding sites (^{3}H-dihydroalprenolol) in crude membranes from ischemic and non ischemic zones of LAD and sham occluded canine hearts (adapted from [12]).

Time	LAD		SHAM	
	n. i. B_{max}	i. B_{max}	n. i. B_{max}	i. B_{max}
15 min	97	110	81	93
1 h	101	163$^{**}_{+}$	94	86
3 h	101	141$^{***}_{++}$	85	68
8 h	124(*)	154$^{*}_{+}$	89	93

B_{max}-values represent the mean ($\overline{X}$) calculated from the Scatchard plots.
B_{max} = fmol/mg protein.
Significance levels: (*) = p < 0.1, + or * = p < 0.05, + + or ** = p < 0.01, *** = p < 0.001.
* = comparison between LAD and sham occluded, + = comparison between ischemic and non-ischemic zone.
Abbreviations: LAD = occlusion of the left anterior descending coronary artery, sham = sham occluded, i. = ischemic and n. i. = non ischemic zone.

an increase of 100%. Interestingly, the number of binding sites was also increased significantly in the non-infarcted tissue.

A definite correlation to the degree of regional NA depletion could not be established.

Since the number of cholinergic receptors was unaltered, both in the infarcted and non infarcted areas, an increase in the number of β-adrenoceptors due to protein biosynthesis was excluded. The induction of protein synthesis by catecholamines, moreover, is a delayed process and, as shown by Zimmer and Gerlach (24), will only become marked about 48 h after exposition to catecholamines.

The elevated number of β-adrenoceptor binding sites in the dog was functionally coupled to a heightened frequency response of the hearts towards isoproterenol (13).

Results opposite to those of Mukherjee and coworkers (12, 13) have been presented by Baumann et al. (1), who observed a reduction in β-adrenoceptor binding number 3 days after experimental infarction in guinea-pigs. The binding assay, also performed with ^{3}H-dihydroalprenolol, was, however, conducted on membrane preparations of the non-infarcted right ventricle. In full agreement with the binding data, the hearts which had undergone infarction showed reduced response to isoproterenol in comparison to controls, isolated Langendorff preparations being used.

In our own experiments with rats (Sprague-Dawley, IVANOVAS, strain SIV 50) the changes of myocardial β-adrenoceptors were followed over a wide range of time after experimental infarction.

Initially, we determined the number of β-adrenoceptor binding sites with ^{3}H-dihydroalprenolol according to the method of Williams and Lefkowitz (23), precise details to be found in Takeda et al. (21), in membrane preparations of the whole heart tissue.

Two hours after ligation of the great cardiac vein, the binding sites had risen by 26% in comparison to sham operated control hearts (Fig. 4).

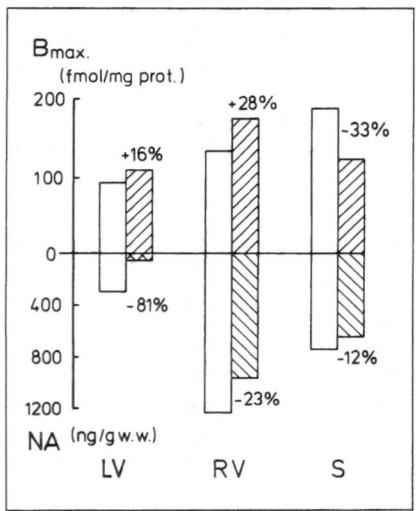

Fig. 4. β-adrenoceptor binding sites (B_{max}, fmol/mg protein, ^{3}H-dihydroalprenolol) in crude membranes from rat myocardium, 2 hours after experimental myocardial infarction (occlusion of the great cardiac vein) or sham operation. B_{max}-values were calculated from the Scatchard plots and represent the mean of 4 experiments respectively. Open column = sham operation (open columns, n = 8).

Abbreviations: LV = ischemic left ventricle, RV = right ventricle and S = interventricular septum.

In a second series of experiments, we measured the number of β-adrenoceptor binding sites (^{3}H-dihydroalprenolol, according to the method of Mukherjee et al. (13), in highly enriched sarcolemmal membrane fractions after occlusion of the left coronary artery. Binding was determined in the infarcted free wall of the left ventricle, in the right ventricle and in the interventricular septum, the latter two regions being non-ischemic.

The measurements revealed an elevated number of binding sites in the infarcted left ventricle (+ 16%) and in the right ventricle (+ 28%), but a reduction of 33% in the septal tissue (Fig. 5). As already related by Mukherjee et al. (12) for the dog, we also were unable to detect a firm relationship between the regional NA content and the binding site density in the rat heart (Fig. 5).

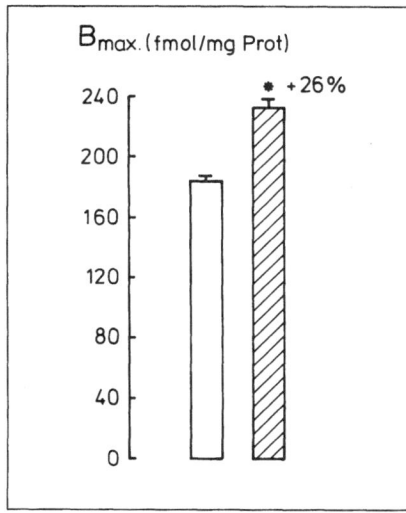

Fig. 5. Upper part: β-adrenoceptor binding sites (B_{max}, fmol/mg protein, ^{3}H-dihydroalprenolol) in highly enriched sarcolemmal membranes from different parts of rat myocardium, 2 days after experimental myocardial infarction (occlusion of the left coronary artery, hatched columns) or sham operation (open columns). B_{max}-values were calculated from the Scatchard plots and each column represents the mean of 4 experiments respectively.

Lower part: noradrenaline content (NA) in different parts of rat myocardium, 2 days after experimental myocardial infarction (hatched columns, n = 8) or sham operation (open columns, n = 8).

Abbreviations: LV = ischemic left ventricle, RV = right ventricle and S = interventricular septum.

How can the discrepant results of these various binding studies be interpreted?

To begin with, there is agreement between the results of the binding studies carried out on dog and rat hearts shortly after acute myocardial infarction. Although a considerable release of catecholamines takes place following infarction (see Figs. 1, 2 and 3 and [12]), the number of β-adrenoceptor binding sites is increased, a phenomenon ascribed to the externalization of adrenoceptors from the light vesicle (intracellular) fraction (11, in this paper the authors report an increase in the number of β-adrenoceptors in guinea-pig hearts 15–90 min after experimental myocardial infarction). The total number of cellular β-adrenoceptors is not supposed to be altered by this process, only the distribution of specific receptors between cytoplasm and membrane. Because the internalized adrenoceptors are physiologically inactive, their interaction with agonists is precluded, as is the coupling between β-adrenoceptor and adenylate cyclase, and thus the formation of the second messenger cAMP.

Possibly, the increase in externalized β-adrenoceptors following myocardial infarction is a compensatory mechanism in response to the drop in cardiac performance. The enhanced release of catecholamines is also often seen in this light. In addition, the potentiated automaticity of the heart after fresh infarction would be well explained by a rise in β-adrenoceptor density, all the more, since the ensueing arrhythmias are very susceptible to therapy with β-adrenoceptor blocking agents (2). Not-with-standing, the precise stimulus leading to externalization of β-adrenoceptors is still unknown.

The results of Baumann et al. (1) are conclusive in themselves, as far as the reduced number of β-adrenoceptor binding sites and the reduced effect of isoproterenol on the hearts is concerned. However, several aspects remain unclear, for instance, the pronounced elevation of the receptor dissociation constant K_D measured after infarction. Furthermore, the binding studies were carried out on isolated hearts which had just previously been stimulated with isoproterenol. It is more than likely that the conditions after in vitro stimulation with catecholamines will not be the same as in vivo, thereby restricting comparability to other studies.

A species dependent variation of the behaviour of β-adrenoceptors is not likely because in the previously cited paper of Maisel et al. (11) the authors demonstrated an increased number of β-adrenoceptors subsequent to myocardial infarction also in guinea-pig hearts. The only possible explanation might be the different times after experimental infarction at which the binding studies were performed.

In addition to the problems extensively discussed here, there is further evidence in the literature for discrepancies between the results of binding studies and functional experiments (21, 22). However, the fact that β-adrenoceptor translocation appears to be a rapid process, could well offer an explanation for receptor binding studies with – at first sight – seemingly contradictory results.

References

1. Baumann G, Riess G, Erhardt WD, Felix SB, Ludwig L, Blümel G, Blömer H (1981) Impaired beta-adrenergic stimulation in the uninvolved ventricle post-acute myocardial infarction: reversible defect due to excessive circulating catecholamine-induced decline in number and affinity of beta-receptors. Am Heart J 101: 569–581
2. Benfey BG, Elfellah MS, Ogilvie RI, Varma DR (1984) Anti-arrhythmic effects of prazosin and propranolol during coronary artery occlusion and re-perfusion in dogs and pigs. Br J Pharmacol 82: 717–725
3. Brodde OE, Prywarra A, Daul A, Anlauf M, Bock KD (1984) Correlation between lymphocyte beta$_2$-adrenoceptor density and mean arterial blood pressure: elevated beta-adrenoceptors in essential hypertension. J Cardiovasc Pharmacol 6: 678–682
4. Chuang de-M, Costa E (1979) Evidence for internalization of the recognition site of β-adrenergic receptors during receptor subsensitivity induced by (–)-isoproterenol. Proc Natl Acad Sci USA 76: 3024–3028
5. DaPrada M, Zürcher G (1976) Simultaneous radioenzymatic determination of plasma and tissue adrenaline, noradrenaline and dopamine within the femtomole range. Life Sci 19: 1161–1174
6. Dominiak P, Grobecker H (1982) Elevated plasma catecholamines in young hypertensive and hyperkinetic patients: effect of pindolol. Br J Clin Pharmacol 13: 381S–390S
7. Dominiak P, Schulz W, Delius W, Kober G, Grobecker H (1981) Catecholamines in patients with coronary heart disease. In: Delius W, Gerlach E, Grobecker H, Kübler W (eds) Catecholamines and the heart. Springer-Verlag, Berlin Heidelberg New York, pp 223–235
8. Dominiak P, Delius W, Grobecker H (1985) Changes in plasma catecholamine concentrations in patients with coronary heart disease during pacing and physical exercise. Clin Cardiol 8: 77–81
9. Kissinger PT, Brüntlett CS, Shoup RE (1981) Neurochemical applications of liquid chromatography with electrochemical detection. Life Sci 28: 455–465
10. Limas CJ, Limas C (1984) Rapid recovery of cardiac β-adrenergic receptors after isoproterenol-induced "down"-regulation. Circ Res 55: 524–531
11. Maisel AS, Motulsky HJ, Insel PA (1985) Externalization of β-adrenergic receptors promoted by myocardial ischemia. Science 230: 183–186
12. Mukherjee A, Wong TM, Buja LM, Lefkowitz RJ, Willerson JT (1979) Beta adrenergic and muscarinic cholinergic receptors in canine myocardium. J Clin Invest 64: 1423–1428
13. Mukherjee A, Bush LR, McCoy KE, Duke RJ, Hagler H, Buja LM, Willerson JT (1982) Relationship between β-adrenergic receptor numbers and physiological responses during experimental canine myocardial ischemia. Circ Res 50: 735–741
14. Nadeau RA, deChamplain J (1979) Plasma catecholamines in acute myocardial infarction. Am Heart J 98: 548–554
15. Nagatsu T, Oka K, Kato T (1979) Highly sensitive assay for tyrosine hydroxylase activity by high-performance liquid chromatography. J Chromatogr 163: 247–252
16. O'Malley K, O'Brien E, Fitzgerald D, Kelly J (1985) Adrenoceptors and hypertension. In: Szabadi E, Bradshaw CM, Nahorski SR (eds) Pharmacology of adrenoceptors. VCH-Publishers, Weinheim, pp 197–204
17. Peuler JD, Johnson GA (1977) Simultaneous single isotope radioenzymatic assay of plasma norepinephrine, epinephrine and dopamine. Life Sci 21: 625–636
18. Schömig A, Dart AM, Dietz R, Mayer E, Kübler W (1984) Release of endogenous catecholamines in the ischemic myocardium of the rat. Part A: locally mediated release. Circ Res 55: 689–701

19. Sibley DR, Lefkowitz RJ (1985) Molecular mechanisms of receptor desensitization using the β-adrenergic receptor-coupled adenylate cyclase system as a model. Nature 317: 124–129
20. Stiles GL, Caron MG, Lefkowitz RJ (1984) β-adrenergic receptors: biochemical mechanisms of physiological regulation. Physiol Rev 64: 661–743
21. Takeda N, Dominiak P, Türck D, Rupp H, Jacob R (1985) The influence of endurance-training on mechanical catecholamine responsiveness, β-adrenoceptor density and myosine isoenzyme pattern of rat ventricular myocardium. Basic Res Cardiol 80: 88–99
22. Takeda N, Dominiak P, Türck D, Rupp H, Jacob R (1985) Myocardial catecholamine responsiveness of spontaneously hypertensive rats as influenced by swimming training. Basic Res Cardiol 80: 384–391
23. Williams RS, Lefkowitz RJ (1978) Alpha-adrenergic receptors in rat myocardium. Identification by binding of ^{3}H-dihydroergocryptine. Circ Res 43: 721–727
24. Zimmer H-G, Gerlach E (1980) Early metabolic alterations during the development of experimentally induced cardiac hypertrophy. Drug Res 30: 2001–2007

Authors' address:

Prof. Dr. med. P. Dominiak, Physiologisches Institut, Universität München, Pettenkoferstraße 12, D-8000 Munich 2 (F.R.G.)